Cry for Health
VOLUME 1

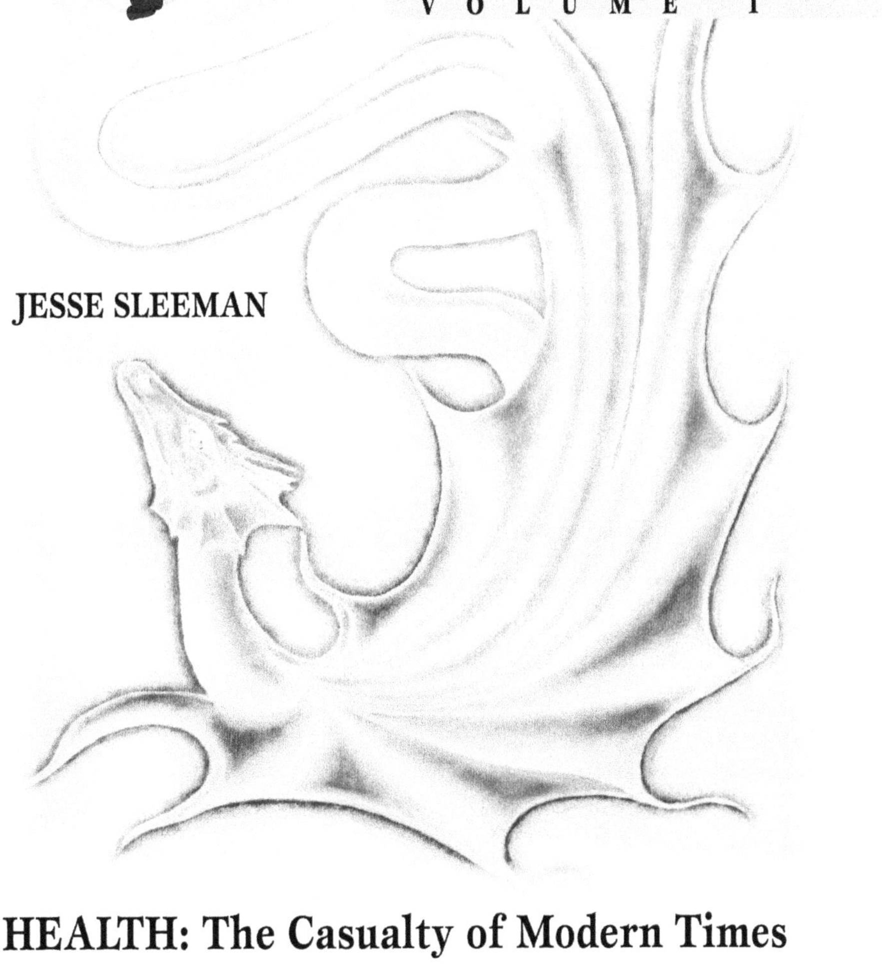

JESSE SLEEMAN

HEALTH: The Casualty of Modern Times

Dedication

This book is dedicated to my late parents, Gay and Ces; my children, Tehani, Kane, Phoebe, Jake and Daisy; my stepchildren, Amalie and Michael; my grandchildren, Zac, Jude and Dashiella; my mother-outlaw, Heather; and my partner and soulmate, Carola.

Published by
Dragon Lair Publishing
PO Box 553 Mt Barker, SA 5251, Australia

http://www.dragonlairpublishing.com.au
http://www.cryforhealth.com.au

First published in Australia in 2010.
This Lulu Printed edition first published February 2011.

This Book is sold subject to the condition that it shall not be lent, resold, hired out or otherwise circulated without the publishers permission by way of written confirmation and consent in any form of cover or binding other then which it has been originally published.

© Jesse Sleeman. All rights reserved.

National Library of Australia Cataloguing-in-Publication entry

Sleeman, Jesse.

Health the casualty of modern times/Jesse Sleeman

ISBN: 978 0 646 55216 3(pbk.)

Cry for health; v. 1

Includes bibliographical references and index.

Public Health – 21st century.

Diseases – 21st century.

Human beings – Effect of technological innovations on.

Chemicals – Physiological effect.

362.1

Printed by Lulu

Commentary on cover page design:
The Fallen Dragon, by Carola Maier

In modern times, two symbols are associated with medicine and the healing arts: one, the caduceus, the other the staff of Aesculapius. The most popular symbol, particularly amongst commercial organisations, is the caduceus; it's a staff with two serpents encircling it, and is topped by a pair of wings.

In ancient Greece, however, the caduceus had nothing whatsoever to do with healing. It was the magic wand of Hermes, the messenger of the gods and the guide to the underworld. As the patron of border crossings, travellers, thieves, sports, literature, invention, hidden meanings, and commerce in general, this Olympian god and his staff came to be associated with the hidden arts of alchemy during the 7th century AD. And from the 16th century onwards the caduceus came to be associated with medicine.

But the traditional Greek symbol of medicine and the healing arts was the staff of Aesculapius, which had a single sacred serpent coiled around a wooden rod. Aesculapius (Asclepias), not Hermes, was the patron of medicine. The origins of this symbol date back to at least 3000 BC, to ancient Sumer, seen in the symbol of a fiery dragon encircling a staff.

A dragon is a snake with wings: the winged serpent. In earlier times in all cultures it symbolised the unity of matter and spirit (beast and bird). It has been variously known as the Earth Mother, Dana, the Great Serpent, Lindworm, the Mother of Waters, Tiamat, the warrior sun god, Kulkulkan, Quetzalcoatl, Amaru, Boi-tata, Quiche Gukumatz, Makara the sea-goat or elephant-headed god, Loong, Naga, Ryu, Yong, Lac Long Quan, Bakonawa. And in Australia, Aboriginal people still relate the story of how the Rainbow Serpent, the biggest of the Dreamtime Beings, shaped the earth, and that to this day it inhabits permanent deep waterholes.

Being a manifestation of the unity of life-giving water and the breath of life, the dragon was the first of the sky gods and earthly masters, and hence came to be associated with emperors and kings. In indigenous American and Indian traditions the dragon was thought to control the rain, clouds, thunder, lightning, vegetation, and fertility in general, and was associated with the tops of mountains. In Egypt, Babylonia, China, Japan and India the dragon was considered to be not only the controller of water, but also the very impersonation of water and its life-giving powers that give, maintain, and prolong life and guard against all kinds of danger to life. On the one hand, the dragon was the guardian of treasures and of the portals of esoteric knowledge; and on the other, it was a symbol of untamed nature, of wildness and wild animal instincts. In other words, the dragon is nature's bringer of good luck, the rejuvenator of mankind, and the giver of immortality.

For the Christian Church, however, the dragon, and it's wingless cousin (the snake) were symbols of evil, darkness, the Devil, the Temptor, death, paganism and heresy. Hence, in the West, dragons have had a bad press for two millennia, and dragon slayers have been lauded as heroes.

The cover design by Carola Maier represents the fallen dragon of life and health swirling around a leafless tree in the darkness of a wintry night. But, as the ancient traditions tell us, it is only in the darkest places that we can see the brightest lights. And hopefully the dragon, together with its associated energies, is beginning to rise to its rightful place to heal all life on Earth.

Disclaimer

This book is a reference work not intended to treat, diagnose or prescribe. The information contained herein is in no way to be considered as a substitute for consultation with a qualified health-care professional.

Experts in the field of health hold widely varying views. It is not the intent of the author to replace the guidance of a qualified health-care practitioner, and anyone who believes he or she is ill should seek their professional advice. The intent is only to offer health information to help you cooperate with your health-care practitioner in your mutual quest for health. In the event you do use this information without your practitioner's approval, you are prescribing for yourself, which is your right, but the publisher, editors and author expressly disclaim liability to any person for the consequences of anything done or omitted to be done by any such person in reliance, whether whole or partial, upon any part of the contents of this publication.

While every effort has been made to ensure the accuracy and authenticity of the information contained in this book, the publisher, editors and author accept no responsibility for or liability arising from any part of the contents contained herein.

Jesse Sleeman

For the past 25 years Jesse Sleeman has been the court jester of natural therapies in Australia, playfully challenging the established beliefs of public audiences, as well as complementary medicine practitioners and students alike with his oftentimes apparently radical ideas.

He was born in Christchurch, New Zealand in 1949; it was a time when nearly everyone's mum was at home when the kids got home from school, when children made billy carts and transformed their bikes into motor cycles with cigarette cards in the spokes. In the early '60s his family migrated to Sydney, Australia, where he soon took to surfing the wild winter waves off Sydney's northern beaches. By the late 1960s, with a Commonwealth Scholarship to his credit, he was a student at Sydney University, embroiled in the anti-Vietnam protest movement (the 'flower power generation' considered that making love, not war, was a far more intelligent pursuit, and certainly more fun), a reporter for the student newpaper *Honi Soit*, and learning the art of Method Acting from Hayes Gordon and Zika Nester at the Ensemble Theatre, and the art of film making from Phil Noyce.

To surf for hours at a stretch, and without a wetsuit, required superb health and fitness. This sparked his interest in health, and particularly in what was then called Fringe Medicine. By the early 1970s he had graduated with a Bachelor of Arts, majoring in English, Psychology and Philosophy, and went on to gain a Master of Arts in Psychology, specialising in Social and Abnormal Psychology. He would later apply this knowledge to health matters.

Soon after he and his new wife moved to Bath in Britain, he began a course in medical herbalism with the prestigious National Institute of Medical Herbalists. Over the following 10 years, working as a carpenter by day and studying herbal medicine by night, he completed the course to achieve membership of the Institute; and, later, managing to juggle time for a carpentry business together with a busy herbal practice in Bath and Chippenham, he fathered and, together with his wife Su, raised five children, none of whom were vaccinated, and all of whom maintained excellent health through dietary and herbal means. By this time, because of increasing public disenchantment with convention medicine, Fringe Medicine had become known as Alternative Medicine.

Upon the family's return to Sydney, he established a herbal practice in Dee Why, and then later in Balmain, began lecturing at various colleges of natural therapies, and added both Traditional Chinese Medicine and Ayurveda to his medical repertoire. At that time, with increasing numbers of people beginning to abandon conventional medicine in favour of traditional therapies, Alternative Medicine was becoming known as Complementary Medicine. Then in 1989 the family moved to the tranquil city of Adelaide where he established herbal practices in Adelaide City and the Adelaide Hills. He ceased practising as a full-time medical herbalist in 1995 to devote more time to writing and lecturing.

Over the past 25 years he has been a lecturer in herbalism and medical philosophies at the NSW College of Natural Therapies, the Australasian College of Natural Therapies, the Sydney College of Natural Therapies, Southern Cross School of Herbal Medicine, Nature Care (as an occasional lecturer), the SA School of Herbal Medicine (for which he designed and wrote a correspondence course), the SA School of Natural Therapies, the Adelaide Training College of Complementary Medicine (for which he designed and wrote, and was the course coordinator for, a four-year full-time course in Western Herbalism), Health Schools Australia, the Perth Academy of Natural Therapies, and the Australian Institute of Holistic Medicine.

During the late 1980s and early 1990s, Jesse Sleeman was a member of the Executive of the National Herbalists Association of Australia, and one of its Vice Presidents between 1992 and 1993. He represented the Australian Traditional Medicine Society on the Profession and Industry Committee for Liaison, an organisation that liaised with the Commonwealth Government regarding the Therapeutics Goods Act, which was enacted in 1989. He has presented talks on health matters at numerous professional meetings and conferences, and at public meetings, including training sessions to members of Neways International, and to participants in his lectures on the Buteyko Method at the WEA in Adelaide. He has also developed and written many original research articles for professional journals, as well as for newspapers and magazines.

Today, he continues to write, having completed an Advanced Diploma in Professional Writing, lectures at Endeavour College of Natural Health in Adelaide, and runs Buteyko Breathing courses, a therapy he learned from his partner Carola Maier, who trained with Dr Konstantin Buteyko in Moscow.

Acknowledgements
In writing this book over the past 17 years, I am indebted to numerous individuals without whose help and inspiration this book would never have come to fruition.

To my colleagues and friends at the National Institute of Medical Herbalists in Britain, particularly Kristin Jeffs and Janet Hicks, I thank you for starting me on the health road all those years ago and inspiring me with your knowledge and dedication to health care. Thank you to my colleagues and friends at the National Herbalists Association of Australia, and the Australian Traditional Medicine Society, and particularly to my good friend Raymond Khoury, one of the unsung heroes of complementary medicine in Australia, whose encouragement kept me going, and whose hospitality has always been second-to-none.

I am also indebted to the many students I have taught over the past 24 years, at eleven colleges of natural therapies across Australia, for challenging me about some of my ideas, for providing me with new ideas about health promotion and disease prevention; and for confirming that the student can also be the master's teacher.

Thanks to the many academics and health care professionals with whom I have corresponded, including Ms Sandra Russo, Ms Wendy McMahon, Dr Raj Thalluri, Mr Vincent di Stefano, Mr Ken King, Ms Sandra Sebelis, Ms Hilde Hemmes, Professor Andrew Tonkin, Professor Kevin Norton, Dr Lisa Landymore-Lim, Dr Norman Swan, Dr Peter Baratosy, Dr Viera Scheibner, Mr Robert Iseman, Dr Garrett Cullity, Dr Philip Gerrans, Dr George Couvalis, Professor Kerin O'Dea, Ms Joan Gibbs, Dr Duncan Mackay, Professor José Facelli, Dr John Conran, Dr Arnold Mindell, Professor Alfred Poulos, Professor Philip Landrigan, and Professor Peter Dingle.

I acknowledge the efforts of the thousands of academics, researchers, and writers, from both government and non-government organisations, whose evidence, individually and collectively, provided the backbone for the arguments presented in this book. Thank you to the publishers of the books, and scientific and medical journals who published their works, and to the many librarians who hunted down books, articles and academic treatises cited herein; to Google for providing a superb search engine; and to Apple for making superb, user-friendly computers.

I also wish to extend my thanks to students and staff in the Professional Writing Unit at the Adelaide Institute of TAFE for vetting the early drafts of this book. And I especially want to thank Dr Barry Westburg, my writing mentor; Jonathon Stone, a genius wordsmith; and the coordinators of the unit, Jim Roberts and Kate Deller-Evans; and Roger Zubrinich, who approved the book as a negotiated project and whose appetite for my undertaking was whetted after reading the section in Chapter 1, where I wrote that when physicians went on strike in Israel in 1973, and in Britain and California in 1978, the death rate fell by between 35 and 50 per cent; his comment, as I recall, was 'Bloody hell!'

To my editors, Ms Leticia Supple from Brascoe Publishing, who sifted through my drafts with a fine toothcombe, challenging me to clarify issues and arguments I presented, and Ms Gail Weaver from Weaverworks who took up the baton at the last moment; I am eternally grateful to you both for your advise, hard work, and dedication to the project. And to Gary Tonge Latimer, Jake Sleeman, and Greg Turra for the artwork.

To my psychological mentor who helped me chart my way through stormy waters after my divorce, Jackie Marlu, a huge thank you to you too.

And because my family have been waiting patiently for many years for this book to appear, my heartfelt thanks go to all of you; and to my dear friends who gleaned progress reports as the years passed and never doubted that the book would be completed … one day; and particularly to my partner, Carola, without whose financial support, encouragement, feedback, and love, I would never have finished the monumental task I had undertaken.

CRY FOR HEALTH

VOLUME 1

HEALTH: THE CASUALTY OF MODERN TIMES

PART ONE—SICK SOCIETY, AILING MEDICINE 14

    Introduction 15
        Our most priceless possession   15
        The unsung story   16
        The flawed argument on ageing   19
        The band-aid solution   21
            What on earth is stopping us from changing?   22

CHAPTER

1   Death by Doctoring 23
        The unfolding story   23
        The truth revealed   24

2   Tools of Medicine 27
        Where are we going? A summary   27
            Two clues   27
        The perennial tools of medicine   27
        The new tools of medicine   29
            Why create new tools?   29
            Patents   30
            Drug companies   30
            Making sense of drugs   31

3   Why Modern Medicine May Be Harming You 33
        Doctors and drugs—a dangerous mix   33
            A common scenario   33
        Drugs   35
            Pushing and pulling   35
            Ignoring our uniqueness   36
            Drug interactions   37
            Clinical tests   37
        Why trust drugs?   41

4   Drug Hype 43
        Did drugs rid the world of infectious diseases?   43
            A brief history of human illness   43
            Why the death rate declined   44
            Are we really living longer?   45

5   To Vaccinate or Not to Vaccinate 47

The hype	*47*
If not for vaccines	*49*
The first vaccine to fail	*49*
The second vaccine to fail	*53*
The emperor's new clothes and the medical courtiers	*58*
Tetanus	*59*
Whooping cough	*61*
Measles	*64*
Mumps	*68*
Rubella	*69*
The polio scam	*73*
The culprit: poisons or germs?	*74*
The quest for the saviour	*80*
The first shots in the war on polio	*82*
A rose by any other name	*83*
The living virus lurking in the Salk vaccine	*85*
Out of Africa	*86*
The Sabin vaccine's fall from grace	*88*
Polio's great disappearing act	*88*
The aftermath	*89*
Revelations	*93*
The legacy	*95*
The charade, the subterfuge and the propaganda	*97*
Whistle-blowers	*98*
The importance of infections	*102*
Hidden footnotes to the vaccination saga	*103*
AIDS	*103*
The Gulf War Syndrome	*108*

PART TWO—BLINKERED SCIENCE AND THE VITAL FORCE 110

CHAPTER

6 How Do We Know? 111

Where are we going? A summary	*111*
Science	*111*
Two modes of consciousness, two kinds of knowledge	*112*
The waxing and waning of knowledge	*115*
The dream of a certain Descartes	*116*
Life seen through the prism of modern science	*117*
A slice of Bacon	*118*
Science's failings	*118*
The challenge	*120*
Why science is not scientific enough	*122*

7 Two Ways to View Health and Disease 123

A modern perspective	*123*
A vitalistic approach	*124*

8	**Vital Force, 1: Stuck in the Whole** 127	
	Where are we going?—a preview	*127*
	The universal glue	*128*
	Acausal connections	*129*
	Foucault's pendulum	*129*
	The Hundredth Monkey Phenomenon	*130*
	Common acausal connections	*130*
	Causal and acausal connections, and health	*131*
	Table 1: Concordances of humours in Traditional Chinese Medicine	*133*
	Table 2: Concordances of humours in Greek Medicine	*134*
	Table 3: Concordances of humours in Ayurveda	*135*
	Table 4: Concordances of humours in Astrology	*136*
	Figure 1: Chinese Medicine—five phases (Wu Xing)	*138*
	Figure 2: Greek Medicine—four elements and humours	*138*
	Figure 3: Ayurveda—five elements, and three humours (doshas)	*139*
	Figure 4: Astrology—four elements, twelve signs, and three qualities	*139*
	What modern science says about connections	*140*
	Beyond your doctor's philosophy	*141*
9	**Vital Force, 2: Spinning Energies** 143	
	A Chinese perspective	*143*
	Yin and yang	*143*
	Table 5: Yin-Yang attributes	*145*
	How yin and yang dance together	*146*
	Divisions all the way down	*146*
	Control and balance	*146*
	Smooth qi	*147*
	Using yin-yang polarities to assess and treat illness	*147*
	Figure 5: Approach to treatment	*150*
	Indian and ancient Greek perpectives	*151*
	Throwing light on spinning energies	*151*
	The eyes have it	*152*
10	**Vital Force, 3: Signs of Intelligence** 153	
	Of one mind	*153*
	Babble or communication?	*153*
	Stability in the midst of apparent chaos	*155*
	Life finds a crafty way	*157*
	Made to order	*157*
	Accident or design?	*158*
	The odds of the random formation of life	*158*
	Other explanations	*160*
	Does intelligence jump ship when we're sick?	*161*
11	**Health and Disease Revisited** 163	
	What is health?	*163*
	What is disease?	*164*

    The two phases of disease   165
    Positive, tolerant and negative disease processes   166

PART THREE—THE HUMAN CONTINUUM AND BEYOND 168

CHAPTER
12 The Human Continuum 169
    Time to take stock   169
    The setting   170
    Primed for the wild   170
        Trial and error, or instincts?   171
        Stone age instincts   174
        Babies, stone-agers, and wild animals   176
    The health of hunters and gatherers   177
        Aboriginal health   177
        Yekuana health   178
        Moving beyond the continuum   179
        Table 6: Lessons from the human continuum   180

13 Beyond the Continuum 181
    An idea whose time had come   181
        The benefits   181
        The costs   182
        Adaptations   184
        Moving towards the cusp   186
    The Chemical Deluge   186
        An ingenious idea   187
        The war on pests   188
        The war on weeds   190
        Life fights back   190
    Drowning in man-made chemicals   192
        The tip of the toxic iceberg   192
        Scientific uncertainty   194
        The trade-off between health and profits   195

14 Drowning in a Sea of Electropollution 199
    Basking in electromagnetic fields   199
        Awash in a sea of electropollution   199
        Table 7: Characteristics of electromagnetic radiation   201
        Table 8: Comparison of intensity of EMFs from various sources   202
    A cautionary tale   203
        Table 9: Biological effects of radiofrequency/microwave electric fields   205
        Table 10: Biological effects of ELF magnetic fields   206
        Harm by any other name   208
        Harm at work   209
        Harm at home   210
        Harm in the shadow of broadcasting towers   211

Harm in the lab	*213*
The smoking phone	*215*
The birds and the bees	*218*
In the shadow of the phone towers	*219*
Standards for safety or for profits?	*221*

15 The Rape of Life 223
    Vanishing varieties   *223*
        The rise of the food barons   *224*
        The grocery grab   *225*
        Strength in diversity   *228*
    Frankenfoods   *229*
        The genie of life   *229*
        The procedure: raping the genie   *230*
        The lie   *231*
        GE glee   *233*
        GE gloom   *233*
        Chilling warnings   *235*
        Hogwash for the hungry   *237*
    Nuking foods, and nanotech nonsense   *238*
        Irresponsible irradiation   *238*
        Nanoed be thy name   *242*
    Who speaks for life?   *244*

References 245
Index 341

PART ONE

SICK SOCIETY, AILING MEDICINE

Introduction

Duirt me leat go raibh me breoite (Celtic)
(I told you I was ill).
Epitaph on Irish comedian and playwright Spike Milligan's headstone
(1918–2002).

Our most priceless possession

Our most priceless possession, though we often take it for granted, is health. Our very lives depend upon it. So does our enjoyment of life, our work and our relationships. This a two-volume book about how you can enhance or even recover that priceless possession.

There's a lot of good news about health:
- Each of us possesses an incredibly intelligent body that knows how to heal itself. If we give it what it needs it will do the rest.

- By making changes in any part of our lifestyle, our health will begin to improve. The more things we supply to meet the needs of our body and mind, the more our health flourishes.

- When our health flourishes everything else in life is a bonus.

And yet most people ignore their health. That is, of course, until they become sick.

So, if you're ill, welcome. You're in the same boat as at least 80 per cent of the population. If it's any comfort, the Chinese have a saying: 'Illness is part of the journey to perfection.' Everyone in our culture, doctors included, takes the opposite view: that when we're ill something has gone wrong with us.

But what if our doctors are wrong? What if our bodies are doing the right thing, what if they're responding appropriately to the impact of things they don't need? It would mean that we'd have to take a radically different look at how we treat illness. Instead of rushing to use drugs that mask our symptoms we might learn to read the language of our body, in sickness and in health. It would also mean that we'd learn to respect its needs; and avoid the very things that not only does it not need, but indeed harm it.

Most of us don't though. In our turbo-charged world we focus on other things, like making money, working hard and cramming some fun into the remaining time. We hope, like gamblers at a roulette wheel, the dice will deal us winning health, that we won't be attacked by some vicious germ, that our genes aren't flawed. And if we lose, well, it's just bad luck.

If we can blame our illnesses on germs or faulty genes or even bad luck, why bother changing? Such a fatalistic approach means we don't have to take responsibility for our health. And in many ways, that's what we've been taught.

Since the time of Louis Pasteur we've been told that germs alone are to blame for many diseases. What we haven't been told is that germs don't attack and proliferate unless we're already unhealthy—call it a weak immune system, if you like. And armies of germs can't survive when our environment is healthy. One component of that is sanitation and hygiene. But only one.

Many of those diseases that didn't succumb to the onslaught of modern drugs can now be blamed on our genes. For that you can thank the modern quest for the holy grail of life—unraveling the human genome through the Human Genome Project. You're not told this, but genes don't work in isolation from the rest of our body or our environment.

So the message is, if you can't change your genes, or eradicate all germs, change yourself. How? Through your mind and through the things you do and expose yourself to. In essence, it's all about your lifestyle. This then is the focus of Volume 2. It's about identifying and meeting your human needs: your psychological and spiritual needs, your bodily needs, and most importantly the need for connecting with yourself, with those around you, and with the world at large. Health does, after all, demand that we're connected.

But in Volume 1 we'll investigate the reasons for our rapidly declining health. In Part One, we'll investigate how modern medical science undermined and hijacked our health. In Part Two we'll examine how the institution of science failed us because it buried its head in the microscopic world and forgot that life, and hence health, is far more than the workings of an incredibly complex chemical factory; how modern science, unlike every previous cultural approach to health and healing, has ignored the life force itself. And in Part Three, we'll present the shocking revelation that governments, the media and the institutions of science and technology continue to conceal from the public, that the cause of many modern diseases is known; that, in essence, we've drifted far from the lifestyles we are adapted to living and have exposed ourselves to new dangers. The result is that the health of the planet and all life, human included, is paying the price for the stampede to adopt many modern technologies.

The unsung story

For the past half century, the refrain in the modern fugue that has thumped out our lifestyles has been 'Let the Good Times Roll.' We in the affluent West certainly live in superlative times. But in our stampede to 'live the good life' and have more of the 'good things in life'—a stampede that pulses to the cultural beat of economic growth, corporate profits and unfettered market forces—we've been distracted from realising how poor our collective health has become; and, more importantly, from changing our lifestyles to improve our health.

To further distract and confuse us has been the popular spin that our health has never been better. Gone are the epidemics of infectious diseases. Infant mortality has dwindled. Even deaths from cardiovascular disease and cancer are declining. And our life expectancy has never been higher. All that's true.

But there's another side to the story, down-played by all governments: though we're living longer, more of our lives are spent burdened with disease. Our health, in fact, has never been worse. Worldwide, across all age brackets, increasing numbers of people are falling prey to the so-called diseases of modern civilisation. And this is despite skyrocketing health budgets and advances in medicine.

Australia's experience is typical. It's just that we, together with other English-speaking nations, are leading the pack.

Cardiovascular disease, for example, which is still Australia's leading killer, now affects one in six people, 20 per cent more than it did 10 years ago.[1] According to Professor Andrew Tonkin, chief medical adviser of the National Heart Foundation of Australia, even young people are showing signs of the disease.[2]

The incidence of cancer is also increasing. According to the Cancer Council of South Australia, new cases of cancer in that state, which typify the national trend, rose by nearly 30 per cent during the last quarter of the 20th century.[3] Today only the US and New Zealand surpass that figure.

Admittedly, half of those with cancer survive because of medical treatments. And the incidence of some cancers, notably cervical cancer, and lung cancer (in men), has dramatically declined thanks to such preventive programs as the Quit Campaign, bans on tobacco advertising, and the National Cervical Screening Program.

But during the past 25 years, according to the Cancer Council's figures, the age-standardised annual rate for new cases of bowel cancer has risen by 16 per cent, myeloma by 20 to 30 per cent, leukaemia by nearly 40 per cent, breast cancer and non-Hodgkin's lymphoma by 60 per cent. And the incidence of melanoma and prostate cancer has doubled.[3–7]

Per capita, Australia leads the world in the incidence of melanoma, ranks second for bowel cancer, second alongside Canada for breast cancer, second alongside New Zealand and Canada for non-Hodgkin's lymphoma, third for prostate cancer, and third alongside New Zealand for childhood cancers.[8,9] And South Australia leads the world in the incidence of adult leukaemia, myeloma and brain cancer.[5,10]

Diabetes follows the same trend. According to AusDiab, the first national study on the prevalence and impact of diabetes, commissioned by the Federal Government and conducted in 1999–2000, the number of adults with diabetes has more than doubled during the past 20 years.[11,12] Today a quarter of the population has either diabetes or impaired glucose metabolism, which is itself a precursor to diabetes.

Our rapidly declining health is reflected in a doubling in the prevalence of arthritis over the past 25 years. The Access Economics publication, *Arthritis–The Bottom Line*, reports that a third of the adult population now suffers from arthritis or other musculo-skeletal problems such as osteoporosis and chronic back pain.[13]

Autoimmune diseases, which first came to prominence during the 1950s, are now estimated to affect 1 in 15 people, predominantly women.[14] The prevalence in the United States is 1 in 12, according to the National Institutes of Health,[15] but the American Autoimmune Diseases Related Association estimates that the figure is closer to 1 in 5.[16] Type I Diabetes, one of more than 80 autoimmune diseases, is known to have increased by 50 per cent during the past 20 years.[17–19] The highest incidence occurs in Finland, Sweden and Norway followed closely by the United Kingdom and Australia.[19,20] Indeed, according to Diabetes UK the incidence of Type I Diabetes in the United Kingdom has doubled every 20 years since 1945.[21] And a 35-year study on multiple sclerosis found that between 1961 and 1996, the incidence of this nerve disease among residents in the Newcastle region in Australia had doubled.[22]

Asthma, which is one of the main reasons children miss school or are hospitalised, has also reached epidemic proportions. Twenty-five years ago 1 in 20 children had asthma.[23,24] Today it's closer to 1 in 6, over a three-fold increase. Some studies indicate that in some parts of Australia the prevalence of asthma among primary school children is as high as 1 in 4. Again, Australia and New Zealand are world leaders, with Britain in hot pursuit.

Twenty-five years ago, severe food allergies and anaphylaxis were rare. Since then their prevalence and severity have skyrocketed. According to the Australasian Society of Clinical Immunology, food allergies now affect 1 in 20 children, and anaphylaxis occurs in 1 in 200 school-age children.[25] European researchers even predict that if current trends continue, by 2015 half of all Europeans may be suffering from some sort of allergy.[26]

Autism was first identified during the 1940s.[27] Then, paralleling the introduction of mass childhood vaccination programmes in the 1950s, the numbers of children diagnosed with the syndrome began to soar.[28] By the 1960s, British and Danish researchers estimated that about 1 in every 2000 children had the condition.[29,30] By the mid-1970s the estimates were about 1 in 250.[31,32] Between 1976 and 2001 the incidence of autism doubled every two years. Today, autism affects 1 in every 160 Australian children.[33] In the US it's 1 in 150.[34] And if the less severe forms of autism, such as Asperger's Syndrome, are included in what is now called the autistic spectrum, then about 1 in 100 of Australia's population are affected.

Disturbances in human fertility also came to light during the middle of the 20th century. By the mid-1990s, a Danish study that had reviewed over 60 international papers on fertility, estimated that the quantity and quality of sperm in males worldwide had halved since the 1940s.[35] Low sperm counts and defective sperm are linked to miscarriages and birth defects. Today it is estimated that between 1 in 7 and 1 in 15 couples of reproductive age are unable to conceive.[36]

Even our psychological health is in crisis. An Australian Bureau of Statistics (ABS) survey in 1997 found that 1 in 5 adults in the preceding year met the criteria for a mental health disorder.[37] Nor are children spared. Within any six-month period, 1 in 7 of them have also been identified as having a mental health problem.[38] More recent surveys have estimated that 1 in 10 Australians have long-term psychological disturbances,[39] and that almost half the adult population has had a mental disorder at some stage in their lives.[40] One British psychiatrist, Bruce Charlton, commenting on his nation's health, claimed that 'mental health and well being are so rare as to be remarkable'.[41]

As for suicide, almost as many Australians kill themselves as die in road crashes. And according to UNICEF, in 1994 Australia had the highest youth suicide rate of all industrialised countries, with 16.4 suicides per 100,000 among 15 to 24-year-olds.[42] The rate peaked in 1997, with 19.3 per 100,000.[43]

The extent of the population's declining health was highlighted in an ABS survey in 2001 which found that a staggering 87 per cent of respondents reported having one or more long-term health conditions, that 20 per cent had some form of disability, and that nearly 20 per cent experienced pain every day for at least three months.[44]

So much for the spin that our health has never been better.

Tellingly, despite the ability of governments to cull statistics through the ubiquitous computer, data banks and government bureaucracy, the only disease they classify as 'notifiable', apart from infectious diseases, is cancer.[45,46] From periodic surveys alone do we glean any idea about the sweeping landscape of disease. Quite simply, there is no political will to discover and disclose how bad our health really is.

The flawed argument on ageing

Though many factors have been blamed for these epidemics, the popular culprit, particularly for heart disease, cancer, and diabetes, is the ageing of the population. The unfounded argument goes like this: People in the past would have got heart disease or cancer or diabetes if they'd lived long enough, but contagions and pestilence got them first.

Modern evidence, however, emphatically belies this claim. Cardiovascular disease, for instance, was virtually non-existent in the 1960s among rural communities of China, even in the elderly.[2,47] Nor did these rural dwellers have any of the known risk factors, such as high blood pressure, high cholesterol or obesity. The same for the people living traditional lifestyles on the Trobiand Islands of Papua New Guinea.[48]

Cardiovascular disease, diabetes and bowel cancer were very rare in the 1960s in the rural communities of equatorial Africa, South Africa and India.[49] The surgeons from the Royal Berkshire Hospital who conducted the study also noted the rarity of appendicitis, diverticular disease, gallstones, dental caries, haemorrhoids, varicose veins and deep vein thromboses.

In the first half of the 20th century, cancer was remarkably rare or non-existent among the Inuit, the Hunzakuts, West and Central Africans, and the people of Papua New Guinea, Brazil, Ecuador, and Bolivia.[50–60]

But as hunter-gatherer and rural communities began switching to modern lifestyles and diets, adopting modern technologies and being exposed to many of the 80,000 or more chemicals that have been unleashed on the world since the 1940s, they too began to succumb to the diseases of civilisation.[54,57,61–68]

Multiple sclerosis, for example, was thought to be non-existent in the Bantu people of Kenya during the 1970s.[69,70] By the 1990s the first cases were coming to light.[71–75] Today the incidence is increasing.[76] Asthma, which was extremely rare among the highland people of Papua New Guinea in the 1970s,[77] had become common within 10 years of contact with the outside world and adoption of Western lifestyles.[78] And today the incidence of cancer is no longer remarkably rare among the Inuit and the people of Bolivia, Brazil and Ecuador.[63,79–83]

The robust health of the indigenous peoples of North America, Australia and New Zealand had also been chronicled, though long ago. A few of the first Europeans to encounter these people had written that their health seemed far superior to that of Europeans.[84–91] But alas, today their collective health is far worse than that of their non-indigenous compatriots.[92]

The prevalence of Type II Diabetes amongst New Zealand's Maoris, for example, is double that for the non-indigenous Pakehas.[93] Amongst the indigenous people of the US and Canada, it's three times higher than that for their non-indigenous compatriots.[94,95] Amongst the Pima Indians of the America's south-west, it is 19 times higher.[96] And in Australia, Aboriginal adults are almost four times more likely to have the disease than their non-indigenous mates.[64,98] For those aged 20 to 50 the prevalence is 10 times higher. In fact, 1 in every 10 Aboriginal adults between the ages of 35 and 44 has diabetes; and for those over 55, one in three is afflicted. Adding to Aboriginal woes is the fact that compared with their non-indigenous compatriots they have a 10-times greater incidence of kidney disease, which is one of the complications of diabetes.[98]

Tellingly, a study conducted by Australian researcher Kerin O'Dea on a group of overweight, middle-aged, diabetic Aboriginal men revealed that after seven weeks of them reverting to their traditional hunter-gatherer lifestyle, the men had marked improvement in their blood glucose and triglyceride levels, and a dramatic reduction in insulin resistance.[99]

The band-aid solution

To counter the rising tide of modern diseases, governments have pinned their hopes and placed their bets on advances in medicine, on disease management and, for some diseases, on cure. Often, government initiatives provide 'band-aid' solutions at best. Australia's track record on band-aid solutions is typical of nations that have gone down this path instead of providing real solutions.

When the Pharmaceutical Benefits Scheme began 61 years ago, only one person in every 30 was prescribed one of the 139 listed drugs, at a cost (then) of $300,000.[100] Ten years later the prescription rate was two per capita per year, costing $38 million. Today, of the 700 listed drugs, eight prescriptions are written each year for every man, woman and child. And the cost? A staggering $7 billion.[101]

There is no doubt that band-aid treatments have been effective in reducing death rates from cardiovascular disease and cancer, and in relieving the symptoms of many diseases. Unfortunately, this approach hasn't stemmed the rising tide of modern diseases. Nor has it removed the known risk factors, even for cardiovascular disease.

Today half the adult population has high cholesterol levels, 30 per cent has high blood pressure, a quarter still smokes, half doesn't exercise enough, and 60 per cent of adults and 20 per cent of children are overweight.[1] And yet even from the medical perspective, about 85 per cent of cases of cardiovascular disease are preventable, through lifestyle changes and improved nutrition.

Government funding on health promotion, however, has been abysmal. Of the $51 billion spent on Australia's health budget in 2003, less than half of one per cent was spent on health promotion;[102] less than one tenth of that was spent on promoting exercise. And yet physical activity is known to be the most successful factor in preventing disease, apart from quitting smoking. Exercise reduces the incidence of bowel and breast cancer, heart disease, Type II Diabetes, and depression.

Governments have also turned a blind eye to the many other known and suspected disease factors we live with, but which were non-existent in hunter-gatherer and pre-industrial rural communities.

For at least 99.9 per cent of humanity's existence, from Stone Age times until the 20th century, people lived without toxic chemicals being sprayed on foods, without food additives, and without genetically manipulated foods. Nor did people drink water polluted with industrial chemicals or xenoestrogens, or deliberately adulterated with chlorine, or fluoride; the latter is one chemical which, incidentally, most European nations have banned because of its toxicity.

Past generations did not breathe chemically polluted air. They were not exposed to electromagnetic radiation from power lines or mobile-phone towers. They did not take synthetic drugs. Nor were their children spared childhood infections by being inoculated with vaccines—still a controversial issue in British medical circles. And few people endured the relentless stresses and social isolation so typical in our global village.

What on earth is stopping us from changing?

Though we can't return to the Stone Age, we can change our lifestyles and reduce or avoid many risk factors; but if we continue down the band-aid path, then current trends are unlikely to change. Ten years ago, the prediction was that 1 in 3 men and 1 in 4 women would get some form of cancer in their lives.[103] Today, predictions are that 1 in 2 men and 1 in 3 women will get some form of cancer,[104] and that by 2050 a quarter of Australia's population will have cardiovascular disease.[1]

This bleak outlook then begs the question: What on earth is stopping us from changing?

The answer, perhaps, is that we know neither what nor how to change. Or maybe it's just that we've pinned our hopes on advancements in medical science but are blind to the harm it has already caused.

Like the townsfolk in Hans Christian Andersen's story 'The Emperor's New Clothes' we have been fooled into thinking the emperor's new clothes are resplendent.[105] The courtiers from government, science and technology, and the media tycoons, have made sure of that. The whole charade is symptomatic of a global palace gone mad for they've failed to admit that the emperor is covered with festering sores. No one has dared to reveal that health has become a casualty of modern times, that we, like the planet, are ailing. No one has dared to cry for health.

Chapter 1

Death by Doctoring

For, medicine being a compendium of the successive and contradictory mistakes of medical practitioners, when we summon even the wisest of them to our aid, the chances are that we may be relying on a scientific truth, the error of which will be recognised in a few years' time.
Marcel Proust, French novelist (1871–1922).

The unfolding story

Imagine the newspaper headlines and the political furore if, in the US alone, six jumbo jets crashed every day. Or if, in Australia, one crashed every two days. And yet in the same time frame the equivalent number of people are dying because of modern medicine.

You won't find this emblazoned in the headline news, and rarely is it identified in the statistics on diseases and deaths. That's because up until the 1990s no nation had dared to investigate the extent of the silent epidemic of iatrogenic (caused by medicine) sickness and deaths.

Harm or death caused by medicines has always been the nemesis of physicians. The principle of 'primum non nocere', of 'first, do no harm', has been one of the basic tenets of all traditional systems of medicine—in the Jewish 'Prayer of Maimonides', the Indian 'Oath of the Hindu Physician', the Persian 'Advice to a Physician', the Japanese '17 Rules of Enjuin', and it is embraced in the 'Hippocratic Oath', directing the physician to 'abstain from whatever is deleterious or mischievous', which, until the beginning of 20th century, Western-trained medical students would swear.[1-3]

Death by doctoring claimed many lives in the past, including those of King Charles the Second and George Washington. If the stroke the King suffered didn't kill him, then the barrage of herbs and chemicals and the blood-letting administered by 14 royal physicians did.[4] And the first US president, who apparently had quinsy, not surprisingly died after two physicians drained away a third of his blood.[5]

The litany of harm caused by modern drugs was first identified half a century ago when US Army Major (later Lt. Colonel) Robert H. Moser published his findings from a survey of existing medical literature on iatrogenic disease. He warned colleagues of the dangers of hundreds of drugs, as well as from surgically-induced and radiation-induced diseases.[6,7]

The unsuspecting public, however, were not alerted to the epidemic of iatrogenic injury and fatalities until 1976, when Ivan Illich published his book *Limits to Medicine*. He claimed that 1 in 5 Americans entering a typical hospital at that time would acquire some sort of iatrogenic disease. He warned: 'The impact of modern medicine [is] one of the most rapidly spreading epidemics of our time'.[8]

During the 1980s and '90s other medical writers were warning us of the rising epidemic.[9-12] We learned, for example, that when physicians went on strike in Israel in 1973, and in Britain and California in 1978, the death rate fell by between 35 and 50 per cent.[12]

Undoubtedly, doctors were also becoming aware that many of the new drugs they were prescribing, though advertised in glowing terms by pharmaceutical companies, and hailed as miracle cures by the media, were in fact harming their patients.[13]

Dr Norman Swan, producer and presenter of the Australian Broadcasting Corporation's Health Report, recalls that when he was in medical school, terribly sick and elderly patients would be admitted to hospital with signs and symptoms that would puzzle medical students.[14] But when consultants took them off all but the absolutely necessary drugs many of their complaints would disappear. The combined actions and interactions of the drugs had harmed them.

Until the 1990s the magnitude and nature of the modern epidemic of death and harm caused by modern medicine had largely been ignored by our medical authorities and the media. An early study in 1964 should have rung alarm bells in the corridors of the medical establishment.[15] It had found that 200 out of every 1,000 hospital patients had been harmed by medical treatment: half of those were harmed by the effects of drugs, and 50 of those harmed subsequently died.

No doubt the alarm bells did ring with the publication in 1991 of the first major study into hospital blunders.[16,17] Conducted in New York State in 1984, the study found that out of every 1,000 hospital patients, 37 had been harmed whilst in hospital; 10 of these were harmed as a result of hospital blunders. Five of these patients—that's 1 in 200 patients—subsequently died, and one was permanently disabled.

The truth revealed

Finally, in 1999, the US Institute of Medicine did acknowledge the size of the problem.[18] Using the figures from the New York study, and the results of another conducted in Utah and Colorado,[19] the Institute estimated that as many as 98,000 patients die each year as a result of medical errors.

However, Dr Lucian Leape, one of the researchers in the New York study, had already estimated that with over 30 million people being admitted to hospitals across the US each year, the figure was closer to 180,000 deaths.[20] That, according to Dr Leape, is the equivalent of three jumbo jet crashes every two days.

Meanwhile, Australia had also conducted an extensive study into hospital errors.[21] The study identified that the number of patients dying as a result of hospital blunders was the same as that estimated in the New York study: 1 in 200. For Australia, this equates to about 14,000 patients per year. Equally alarming was the estimate that each year more than twice that number of patients—over 20 times the US rate—were permanently injured.

While commentators debate the differences between the figures for Australia and the US, some claiming that the American figures underestimate the prevalence of medical injury and error,[22] or are under-reported because of fear of law suits, we can be sure of one thing: hospitals are potentially dangerous places to be in.

And we've only dealt with preventable medical errors in hospital. What about the harm and deaths resulting from unnecessary diagnostic or surgical procedures that are performed in hospital? Or infections that are caught in these factories for the sick? Or the errors made by general practitioners? Or the vexed question of the side effects of drugs, known in medical jargon as adverse drug reactions, that Dr Moser had warned his colleagues about almost 50 years ago?

Again, only estimates are available. This may be because the juggernaut of modern medicine is too cumbersome to adequately monitor or, indeed, to control, for it is thought that only about 10 per cent of adverse drug reactions are reported.[23,24] But it may also be that the political will to do anything about it never existed. Fragments of the picture, however, are emerging from various studies. And it's not a pretty picture.

Ten per cent of the people admitted to hospital in the US are there because of the side effects of the drugs their doctors prescribed.[25,26] For Britain, the estimated figure is 3.5 per cent of admissions.[27] And for Australia, 3 per cent.[28] In the Australian context this means that 30,000–40,000 patients are admitted to acute medical wards every year because of the side effects of prescribed drugs, and that 700–900 of those die.

Even while in hospital, between 6 and 15 per cent of patients in Australian hospitals suffer from an adverse drug reaction,[29] though estimates for US hospitals range from 1.5–43.5 per cent.[26] If we take a low estimate of four per cent, it would mean that over one million Americans are harmed by drugs each year.[25]

A person who would have known the extent of the disaster back in 1984 was epidemiologist Dr Julian Gold, head of the Australian National Health Surveillance Unit of the Commonwealth Institute of Health. He estimated that up to 40 per cent of all patients may be victims of iatrogenic disease.[30] Recent figures from the UK suggest that the level may be as high as 50 per cent.[31]

One doctor who has tallied up the figures for deaths caused by modern medical practice in the US is Dr Matthias Rath, a campaigner against iatrogenic disease.[32] Using the results of existing studies, he estimates that mistakes made in surgery may kill as many as 32,000 patients a year;[33] unnecessary diagnostic and surgical procedures, 37,000;[34] hospital infections, 88,000;[35] adverse drug reactions in hospital, 106,000;[36,37] and adverse drug reactions from those prescribed by general practitioners, 199,000.[22,38]

Adding these figures, and those for deaths from bedsores and malnutrition, to those for medical errors, Dr Rath estimates that as many as 784,000 Americans die each year because of medical intervention, equivalent to six jumbo jet crashes a day, or 42 every week. And if a nationwide poll in 1997 on medical and drug errors is anything to go by, the figure, according to Dr Rath, may be as high as 1 million.[39] That would increase the weekly death toll from the equivalent of 42 jumbo jet crashes per week to 53. That then relegates death by doctoring to the number one position in causes of death, at least in the US. It is unlikely to be any different in other Western nations, since their doctors employ the same medical tools.

Is it any wonder that the principle of 'doing no harm' is conspicuous by its absence from medical oaths written during the 20th century and based on the principles of modern bioethics—the 'Physicians Oath' of the Geneva Declaration and the 'Oath of Lasagna', for example, which some, and only some, medical students swear? Admittedly, 98 per cent of medical schools in the United States and Canada do have some form of declaration that graduating students swear, though in Australia and New Zealand it's about 60 per cent, in the United Kingdom about 50 per cent, and in the Republic of Ireland only about 20 per cent.[40-43]

Nevertheless, the import of such oaths on modern medical practice leaves much to be desired. According to one American doctor, David Graham, writing in *The Journal of the American Medical Association* in December 2000, 'the original [Hippocratic] oath is redolent of a covenant, a solemn and binding treaty. By contrast, many modern oaths have a bland, generalized air of "best wishes" about them, being near-meaningless formalities devoid of any influence on how medicine is truly practiced.'[44]

As the editor of the *British Medical Journal* declaimed about the harm modern medicine is wreaking: 'It's essential that doctors, patients and politicians worldwide grasp the scale of the problem.'[45]

Perhaps more to the point, it's time modern medicine was healed, because it too is very sick. Not only are increasing numbers of people falling foul of the diseases of civilisation, many are also becoming part of the collateral damage of the war on disease.

Chapter 2

Tools of Medicine

> *Marketing a disease is the best way to market a drug.*
> Susan Love MD, American surgeon.

Where are we going? A summary

Drugs, and the mindset of modern medicine, are at the heart of medicine's failure to halt the diseases of civilisation and the swathe of harm and death-by-doctoring it is wreaking. Chapters 3 to 7 will examine that mindset. It favours drugs over natural medicines, and it has trained doctors to focus on pathology, not health and healing; hence it has created a disease-care system. And the general public has been seduced into adopting this mindset.

First, in this and the following three chapters we'll examine the primary tools of medicine: drugs.

Two clues

The first clue to the reason for the modern epidemic of harm through doctoring is the nature of modern drugs. Of the modern pharmacological armamentarium, at least 75 per cent are concoctions that do not exist in nature.[1] The remainder are chemicals that are extracted from plants, or their synthetic equivalents.

The second clue is the brief span of time in which they have been used. It was only one hundred years ago that the first synthetic drug, a compound of arsenic subsequently used in the treatment of syphilis, was discovered by German scientist Paul Ehrlich. Hence only five generations of people at most have been taking these chemical concoctions.

The perennial tools of medicine

Since time immemorial, plant medicines have been the primary tools for healing. Modern scientists assume that the earliest humans discovered the therapeutic effects of various plants by trial and error. It is more likely, however, that our earliest cousins, those members of Homo habilis and Homo erectus who roamed the Earth for about two million years until they died out perhaps 400,000 years ago, instinctively knew which plants in their locales would restore them to health, just as sick animals instinctively seek out certain grasses and herbs.

Certainly much of the early humans' herbal lore would have been based on what they saw in nature: on what animals did or ate when they were sick. The following example illustrates this point.

In 1987, while observing chimpanzees in the Mahale Mountains National Park in Tanzania, Mike Huffman, a researcher based at the Primate Institute of Kyoto University, Japan, watched a clearly unwell adult female chimpanzee lagging behind her troop.[2,3] Her appetite seemed to have vanished; except, that is, for one plant: bitter leaf (*Vernonia amygdalina*). She was plucking the young stems and eating the inner pith. By the next day she was up and running, apparently having made a complete recovery from a gastrointestinal upset caused by parasites. Huffman subsequently learned that the local Tongwe people, when they had stomach cramps and intestinal parasites, used the same plant's leaves, bark and root, though not the pith.

We know that our Neanderthal cousins were using medicinal plants 63,000 years ago, many of which are still prescribed by today's herbalists.[4,5] From the inscriptions on plates of stone and the writings on papyri, we know that physicians in the early civilisations of Mesopotamia, Egypt and China were prescribing herbal remedies; though some, admittedly, were very bizarre remedies that contained odd bits of animals.

No matter where civilisation flourished, whether it was in the South American civilizations of the Mayans and Incas, or the Celtic, Greek and Roman civilizations of Europe, the herbal traditions continued. During the Dark Ages, knowledge of herbal remedies centred on the European monasteries. Using herbs from their physic gardens, monks, who in many areas were the only ones who possessed any medical skills, tended the sick.

Beyond the gates of the cities, generations of wise men and women were also passing their knowledge of plants on to their children and grandchildren. And in the tracts of wilderness, the tribes of hunters and gatherers were keeping their herbal lore alive.

Though medical pundits would like to relegate herbal medicine to a footnote in the history of medicine, it is a fact that even today about 80 per cent of the world's population still relies on traditional medicine as the main source of health care.[1] Indeed, in recognition of this, the World Health Organisation (WHO) established its Traditional Medicine Programme in 1978 to help developing countries integrate traditional approaches to birthing and healing into their primary health care systems. Today, worldwide, there are 19 WHO Collaborating Centres for Traditional Medicine.

Thus, both historically and demographically, herbal medicine is the world's orthodox medicine. Modern medicine is the newcomer on the block.

The new tools of medicine

The sad tale of modern drugs had been foreshadowed over 300 years earlier when the Swiss physician and philosopher Paracelsus introduced laboratory chemicals into European medicine to replace traditional herbal remedies. The medicines began as a spin-off from a revival of the ancient alchemical quest to transmute matter; in particular that of turning base metals into gold. But while Paracelsus, who recognised that every substance can be a poison depending on its dose, had recommended that physicians prescribe very low doses, many of his followers dished out liberal amounts.

For the next two centuries, trained physicians plied their patients with such poisonous chemicals as antimony, arsenic and mercury for fevers, bronchitis, asthma, indigestion, and skin complaints. Today we understand the hideous error of their therapeutics.

But the saga of death by doctoring was far from over. In fact, it was about to explode. This time, the tools would emerge as a spin-off from the gigantic oil industry, which had also spawned the aniline dye and paint industries, and, later, the agricultural chemical industry. This time, not just some, but all, doctors would prescribe them. Under the guise of 'scientific medicine', medical associations, together with medical colleges, would ban the teaching and use of any remedy that had not been scientifically validated for safety and efficacy.[6] Government regulators made sure of compliance.

Herbs, foods, homoeopathic remedies, sunlight, exercise and massage were considered to be neither scientific nor therapeutic. Over the years, the population at large fell into line with this view, so that by the 1970s, when I trained in medical herbalism, these traditional therapies were classified as 'fringe medicine'. Then, as increasing numbers of people became disenchanted with modern medicine, such therapies came to be known as 'alternative' during the '80s. By the 1990s they were classified as 'complementary medicine'.

Why create new tools?

Let's pause for a moment. Why would modern medical science claim that traditional knowledge about healing remedies is not scientific? After all, if we look at the origin of the word 'science' we discover that it means 'to know', from the Latin *scire*. And, as the philosophy of knowledge (epistemology) states, all of our knowledge arises from observation and experience. Tellingly, modern science substituted the word 'experiment' for 'experience' (see Chapter 6: 'A Slice of Bacon').[7,8]

We could therefore conclude that the clinical trials on thousands of plant remedies world-wide have been conducted for tens of thousands of years. If we date the emergence of modern man to between 125,000 and 200,000 years ago, as many palaeoanthropologists, geneticists and archaeologists claim,[9–18] then from 4,000 to 6,500 generations of our ancestors (about 30 years per generation) observed and experienced the effects of various medicinal plants. That's not a bad trial.

And the time-frame for modern medicine? —which began during the second half of the 19th century with the promulgation of Louis Pasteur's germ theory of disease,[19,20] the isolation and extraction of chemical constituents from plants,[21] the publication of the first editions of pharmacopoeia (drug manuals), and the rise of modern pharmaceutical companies.[22] About five generations. And since the onslaught of drugs into the public arena? About two generations.

Moreover, the clinical trials on plants were conducted on all sorts of people. Young people. Old people. Sick people. Pregnant women. Breast-feeding mothers. Not, as modern medical science initially does, on rats or guinea pigs, and then for a short period of time on a select group of supposedly healthy human guinea pigs.

And if the god of science does require that a medicinal plant be peered at through a microscope and subjected to a barrage of tests, and then clinically trialled in double-blind, cross-over tests before its safety and efficacy are proven, then why has this never been done?

Patents

The answer, it would seem, lies with the age-old demons of power and greed, which, for the past 200 years, have been masquerading as corporate ownership, monopoly and profits. The old European system of individual ownership had already deprived the Australian and North American indigenous custodians of their traditional lands. But in the 20th century it was the western system of patent law, now universally applied, that spurred the stampede to own medicines.

Patent law enables any person or organisation that has invented a new product to gain 20-year monopolistic rights to the manufacture and sales of, and profits from, that product.[23] You can patent a new chemical concoction that you've developed in a laboratory. But, up until 1978—when the US Supreme Court granted the first patent on a life form (see Chapter 15: 'Frankenfoods')—you couldn't patent a plant or any other living organism.

Drug Companies

If, as a pharmaceutical company, your motive was massive profits, then you'd opt for a patented medicine. Why would you bother with medicinal plants since they are part of the common domain? And that's exactly what pharmaceutical companies did. They already had a captive market of doctors in developed countries. All they had to do was persuade them that the new drugs they produced were safe and effective. Then the good times would roll.

Further opportunities for profits arose during the latter half of the 20th century with the advent of national health schemes throughout the developed world. These schemes enabled everyone to access subsidised drugs. Australia's experience (as discussed in the Introduction) is typical of the global trend: for doctors to prescribe more medicines to more patients, and for national health budgets to soar to meet the soaring costs of new drugs.

The beneficiaries of the global drug binge have been pharmaceutical companies. In 2002, the combined drug sales of the large drug companies, 15 of which controlled over half of the global drugs market, reached US$430 billion.[24-26] Only 10 nations have gross national product sales (GNP) in excess of this.[27]

Pharmaceutical companies justify the rocketing prices of their drugs by claiming that they must recoup costs and invest in further research and development for newer drugs.[28] The facts belie this claim. More money—two and a half times more in the US, according to Families USA, a US health care advocacy organisation—is spent on marketing, advertising and administration than on research and development.[24,29,30] In fact, in 2000, the pharmaceutical industry spent US$92.3 million on lobbyists in the United States: that is, more than one lobbyist for every member of Congress.[24,28,31]

If you had thought drug companies were on a noble mission to fight disease, hopefully your belief is fading fast. Now, to shatter your belief, consider this: just over one per cent of the drugs developed during the last quarter of the 20th century were targeted at tropical diseases and tuberculosis.[24,32] Most of these drugs were developed in publicly funded, not corporate, laboratories.[24,26] Yet these diseases accounted for 11 per cent of the global disease burden.[24,32] Even now, only 10 per cent of global health research, both corporate and public, is devoted to diseases that account for 90 per cent of the world's disease burden.[24,32]

We know that poverty breeds infectious disease, but poor people would hardly be a target for profit-focused medicine. The goldmine is in the wealthy nations, particularly North America, where over half of all drugs sales are made.[24,33] Thus, the top selling drug in 2002 was Pfizer's Lipitor, with sales of nearly US$8 billion.[25] This drug is a cholesterol reducer.

Perhaps now you can understand why the drug industry spends more money on lobbying US politicians and regulatory authorities than any other industry in the US;[24,30,31] and why it spends nearly A$10,000 a year on each Australian doctor, trying to woo them into prescribing their latest magic bullets.[34,35]

Making Sense of Drugs

For a profit-driven industry it makes sense to focus on creating drugs for disorders of affluence, like high cholesterol levels and high blood pressure. It makes sense to medicalise risk factors. It makes sense to create drugs for imagined diseases like menopause or obesity.

And it makes sense of why, out of all industries, the drug industry, up until 2003, had the highest profit margins, outstripping commercial banks and oil and mining giants.[24,36] And, perhaps it begins to make sense of why many of the drugs it peddles are not safe.

Chapter 3

Why Modern Medicine May Be Harming You

*Doctors are men who prescribe medicines of which they know little,
to cure diseases of which they know less,
in human beings of whom they know nothing.*
Voltaire, French writer and philosopher (1694–1778).

Doctors and drugs—a dangerous mix

In ancient China, the role of doctors was to ensure that people remained healthy. When a person succumbed to an illness, the doctor wasn't paid. Today the opposite is true; if it were otherwise, today's doctors would be penniless. Doctors focus on treatment, not prevention. They get paid for disease care, not health promotion. They're focused on closing the gate after the horse has bolted, not on training the beast in the first place.

Modern medicine approaches the treatment of disease with the same war-like mindset that our politicians apply to things they don't like: the war on want, the war on drugs, the war on terror, and so on *ad nauseam*.

The proof of this is that prevention programmes (excluding vaccination programmes), such as advice on diet, exercise and lifestyle, comprise less than half of one per cent of 'health' budgets.[1]

Moreover, medicine's focus is on the disease process itself, rather than on the unique individual who happens to have a disease. As a consequence, modern nations employ vast armies of disease-care workers who use weapons that fight our bodies' processes. Symptoms are smothered, bacteria are blitzed, and, if all else fails, offending organs are removed. The problem is compounded by patients' expectations that doctors will fix health problems by prescribing a pill for every complaint.

A common scenario
You're sitting in the doctor's clinic feeling terrible. For months you've tried to ignore the pain, or the lump, or the difficulties you have with eating or breathing or walking; or maybe you're generally feeling unwell. You'd hoped the symptoms would go, but they didn't. So, perhaps under pressure from family and friends, you made an appointment with your doctor. On your first visit your case history was documented, tests were performed. Perhaps your doctor sent you for tissue tests or

X-rays. Perhaps you were prescribed a drug or two but, as you soon discovered, to no avail. Either way you had the tests, the results have come through, the dreaded moment when the doctor delivers the verdict has arrived.

It's cancer, you're told. Or diabetes. Or arthritis. Or Crohn's disease. Or any one of the many diseases that now plague our population. Up until this point in your life, you were in control of your destiny. At least, that's how you felt. The diagnosis is already shattering that belief. Your doctor's explanation of what is happening inside your body, that some function has gone awry, won't endear you to your body. More than likely you'll feel betrayed and curse your body. And, depending on the prognosis, many of your dreams about your future may also be shattered.

Your doctor's answer to your question about why the disease arose won't empower you either: it's part of the ageing process; it's genetic; it's a virus. How can you change your age or your parents? Why did the virus attack me? The answer that reveals the medical profession's ignorance about many diseases, is 'We just don't know'.

So, disempowered and potentially hating your body, you, like millions of others, are now on the medical treadmill. You'll be prescribed some drugs which, although they won't cure you, may help you to soldier on. Rarely will you be informed about their possible side effects; or, if you are, certainly not all of them. You may even be put on the waiting list for surgical removal of the offending part; you might need to have it replaced by some bionic bit. And every few months you'll return for a check-up, a repeat prescription, and perhaps a script for an additional drug to counter a new symptom, which may have been caused by the prescribed medication.

If you're silly enough to ask whether there is anything else you can do—besides taking the drugs, of course—it is likely that your doctor will offer platitudes about a healthy diet and a modicum of exercise, which he or she was taught as part of 'health promotion' training. Mention herbs or homoeopathy, or any of the other so-called alternative therapies and, depending on your doctor's bias, your question will either be palmed off with 'I don't see how it can do you any harm', or dismissed with a quip about not wasting your money on such quackery.

The reason your doctor hasn't got a clue is that his medical training has been focused entirely on the study of disease, not health, and on drugs that fight disease. His library is crammed with textbooks and magazines on disease. But there's nothing on health. He can reel off the signs and symptoms of a thousand diseases. But he can only identify health as the *absence* of disease.

The flood of new information from medical magazines, drug companies, and medical seminars on the latest ideas about how to treat your illness doesn't help your doctor either. Without a traditional approach to treating the sick, he is at the mercy of the latest whims of medical science. A few years ago he was advising mothers to bed their newborn babies on their fronts; now it has flipped 180 degrees, to laying them on their backs. Last year he was confidently prescribing hormone replacement therapy to his menopausal patients; this year he's not so sure.

Today your doctor will be endorsing a therapy that, in hindsight, may turn out to have been a mistake.

Drugs

Now let's identify some of the specific reasons why modern drugs harm so many people. We'll start with the actions of drugs.

Pushing and pulling

Medicines that push and pull and counter our bodily processes were known to ancient Greek physicians as contraries, or opposites. You'll recognise this with any drug that has an 'anti-' or opposite action. For example, inflammation is treated with anti-inflammatories, depression with anti-depressants, bacterial infection with antibiotics, high blood pressure with anti-hypertensives, bronchoconstriction with bronchodilators, and so on.

Such medicines have always been central to the treatment of acute illnesses that are likely to kill or result in irreversible damage to organs. Using contraries for these conditions is known in traditional Chinese medicine as 'stem treatment'. Just as a gardener may apply a spray to kill off a pest that is threatening to destroy a plant, so too do doctors prescribe drugs to treat 'the stem' of their patients' illnesses.

Stem treatment is certainly the forte of modern medicine, as is surgery. Many people who have had life-threatening diseases, like bacterial meningitis or pneumonia, would be dead but for modern drugs. Such treatment has also saved organs that would otherwise have been irreparably damaged: for example in treating infections of the inner ear or retina with anti-inflammatories and diuretics. And certainly many people with chronic and degenerative diseases are being kept alive, and in many cases symptom-free, thanks to modern drugs.

But the 'root' of the problem—the underlying reason why people get the illness in the first place—is ignored. And that is the key blind spot of medical science.

Though restoring and maintaining health will be explored in Volume 2, it is important to understand here that the use of contraries is based on the medical assumption that when we are sick our bodies have gone wrong, that they are malfunctioning, that things inside have gone awry. Understandably, you'd probably agree. The symptoms of asthma, influenza, depression or insomnia are unpleasant, to say the least. We'd like to be rid of them or, at the very least, to 'soldier on' as one drug company claimed for its flu remedy.[2] And contraries do oblige.

However, the indiscriminate use of contraries for almost every illness, both acute and chronic, regardless of whether or not they are life- or tissue-threatening, is one of the central reasons for iatrogenic disease. The indiscriminate use of antibiotics for every infection, for instance, has not only spawned antibiotic-resistant superbugs, but can also lead to gastrointestinal disturbances, including fungal infections. In developing countries, indiscriminate use of anti-tubercular drugs has produced the XRD strain of drug-resistant tubercular bacillus. Even DDT-resistant mosquitoes have been spawned.

And paradoxical, even ridiculous, though this statement may seem to you now, many disease processes are essential to our health. By thwarting these processes, contraries interfere with our health.

Ignoring our uniqueness

Another reason for the current iatrogenic disaster is the failure of modern medicine to recognise the uniqueness of the individual. Even if we disregard our differences in general health, age, personality, lifestyles and dietary habits, we still have physiological differences.

The science of pharmacokinetics, which is the branch of pharmacological science that deals with the movement of drugs within the body, has shown that for any one drug each of us differs in digestion, absorption, distribution, tissue and plasma protein binding, immune response, tissue sensitivity, metabolism and excretion. In fact, within the population at large there is a 9- to 10-fold difference in the availability and efficacy of a drug.[3-5] Hence, predictability of your response to a drug is an illusion.[6]

Nevertheless, in the clinical trials of their magic bullets, drug companies use sophisticated analyses to 'average out' the dose needed to affect the targeted tissues. Admittedly, side effects are documented. But this clearly makes standard doses rather meaningless and, for some drugs, deceptively dangerous.

What doctors prescribe are standardised drugs for standardised diseases. The only guides they have are drug manuals that identify the known side effects of each drug. Moreover, only those adverse effects that occur more frequently than one in 1,000 patients in the pre-marketing clinical tests are listed.[7]

Most adverse drug reactions arise from the known pharmacologic effects of drugs, the main offenders being antibiotics, anticoagulants, chemotherapy and cardiovascular drugs.[7] Though the incidence of adverse drug reactions from the known side effects are more prolific than the unknown side effects, luckily for us they are less likely to be lethal.

However, the occurrence of unknown or inexplicable side effects reveals that not only is medical science unable to fully understand the actions of drugs and the cascading effects they have on our bodies, but also that we the public are, in a sense, the experimental guinea pigs.

Aspirin, for example, had been marketed as the universal pain reliever since 1899. Not until the 1988, 89 years later, was it linked to Reye's syndrome in children, a non-inflammatory condition that produces pressure on the brain and damages the liver. Only then was baby aspirin removed from pharmacy shelves.

And only in the past 10 years have national surveillance systems been implemented whereby doctors can report—but only if they choose to—serious adverse effects of drugs.

Drug interactions

The third reason for iatrogenic harm arises from drug interactions. Before a medicine is released onto the market it is tested on animals and then human subjects for its safety and efficacy. Doctors, however, often prescribe drug cocktails, particularly to their elderly patients.

The practice of prescribing a drug to counter the side effects of another is also typical of modern medicine. It is reminiscent of the song that begins: 'There was an old lady who swallowed a fly that wiggled and jiggled and tickled inside her, perhaps she'll die ... '.[8] Then she swallowed a spider to catch the fly, a bird to catch the spider, and by the time she'd successively swallowed a cat, a dog, a cow and a horse, she died, of course.

Clearly, drug interactions can be a recipe for disaster.[9] Drugs can also interact with disease processes themselves, as well as with foods and herbs. But rarely are such interactions tested by pharmaceutical companies. Ironically, while much of the medical profession on the one hand dismisses alternative therapies as quackery, on the other hand it blames alternative treatments, particularly herbs, for causing adverse interactions with drugs. Ginkgo, garlic, and dong quai, for example, have been cited as magnifying the effects of anticoagulant drugs, leading to bleeding; and the laxatives senna, cascara and psyllium seeds have been blamed for decreasing the absorption of drugs.[10]

Clinical tests

Which brings us to the most contentious issue of all: clinical testing. When a new drug is developed, it is initially tested on animals. Why? Are all creatures really the same? Can we assume that because rabbits relish the fly agaric toadstool then we can readily eat it?[11] And, because koalas thrive on eucalyptus leaves, we can do the same? Of course not. For us the toadstool is a deadly poison. And should we eat more than one or two eucalyptus leaves our kidneys become irritated, and if we were to eat higher amounts we'd die from respiratory failure.

Similarly, whereas cats have no problems eating food contaminated with botulin toxin, we're more than likely to suffer an agonising death.[11] Morphine will sedate us as it does many animals. But as veterinary surgeons know, it sends cats into a frenzy. Again, penicillin kills many bacteria, but if given to guinea pigs it will kill them too. And arsenic kills us, but is harmless to guinea pigs, chickens and monkeys. We could go on providing example after example, but the simple fact is that one creature's food is another creature's poison.

A sad example of the absurdity of testing drugs on animals is the drug thalidomide. Scientists had subjected a host of animals, including rats, mice, rabbits, hamsters, ferrets, armadillos, pigs, dogs, cats, and primates to the drug.[12] Only occasionally did it cause malformed foetuses. On the basis of those animal tests, government regulatory bodies approved the drug for use by pregnant women who had morning sickness. As we now know, it was a human disaster.

We can conclude, as do many medical academics, that assessing a drug's safety on the basis of animal tests is not only unreliable and misleading, indeed meaningless, it is also scientific fraud.[11,13-23] As Dick Smithells—Professor of Paediatrics and Child Health at Leeds University, UK, during the 1980s, and a former member of the UK Committee on the Safety of Medicines, and the man who discovered that lack of dietary folic acid in pregnancy was linked to spina bifida—was driven to comment: 'The extensive animal reproduction studies to which all new drugs are now subjected are more in the nature of a public relations exercise than a serious contribution to drug safety.' He continued, 'The illogicality of the situation is demonstrated by the continued use of well-established drugs which are known to be teratogenic [leading to foetal abnormalities] in some mammalian species (e.g. aspirin, penicillin/streptomycin, cortisone). Conversely a new drug comes through its animal reproductive studies with flying colours may nevertheless be teratogenic in man.'[13]

Moreover, subjecting animals to the misery of laboratory testing also calls into question the assumption that our society is ethical, compassionate and intelligent.[22-24] Animal tests have nothing whatsoever to do with ensuring the safety of drugs. The real reason for animal testing is the legislative requirements that protect official regulatory bodies and corporations from legal liability should a drug later be found to be harmful.[11,15,20]

As for human tests, only about 2,000–3,000 subjects at best are tested in typical clinical trials.[25,26] Some researchers claim that at least 16,000 subjects should be tested to determine whether there is likely to be an adverse reaction in one out of 10,000 patients.[7] Moreover, people with complicated medical histories or medication regimes are often excluded from the trials, and most trials also exclude children, the elderly, and pregnant or breast-feeding women.[27] The upshot is that the human subjects taking part in tests do not represent those who will use a drug after its approval.

Marcia Angell, a former editor of *The New England Journal of Medicine*, is scathing in her criticism of pharmaceutical companies, particularly on the topic of how they conduct clinical trials in America.[28-30] As the author of *The Truth About Drug Companies: How They Deceive Us and What to Do About It*, she has documented how pharmaceutical companies design tests to guarantee favourable results for their drugs, in terms of both safety and efficacy. Any negative findings are simply not published. She has even speculated that 'perhaps most' clinical trials in the US are considered by medical critics to be 'excuses to pay doctors to put patients on a company's already-approved drug.'[31]

Equally reprehensible is the trend for drug companies to use poor countries as testing grounds for unapproved drugs, drugs that will eventually be prescribed in the wealthy West for such First World medical conditions as obesity, high blood pressure, and raised cholesterol levels.[32-34] Angell estimates that close to half of all clinical trials today are conducted in the Third World.[32] The reason? It's cheaper, and in many respects easier and faster to conduct them there. This ploy enables drug companies to circumvent ethical committees, avoid the necessity of obtaining 'informed' consent from subjects, and bypass other drug-testing protocols stipulated by regulatory authorities in the developed world. Even more enticing to drug companies is the fact that in poor regions of the world, they can more readily get away with distorting research to make their drugs look safer and more effective than they really are.

Vaccines are not even subject to the standard double-blind, placebo-controlled tests required for every other drug. A placebo is a biologically inert substance; ingesting a sugar pill, or being injected with a sterile saline solution is to be given a placebo. But to compare an experimental group that is injected with the new vaccine with a control group that is injected with either another vaccine or with the experimental vaccine from which the biological antigens have been removed is to guarantee that harm from the experimental vaccine will never be identified.

It is little wonder that investigators at the prestigious Cochrane Collaboration, a global organisation that provides independent systematic reviews of research into various healthcare interventions, should report that for many vaccines the design of experiments and the reporting of safety outcomes was 'largely inadequate', 'scarce and incomplete', and indicated 'reporting bias' and 'lack of standardisation'; and for some vaccines tested, that 'no studies reported on adverse reactions.'[35–38]

Indeed there are no true placebo groups in any vaccine trial because the experimental vaccine is tested on one group of previously vaccinated children and compared with another group of previously vaccinated children. This is despite research indicating that vaccinations have been implicated in brain damage, meningitis, encephalitis, autism, Guillain-Barré syndrome, attention deficit/hyperactivity disorder (ADHD), asthma, arthritis, and multiple sclerosis (see Chapter 5).

And, according to the American drug manual, the *Physician's Desk Reference*, not a single vaccine has been evaluated for its potential to cause cancer, mutagenicity (gene mutation) or infertility.[39]

Despite the controversy surrounding a possible link between autism and vaccines, and the fact that the prevalence of autism spectrum disorder in America's 8-year-old children increased by 57 per cent between 2002 and 2006 (from 1 in 150 to 1 in 110),[40] and that the estimated US national prevalence amongst 3- to 17-year-old children is now 1 in 91,[41] not a single official study has ever been conducted to compare the prevalence of autism in vaccinated versus unvaccinated children. The reason? Medical officialdom blames autism on people's genes, together with 'some environmental factor', and vaccines, it claims, are certainly not to blame. Hence the standard reply is that there are too few unvaccinated children in the US to use as a comparision.

But given that a study by the US Centers for Disease Control and Prevention found that in 2004 about 17,000 American children aged between 19- and 35-months-of-age were unvaccinated,[42] it would mean that close to 200,000 American children up to the age of 17 years would be unvaccinated; and they would provide the perfect comparison group.

One person who did dare to investigate the issue was investigative journalist

Dan Olmstead, a former senior editor with United Press International in Washington, DC. Between January 2005 and July 2007 he wrote 113 reports, collectively entitled 'The Age of Autism', about his findings. And where better to find unvaccinated children than among Amish communities in which the vast majority of parents obtain exemptions on religious grounds from otherwise mandatory vaccinations.

His starting point was among the Amish community in Lancaster County, Pennsylvania. From talking to medical practitioners, public health officials and residents, and from the e-mails he received thanks to his nationwide syndicated articles, he learned that autism was almost non-existent among Amish children; in a population of 22,000 there should have been dozens of autistic children in Lancaster County, based on the CDC's then-estimated prevalence nationwide of 1 in 166.[43–46] But Olmstead had heard of only three, possibly four cases, and tellingly at least two of them had been vaccinated.

Olmstead then turned to Ohio, the state with America's largest Amish population. He learned from Dr Heng Wang, medical director, physician and researcher at the Das Deutsch Center Clinic for Special Needs Children, in Middlefield, Ohio, that the prevalence of autism in the Amish community in that area of north-eastern Ohio, was 1 in 15,000, literally—there was only one child, a boy, with autism in a population of 15,000, and ominously he had received routine immunisations.[47] Olmstead unearthed similar patterns from his investigations among the Amish populations of Kentucky and Indiana.

Chicago was Olmstead's next port of call. There, many of the city's parents took advantage of Illinois' relatively permissive immunisation policy to avoid having their children vaccinated. Perhaps not surprisingly, the incidence of autism in Illinois in 2005 was 1 in 263, 37 per cent lower than the prevalence in the rest of the nation.[48] Olmstead learned from Dr Mayer Eisenstein, medical director of Homefirst Medical Services in Chicago—a large practice that provides a service to 30,000 to 35,000 children, many of whom have never been vaccinated—that he was aware of only one case of autism (and one case of asthma) amongst any unvaccinated children.

In essence, Olmstead had discovered that among America's Amish population of approximately 100,000 people, there were fewer than 10 cases of autism.[49] No, it wasn't a scientific study, but it did unearth something that regulatory watchdogs refused to investigate … and still refuse to investigate to this very day.[50,51] It's an issue that would never have arisen in the first place if there had been rigorous clinical trials on vaccines.

But there is one organisation that did investigate the issue, and it wasn't a government agency. Rescue Generation, a public advocacy organisation founded by parents of children with such neurological disorders as ADHD and autism, commissioned a telephone survey in 2006 to study the prevalence of neurological disorders among 17,600 4- to 17-year-old children in nine counties of California and Oregon; 991 of the children were described as never having been vaccinated.[52]

Just as many parents with neurologically damaged children had suspected, the survey did indeed find a strong correlation between neurological disorders and vaccinations. Vaccinated boys aged 4 to 17 years, were two-and-a-half times (155 per cent) more likely to have neurological disorders compared with unvaccinated boys of the same age. The risk of having ADHD was 224 per cent higher in vaccinated boys, and the risk of having autism was 61 per cent higher. But the 11- to 17-year-old boys fared far worse. They were 317 per cent more likely to have ADHD than their unvaccinated counterparts, and 112 per cent more likely to have autism.

That's certainly something many American parents might have wanted to have known before they had had their children vaccinated, given that 1 in 91 American children today have autism,[41] and that 1 in 13 have ADHD;[53] and that for 16-year-old boys the figure for ADHD is 1 in 7.[53]

Why trust drugs?

When we add all of the above to the fact that the only long-term 'drug tests' are conducted on the population at large, we are led to ask, why would anyone trust modern drugs? Perhaps it's because we think they are so effective in the fight against disease. But, are they really?

Chapter 4

Drug Hype

I firmly believe that if the whole materia medica, as now used,
could be sunk to the bottom of the sea,
it would be all the better for mankind,
and all the worse for the fishes.
Dr Oliver Wendell Holmes Sr. MD, poet, physician and essayist (1809–1894).

Did drugs rid the world of infectious diseases?

An old axiom of medicine states that if you have the flu and don't bother to treat it, it will last two weeks. But if you do take a medicine the illness will last only a fortnight. In other words, flu remedies don't work; at best they relieve symptoms. The same applies to many other drugs for a raft of illnesses. In fact, according to some studies, about 80 per cent of people who seek medical care have conditions that will either get better without any medical treatment, or cannot be improved by medical care.[1,2] That is an abysmal failure rate for a medical system that purports to have proven the efficacy of its drugs.

Now you may be asking yourself, what about infectious diseases? Haven't antibiotics and vaccinations rid the world of the past scourges of smallpox, tuberculosis, and many other communicable diseases? Aren't we living longer thanks to the power of modern drugs to conquer these pestilences?

To answer this, let's take a brief look at the history of human illness.

A brief history of human illness

Medical historians believe that from the time when people began domesticating plants and animals, beginning about 10,000 years ago until the late 1700s, as many as half of all people died before reaching adulthood.[3]

Some evidence suggests that in earlier times, however, many hunter-gatherers did reach grand-parenthood.[3,4] Indeed contrary to the popular myth that the lives of people in pre-historic times were characterised as 'nasty', 'brutish' and 'short', there is evidence to show that this is simply that: a myth.[5] Certainly in the 1800s, the health of Aboriginal hunter-gatherers, many of whom were elders, had been documented.[6] Admittedly, the term 'elder' in indigenous cultures refers not to an elderly person per se but to a person who, from his or her experience and wisdom, becomes a custodian of traditional knowledge and lore; nevertheless, many 'elders' would have been grandparents.[7,8] In the 20th century, studies of the world's last remaining hunter-gatherers—those in Tanzania, Botswana and Namibia,

Venezuela, Paraguay, and the Philippines—had found that although only about 60 per cent of children survived to adulthood, those that did had a lifespan of between 68 and 78 years.[5]

Living in settlements may have offered villagers and townsfolk such benefits as better shelter, a regular supply of food—though less variety of foods than in earlier times—and a broader distribution of skills not afforded to the smaller clans of hunters and gatherers. But such close-knit communities did increase people's exposure to infectious diseases.

You may be inclined to think that the high death toll in villages and towns was the result of such pandemics as the bubonic plague, which wiped out a quarter of Europe's population in the 14th century; or cholera and typhus, which ravaged populations during the 19th century. Such mass epidemics, together with harvest failures and wars, certainly wreaked havoc on populations from time to time, but it was in day-to-day life that the relentless toll from epidemics of infectious diseases occurred.[3] Poor people, peasants, serfs, slaves, and babies and children in particular, bore the brunt. We are familiar with many of these diseases today: they included gastrointestinal and lung infections, influenza, diphtheria and measles, and tuberculosis and malaria.

Consequently, life expectancy at birth was low, estimated to be just over 22 years in ancient Egypt, and between 25 and 35 in ancient Greece and Rome, and throughout Europe, up until about 1800.[9] It is thought that those who survived into adulthood could expect to live at least into their 30s or even 40s, though some, particularly the wealthy, reached the old Biblical yardstick of three score years and ten. Confucius, for example, was 72 when he died, Plato 82, and Elizabeth the First 70. According to the inscription on his small white marble gravestone in the centre of the south transept of Westminster Abbey in London, old Thomas Parr, an agricultural worker from Shropshire in England lived through the reigns of 10 monarchs during the 15th, 16th and 17th centuries to reach the grand old age of 152 years and 9 months.[10]

Then, at about the time when Shakespeare was churning out his plays, epidemics of bubonic plague and typhus began retreating from north-western Europe.[3] During the 1700s other communicable diseases, such as scarlet fever, small pox, typhoid fever, diphtheria and whooping cough, also began to decline—though not for babies—initially in rural populations and then during the 1800s amongst city dwellers.

Why the death rate declined

Why did these diseases decline? Scholars believe that higher living standards, especially improved nutrition, enhanced people's resistance to infections.[11-15]

The quality, variety and amounts of foods available had increased following improved trade and the introduction of a new method of crop rotation. The latter had replaced the earlier method of three-crop rotation and a year of lying fallow, with a four-year crop rotation that advocated the successive planting of root vegetables, legumes, barley and wheat.

The squalor, filth and poverty of the densely populated cities of Europe and North America, however, continued to provide the ideal breeding ground for such diseases as cholera and tuberculosis, as well as for childhood infections. Not until the late 1800s, after the introduction of public sanitation methods for sewage disposal, drainage, water supply, food storage and building ventilation, did the epidemics of cholera cease, the incidence of tuberculosis decline, and infant mortality rates decrease sharply.[3,14]

The introduction of hygienic birthing and surgical practices, as well as practices introduced by New Zealand's trailblazer in neonatal care, Dr Truby King, drastically reduced infant mortality rates during the first half of the 20th century.

According to the British Association for the Advancement of Science, childhood diseases decreased 90 per cent between 1850 and 1940, well before mandatory vaccination programmes.[16] Infectious diseases, including measles, diphtheria and whooping cough, continued to decline up until the 1950s, after which they levelled out and remain much the same today.[9] Neither antibiotics, which were developed in the 1940s, nor vaccination programmes, which reached only a small percentage of the population, can take credit for the reduction in communicable diseases.[17] Even the polio epidemics, which peaked in Britain in 1950, had already declined by 82 per cent when the Salk vaccine was introduced in 1956.[18]

Nor has modern medicine been a major factor in the decline in disease and death rates in Third World countries in recent years. According to a recent World Health Organisation report, the decline has been the result of improved standards of sanitation, hygiene and diet.[19] Quite simply, infectious diseases thrive where there is overcrowding, filth, poverty, wars and famine. Improve the social, economic, nutritional and sanitary conditions and such diseases rapidly decline.

Are we really living longer?

As for life expectancy at birth, we know that the global average today is 67 years.[20] For people in the developed world it is over 75 years. But the question remains: are we really living longer, as many medical propagandists claim? Or is it simply a statistical illusion generated by the fact that fewer infants are dying?

Russian researchers who investigated the records of 30,000 Russians born between 1700 and 1899, and who then compared these with modern data, found that indeed there has been no increase in human longevity, or life span.[21]

So, despite the purported miracle cures, and the vast armies of carers in our health care systems—which in reality are disease care systems—we are not only *not* living longer, many of us are succumbing to the very medicines that are supposed to be improving our health.

Chapter 5

To Vaccinate or Not to Vaccinate

As we know,
There are known knowns,
There are things we know we know,
We also know
There are known unknowns,
That is to say
We know there are some things
We do not know.
But there are also unknown unknowns,
The ones we don't know
We don't know.
Donald Rumsfeld, former US Secretary of Defense
February 12, 2002, Department of Defense news briefing.

The hype

To vaccinate or not to vaccinate? That is the question every parent must face—unless, of course, you live in a country where the government makes the decision for you. And behind that question are a host of others. Is vaccination safe? Is every one of the 13-odd vaccines, which the government recommends every child should get several times before he or she turns two, really safe? Is there a link between certain vaccines and autism or other disorders? Do vaccinations really work? What if I don't have my baby vaccinated, what will happen?

The medical hype, of course, is that immunisation is one of the most important health interventions of the 20th century; that it has eliminated smallpox infection worldwide, driven polio from most western countries and made formerly common infections like diphtheria, whooping cough, and measles rare occurrences.

So, who do you turn to, who do you trust? The vaccine manufacturers and their scientists, the public health department with its pro-vaccination campaigners, and your doctor who administers the jab? Or do you trust those who warn against vaccinations, claiming that vaccinations are neither safe nor efficacious?

In every country except Australia, doctors have no legal obligation whatsoever to tell you all the issues about any medical procedure. Their advice is based solely on 'medical opinion', and the doctor paternalistically decides what is in the patient's best interests. But in Australia, thanks to a High Court ruling in 1992 (Rogers v. Whitaker), Australian doctors have a legal duty of care to warn patients of all the side effects of all procedures whether the patient asks or not.[1] The problem is, most doctors only know about the pros of vaccinations and have no idea about the cons.

Since your baby's future health is at stake, it's certainly an emotive issue. Indeed the last thing you need in making your decision is to have fear added to the mix. But alas, that's exactly what governments and many doctors do. Hence informed choice flies out the window, the result being that those of us who have children invariably succumb to fear-mongering tactics.

Parents who do refuse to have their children vaccinated are typically condemned as being irresponsible. The professional inquisitors are well armed: 'Do you know how dangerous diphtheria and tetanus and measles and mumps, and all the others diseases for which modern medicine has created a vaccine, are ...?' 'Do you appreciate how miserable your children will be when they contract whooping cough ...?' 'Why would you put your children at risk when a simple shot or two, or thirty (which is roughly the number they'll get before they start school) will protect them from nasty childhood illnesses?'

If such rhetoric fails to convince the parent, there's always the stab to the parent's social conscience: 'Do you know that by refusing to vaccinate your child you're putting other people at risk as well?'

What your doctor doesn't tell you, is that unlike every other drug, not a single vaccine has ever been tested for either its efficacy or its safety in a double-blind, placebo-controlled field trial. No one has dared to compare the health of vaccinated and non-vaccinated children because such a trial is construed as unethical. But in a logical absurdity worthy of *Alice in Wonderland*, it is considered ethical to test vaccines on mass populations of children and adults.

Nor does your doctor tell you that many doctors do not follow their own advice: many refuse to have their own children vaccinated; or won't follow the nation's vaccination guidelines by delaying the administration of certain vaccines until their own child is aged two or more, or by picking and choosing which vaccines their own children will and won't get.

In a rare instance of doctors disclosing their own biases and indeed their own double standards, a Swiss survey sent to 2,000 doctors—roughly half of whom, tellingly, didn't reply—revealed that 15 per cent refused to allow their own children to have certain or all vaccines.[2] Five per cent wouldn't allow their children to have the Hib vaccine (against Haemophilus influenzae type b) or the MMR vaccine (against measles, mumps and rubella). And 10 per cent refused to give, or delayed giving, their children the DPT vaccine (against diphtheria, pertussis (whooping cough), and tetanus).

Similarly, a US survey of paediatricians revealed that 12 per cent of those who were parents hadn't vaccinated their own eligible children against chickenpox,[3] and 4 per cent had refused permission for an immunisation for their own children younger than 11.[4] And a Canadian survey showed that 41 per cent of nurses didn't fully agree with medical claims that vaccines were safe and effective.[5] In fact, 40 per cent of nurses thought that such practices as homoeopathy, good eating habits and a healthy lifestyle can eliminate the need for vaccination. Even the former prime minister of Britain, Tony Blair, whose government was waging a campaign to have all children vaccinated against measles, mumps and rubella, refused to disclose whether or not he had had his young son Leo inoculated with the MMR vaccine.

Chances are your doctor isn't even adhering to the medical profession's vaccination guidelines for health workers. Various reports have shown that half of British doctors in one survey, and less than a quarter of US doctors in another survey, were vaccinated against hepatitis B;[6,7] that only 20 per cent of susceptible physicians were vaccinated against rubella;[8,9] that only one of 11 obstetricians and gynaecologists at the Los Angeles County–University of Southern California Medical Center was vaccinated against rubella;[9] and that only a quarter of the trainee doctors in a US hospital emergency department, and a third of all emergency health workers in four hospitals in Canada, were vaccinated against influenza.[10,11]

Even when doctors are bombarded by campaigns to get themselves vaccinated many seem reticent to comply. A study at a Texas training hospital, where only 32 per cent of doctors and medical students had ever been vaccinated against influenza, found that despite sending out a memorandum, followed by a personal letter, and then a telephone call, and then providing free vaccinations at medical conferences, only 62 per cent of the medical staff decided to be vaccinated.[12]

Which all goes to show that many members of the medical profession, and undoubtedly many politicians, are not convinced by their own propaganda.

Of course, we don't know which aspect of the propaganda each of them didn't buy, for the flagstaff from which the vaccination flag flutters is held aloft by three tangled mainstays: one, if not for vaccinations we'd still be ravaged by deadly diseases that plagued past generations of people; two, each vaccine that is targeted at a specific germ will prevent the vaccine's recipient getting the disease that germ causes—in other words, vaccines work; and three, vaccines are safe.

If not for vaccines ...

For 200 years we have been sold the story that vaccines saved generations of people from such diseases as smallpox, diphtheria, whooping cough, polio, tuberculosis, tetanus and, in recent years, from measles, mumps, German measles (rubella), influenza and hepatitis B. But did they?

Let's investigate the record of the first vaccine to be used, the one that has been hailed as the drug that defeated smallpox, first from Europe and now from the world.

The first vaccine to fail

If Edward Jenner's 'great discovery'—borrowed from a Gloucestershire dairymaid's superstition that the pus from a cowpox infection protected milkmaids from smallpox—was so revolutionary, then why did the prevalence and severity of the disease in Britain increase in the years following the introduction of the vaccine in

1796?

Previously, the worst smallpox epidemic Britain had experienced throughout the 18th century was in 1793. London in particular bore the brunt, with two and a half per cent of the population affected, but only one-half of one percent of these people died.[13] A century before this, the eminent British physician, Dr Thomas Sydenham had noted, '… provided no mischief be done either by physician or nurse, it [smallpox] is the most safe and slight of all diseases.'[14]

But mischief was done. After years of widespread vaccinations, an epidemic in 1837–1840 claimed 42,000 lives.[15] Determined to halt further outbreaks, the authorities in 1853 made vaccinations compulsory for children.

Alas, 17 years later, with over 90 per cent of its population vaccinated, Britain experienced its biggest smallpox epidemic in two centuries. In 1871, during the second year of the epidemic, which had then claimed 10,000 lives, the esteemed medical journal *The Lancet* ran an editorial warning that smallpox had reached plague proportions and that the smallpox vaccine seemed ineffectual in halting it. Of the 9,392 smallpox patients in London hospitals, it noted, 6,854 (or 73 per cent) had been vaccinated.[16] And the journal had calculated that 122,000 vaccinated people throughout the realm had contracted the disease. When the 1870–1872 epidemic finally subsided, it had claimed 44,000 lives.[15]

Until the turn of the century, when public sanitation measures, implemented through various Public Sanitation and Public Health Acts, were completed, smallpox continued to plague the squalid, overcrowded sections of Britain's cities even though well over 90 per cent of their populations had been vaccinated. As one hospital physician, Dr Walter R. Hadwen, chronicled of his experiences: 'The vaccinated and re-vaccinated hospital officials fell before the disease side by side with the vaccinated and the re-vaccinated inhabitants.'[17]

In the city of Sheffield—'the best vaccinated town in the kingdom', Hadwen wrote—where 98 per cent of the population were vaccinated, an eighth of the population contracted the disease.[17] Where did that epidemic of 'beggars disease' spring from? A populated area covered with cesspits. And did the vaccine protect them? No. It was useless.

Yet in Leicester, a city where the population had refused vaccinations because of the high death rate in the 1870–72 epidemic and had instead opted for the tried and tested practice of quarantining those with smallpox, less than one person per year had died from the disease.[18]

But the lie that the smallpox vaccine protected people continued to spread like a contagion through the medical profession. It continued despite damning evidence being presented to the Royal Commission on [smallpox] Vaccinations by Alfred Russel Wallace, the famous British naturalist and co-discoverer (with Charles Darwin) of the theory of natural selection. He had presented statistical evidence showing that in the 1891–93 epidemic, for instance, Leicester, with 0.007 per cent of its population vaccinated, had 19 cases of smallpox, and one death, while Warrington, with 99.2 per cent of its population vaccinated, had 123 cases of the disease and 11 deaths.[19]

Wallace had also revealed that the death rate in the 1871–1872 smallpox epidemic in Prussia had been double that of Britain. And yet 95.7 per cent of the Prussian population had been vaccinated. Similarly, in Sweden, the death rate during the 1874–1876 epidemic had been double that of Britain during its worst epidemic 100 years earlier. And Sweden prided itself on the fact that the whole population was vaccinated.

The fraudulent claims for the vaccine's success were also identified by other academics. In Italy, for instance, Professor Carlos Ruata had noted that even though 98.5 per cent of his nation's population were officially declared to have been vaccinated, it had suffered over 48,000 smallpox deaths in the epidemic of 1887–1889.[20] As Ruata reasoned, why did more men than women die in the epidemic? After all, every man had to undertake army service at the age of 20, and every one of them had to be vaccinated twice a year.[21]

Notwithstanding the warnings from Wallace and Ruata, and from such distinguished epidemiologists as Charles Creighton and William Farr, and from Edward M. Crookshank, Professor of Bacteriology and Comparative Pathology at King's College, London, the lie continued. This led Wallace to later suspect that looming behind the fraud were vested interests.[22]

Something, however, did come out of the citizenry's revolt against compulsory vaccinations, something that would continue down the years: the British Parliament passed legislation that incorporated a 'conscience clause' for parents who refused to have their children vaccinated. Sound familiar?

Thus, by 1919, Britain had become one of the least vaccinated countries in the developed world. And yet that year it had only 28 deaths from smallpox.[23] Tellingly, the best vaccinated country in the world, Germany, had 707 deaths from smallpox that year.

And in that very year the Philippines was being ravaged by its worst smallpox epidemic ever. Throughout the 19th century it had also been plagued by smallpox epidemics. According to reports from the Philippines Health Service, about 10 per cent of those who contracted the disease died.[24] Then in 1898, immediately after defeating the former Spanish rulers, the US began to impose its own rule and set about cleaning up the place and vaccinating the whole population. Initially, the prevalence of smallpox declined although, as a portent of things to come, the death rate for those unfortunates who did contract smallpox soared by between 25 and 50 per cent.

Then in 1917, during a lull in smallpox outbreaks, the US army had another go. In the first round it forced a third of the Philippine population to have the vaccine, yet again. Immediately afterwards, 47,000 people developed smallpox, one third of whom died.[24,25] But true to form, the US army didn't flinch. It then forced vaccinations on the remaining two-thirds of the nation's 10 million population. A further 65,000 people contracted the disease, two-thirds of whom died. In total 60,855 Filipinos died in the worst smallpox epidemic that nation ever had.

Japan's experience was much the same. It too had suffered from smallpox epidemics, and in 1872 had begun a compulsory vaccination programme. But the epidemics kept coming. So in 1885 the government passed a law ensuring that everyone was vaccinated again, and would thenceforth be re-vaccinated every seven years. But the epidemics kept coming. In the following seven years 156,000 people contracted smallpox, of whom 25 per cent died.[26,27] And that was despite the fact that two-thirds of the population had been re-vaccinated.

Obviously dismayed by the vaccine's failure, the Japanese government then passed a law ensuring that everyone was to be re-vaccinated every five years. But the epidemics kept on coming, and with renewed severity. Every year between 1889 and 1908, an average of 8,500 people developed smallpox, 28 per cent of whom died.[26,27] In that 20-year period, a total of 172,000 people contracted the disease, and 48,000 of them died.

In 1908, 'when the Empire should have been reaping the best fruits of its rigorous vaccination laws', to quote John Pitcairn, then President of the Anti-Vaccination League of America, 'the smallpox vaccination cases numbered 18,000—a number not exceeded since 1897—and the deaths were nearly 6,000, or over 32 per cent.'[28]

And yet Australia, which was the least smallpox-vaccinated country in the world, had on average only one smallpox death a year throughout its history.[13] Smallpox eventually dwindled from underdeveloped countries not because of the vaccine, which had been given to less than 10 per cent of the people in those countries, but because of improved sanitation and nutrition.[29–33]

But has smallpox really been eradicated, as the WHO officially proclaimed it had on 10 May 1980? Some researchers suspect that it hasn't. Many other pox viruses exist in nature, and when humans catch such diseases as white pox, camelpox or monkeypox, the clinical signs and symptoms are indistinguishable from those of smallpox. Nor, until the recent advent of gene sequencing, could the pox viruses be distinguished.

Throughout the 1980s, however, there were outbreaks of 'monkeypox' in Cameroon, Ivory Coast, Liberia, Nigeria, Sierra Leone, and, as recently as 1996, in Zaire. Some medical researchers suspect that monkeypox may simply be smallpox renamed.[23,34,35]

As for the first recipients of Jenner's experimental vaccine, his elder son Edward, who had been given swine pox at the age of 18 months and then cowpox when he was 9-years-of-age, was afterwards never well again and died of tuberculosis at the age of 21.[36] James Phipps, the 8-year-old lad who was the first to receive Jenner's cowpox vaccine, and had been given at least 20 cowpox vaccinations during his short life, died at the age of 20, of tuberculosis. If only Jenner had known that cows as well as humans harbour TB.

The second vaccine to fail

The story of diphtheria is not dissimilar to that of smallpox. It too had a notorious history of spreading like wildfire through crowded and impoverished communities. Infants and children in particular bore the brunt of it, estimates being that as many as 70 per cent of those who contracted the disease were under the age of 15.[37] Of course, if they survived they had life-long immunity to the disease. Diphtheria was often deadly, however, because the toxin the germ produces causes swelling of the throat and tonsils, and can thus block airways. Not surprisingly, it was known in some cultures as 'the strangler'.

During the 39 epidemics that swept through squalid European communities between 1557 and 1803, for instance, as many as 80 per cent of those who contracted the disease died.[29] And in the years following the Napoleonic Wars in the early 1800s, as many as 25 per cent of people who came down with the disease died.

During the late 19th century, however, well before the advent of mass vaccination campaigns of the 1940s and '50s, deaths from diphtheria began to rapidly decline. In Toronto, for instance, the death rate of 132 per 100,000 people during the 10-year period of 1886–1895 had halved a decade later, and it continued to halve as each decade went by.[29] When the diphtheria toxoid arrived on the scene in 1924, deaths from diphtheria had declined by over 85 per cent. And by 1940, just before the mass vaccination campaigns for children began, the death rate had declined a further 12 per cent. The United States experienced the same 97 per cent reduction in diphtheria deaths between 1900 and 1940.[38]

In England and Wales, where statistics on deaths had been collated since the mid-1800s, the childhood death rate from diphtheria had declined from 932 deaths per 100,000 children in the 20-year period of 1861–1880, to 293 per 100,000 in the 1921–1940 period.[39]

Why did the death rate drop by only 68 per cent when the US and Canada had much greater declines during this period? Poor nutrition was undoubtedly one factor. But there was another factor, and here's the clue. In 1897, three years after British medical authorities had begun inoculating communities with the anti-diphtheria horse serum, which would have contained horse-protein antigens, deaths from diphtheria began to skyrocket. Indeed the death rates in the ensuing epidemic that lasted until 1910 were 75 per cent higher than they had been 19 years earlier.[40]

In London alone, according to a report by the city's health authorities, 89,445 people contracted the disease during this 15-year epidemic, and 10,837 died.[40] But a closer inspection clearly identifies the culprit: of all the people who contracted the disease 75,310 had been vaccinated, and 10,095, or 13.4 per cent of them had died of the disease; however, of the 13,135 people who hadn't been vaccinated only 742, or 5.65 per cent had died. This means that vaccinated people who contracted the disease—and the vaccine was supposed to protect them—had an approximate 240 per cent greater risk of dying of diphtheria than unvaccinated people.

By the mid-1920s British health authorities had seen the error of their ways and switched to using the new diphtheria toxoid developed by researchers at the Pasteur Institute in Paris. It was the first vaccine to contain the germicidal and carcinogenic chemical formaldehyde; a chemical that would certainly damage the immune system. The vaccine would later be hailed as a godsend in the war on diphtheria. But alas, in 1938 and 1939 yet another diphtheria epidemic struck Britain, killing 32 in every 100,000 children.[41] Steely in their war-time resolve, the British authorities began mass vaccination campaigns in early 1941. After an initial hiccough in 1941 and early 1942, when an epidemic resulted in a considerable increase in diphtheria deaths, the disease began to peter out.

Throughout the war years and up until 1948, health authorities estimated that only 60 to 65 per cent of children had been vaccinated.[41] Nevertheless, despite the fact that the death toll amongst both vaccinated and unvaccinated children in England and Wales declined—in unvaccinated children from 3,000 in 1940, to 551 in 1945, and to 63 by 1949—health authorities proclaimed the diphtheria toxoid a total success. As Lily Loat, then Secretary of The National Anti-Vaccination League of Great Britain, would document, 'Three and half million uninoculated children were as free from diphtheria as five and a half million inoculated children.'

British health authorities ignored the fact that even though diphtheria deaths in England and Wales had declined by 89 per cent since the 1860s, deaths from other childhood infectious diseases had declined even further: whooping cough by 91 per cent, measles by 94 per cent, and scarlet fever, by 99.7 per cent.[41] And all without vaccinations—the whooping vaccine would not arrive on the scene until 1951, the measles vaccine until 1964, and the scarlet fever vaccine … well, there never was a vaccine for that. And they ignored the impact of the social health reforms, particularly the 1944 Education Act which ensured free school milk and subsidised meals for all children at state schools. At the very least, vitamin A from milk and vitamin C from meals would have provided a boost to children's immune systems.

On the Continent, however, the diphtheria vaccine received no kudos whatsoever, particularly from the Germans. After losing the First World War the nation had been ravaged by reparations imposed by the victors, and had then suffered a further blow when the Great Depression struck in 1929. Not surprisingly, poverty and poor nutrition were rife.[42] And as we know, war and its aftermath—social disruption and overcrowding, poor sanitation and hygiene, poverty and poor nutrition—provide the ideal breeding ground for diphtheria bacteria.

Naturally enough, in the 15 years leading up to the Second World War, epidemics did increase in Germany.[41,43] Health authorities countered the onslaught by inoculating people with the new toxoid wherever an outbreak occurred. And in lock-step with that biochemical war on diphtheria, epidemics increased and the death toll rose. Echoing Dr Hadwen's words about the smallpox epidemics in the previous century, Dr T. Crowley, Medical Superintendent of the Wath Wood Hospital and Medical Officer of Health for Wath-on-Dearne in South Yorkshire would write of the whole affair: 'Where they have done the most immunising they are getting the most diphtheria.'[44]

By 1937, as storm clouds gathered over Europe, deaths from diphtheria began to soar. In 1938, on the eve of hostilities, 150,000 Germans (212 in every 100,000) contracted the disease and about 2,500 of them (3.8 in every 100,000) died.[43]

Meanwhile, in France that year—the year French authorities made the vaccine compulsory for children—41 in every 100,000 people contracted the disease.[37] In the Netherlands, which rarely used the vaccine, the rate was 14 in every 100,000. And in Norway and Sweden, neither of which had deployed the vaccine,[41] the incidence of the disease that year was, respectively, 6.3 per 100,000 and 1.6 per 100,000.[37] In other words, the incidence in unvaccinated Norway was 3,300 per cent lower than in vaccinated Germany, and 13,200 per cent lower for unvaccinated Sweden. Indeed, Sweden suffered no deaths at all that year.[45]

Then war broke out. Soon afterwards, the German Reich began to enforce its decree that all children must be inoculated—for adults it was voluntary.[41] And in early 1941, German occupying forces began to enforce the same compulsory ordinance on the children of France, Belgium, Denmark, the Netherlands and Norway.

Did the vaccine protect people? Not one jot. Within a year, the number of diphtheria cases in Germany was 3,000 per cent higher than it had been in the pre-war (1928–1938) years; in France it was nearly 160 per cent higher.[37,46] And as the contagion swept into Belgium and Denmark, and a swathe of other northern European nations, significant increases were being recorded there too.

But the worst affected were the Netherlands and Norway. Though the incidence rates in both nations were slightly less than in Germany at that time, when compared with the levels these countries had had in 1939, they had nevertheless risen: in the Netherlands by 1,500 per cent, and in Norway by 11,700 per cent.[37]

When the epidemic reached its peak in 1943, Germany was still encumbered with roughly the same number of diphtheria cases as it had the previous year: approximately 240,000.[37] France had had a further 150 per cent increase. Denmark and Belgium, and the neutral countries of Sweden and Switzerland had recorded slightly smaller rises. But the populations of the Netherlands and Norway were reeling. Both had had nearly a 300 per cent increase on the previous year's incidence. The sheer scale of the epidemic is readily apparent when we compare their 1943 rates with those in 1939: for the Netherlands 4,400 per cent higher, and for Norway a staggering 32,000 per cent increase.[37]

Soon after the war, the newly-created United Nations estimated that, in 1943 alone, one million people throughout northern Europe, excluding the USSR, had contracted the disease, and 50,000 of them had died.[47]

The epidemic continued unabated through 1944. But by 1945 it was beginning to subside. Why? Were Allied forces inoculating populations as they advanced on the foe, liberating people from the scourge of diphtheria as well as from Nazism? Not at all. US military authorities evidently had little faith in the vaccine for they'd refused to inoculate their own healthy young troops with the toxoid after discovering that it caused moderate to serious reactions in 'an appreciable number' of adolescents and young adults.[48] No, the reason for the epidemic subsiding was that those who had survived the epidemics had acquired lifelong immunity to the disease.

By war's end, possibly as many as two million Europeans had contracted the disease, and as many as 100,000 had died. Aside from war casualties it had been the leading cause of death and disease.[47]

Diphtheria, however, is only one of the consequences of war. Many other infectious diseases also sweep through worn-torn populations. Little wonder that in 12 of the war-torn countries the number of cases of cerebrospinal meningitis, poliomyelitis, typhoid, dysentery, and scarlet fever had doubled.[47]

Pro-vaccination campaigners still argue that the epidemic remained unchecked because of inadequate vaccination coverage. But the evidence belies these claims. Certainly the compulsory ordinance to inoculate children was obeyed in spite of the bombing. In Berlin in 1942, for instance, 70 per cent of the children aged 3 to 5 had been inoculated, as had 85 per cent of the children aged 6 to 13.[41] And in 1943, about half the children of Berlin had received two injections, a much higher number than in London that year.

Even in America, where vaccinations are mandatory for school children, there had been a resurgence of diphtheria in several cities from the late 1960s until 1975. Medical authorities had of course blamed the outbreak on poor vaccination rates. But in Chicago, for instance, of the 16 children who had contracted the disease, 4 had been 'fully immunised', 5 others had received one or more doses of the toxoid, and 2 of them had shown evidence of 'full immunity'.[49] And where did the victims live? In poor, overcrowded communities.

Failures of the vaccine have in recent years also occurred in Sweden, Germany, Portugal, China and Thailand, even though some of these nations have maintained high childhood vaccination rates for at least 30 years.[50] And where did they occur? In poor, disadvantaged groups living in crowded conditions.[37]

As a British adviser to the World Health Organisation had acknowledged in 1975, 'The degree of protection achieved with toxoid immunisation is often less than satisfactory.'[51] The document revealed that the US Communicable Disease Centre [the Centers for Disease Control] regularly admitted that about 7–10 per cent of reported cases of diphtheria in the US occurred in individuals whose medical records indicated that they had been 'completely immunised'. And as recently as 1999, a US researcher identified that both the diphtheria and the whooping cough toxoids produced only about 70 per cent 'immunity' in an individual, and as little as 50 per cent 'immunity' in the community at large.[52]

Clearly the diphtheria vaccine was having an abysmal track record, even by the medical profession's criterion that 'immunity' means having a certain level of antibodies to a particular germ. Public health officials were undoubtedly dismayed for they'd been preaching that the diphtheria toxoid, along with the vaccines for measles and mumps and whooping cough, and German measles, was a godsend.

Something clearly had to be done to head off public concern.

And indeed it was. Public health officials began to preach that a community would only be protected against an infectious disease if a sizeable percentage of them had been vaccinated. 'Herd protection' (the medical profession prefer to call it 'herd immunity') entered the vernacular. Unbeknownst to most people, however, the term had first been used by cattle ranchers in the US to describe the way a herd would naturally fight off an infectious disease and thenceforth be immune to the disease. A young American researcher, Arthur Hedrich, had coined the term to describe the way children in a community would catch measles, fight it off, and then acquire lifelong immunity to the disease.[53] But public health officials had bastardised the term to mean protection by vaccination.

Lack of 'herd protection' would soon be blamed on the epidemic that erupted in Russia and the Newly Independent States soon after the collapse of the Soviet empire. Stretching from Latvia to the Ukraine in the west, and from Georgia to Kazakhstan in the south, and with Russia at the hub, the region, in 1990, was an epidemic waiting to happen. Millions of people were struggling with a partial breakdown of public infrastructure, as well as sporadic civil wars and social upheavals arising from mass movements of people. Public sanitation and personal hygiene were less than ideal, overcrowding and poor nutrition were commonplace, and people were highly stressed. In a nutshell, their health was suffering.

Sure enough, diphtheria did erupt, first in Moscow and St Petersburg, and then it rapidly spread into neighbouring lands. From 1990 until the epidemic subsided in 1997, 157,000 people had contracted the disease and over 5,000 had died.[54]

But unlike diphtheria epidemics in the pre-vaccination era, when about 70 per cent of cases were in children under the age of 15, this one primarily affected adults. Indeed, the figures had reversed: 70 per cent of cases occurred in people over the age of 15.[37] In fact, 76 per cent of the deaths occurred in adults, not children. Another new trend was also emerging: a large proportion of patients, both young and older, experienced complications from the disease, and those most affected were aged 40 to 49.

And who were the people least affected? The people over 50. Only 2.8 in every 100,000 was affected.[37] And the reason? Most had acquired lifelong immunity to the disease when they were children: when airborne diphtheria germs had wafted onto their skin and into their nostrils; and their bodies, perhaps without symptoms, had generated a natural defence against the very source of the toxins, the germ; their bodies would 'remember' that germ for the rest of their lives, and rapidly slaughter it should it waft in again.

Of course, the World Health Organisation and the US Centers for Disease Control readily identified the culprit: lack of 'herd protection'.[37,54] And they clung to that story despite the fact that from 1958 until the early 1980s there had been universal childhood 'immunisation' throughout the Soviet Union.[54] Although childhood vaccination rates had declined thereafter, nonetheless they were sufficient at the time of the outbreak to 'protect' about 60 per cent of the young herd'. This is despite the fact that 60 per cent herd protection against diphtheria is considered by western scientists to be sufficient to well nigh protect the whole 'herd';[55] despite the fact that the same percentage of 'herd protection' occurred in many European nations where diphtheria was virtually non-existent;[50,56] and despite the fact that the highest rate of incidence was amongst adolescents aged 15 to 17, a group who were certain to have received their full quota of vaccines, not to mention a veritable cocktail of the aluminium and mercury compounds, and formaldehyde, that accompany them.

No doubt the great purveyors of vaccines had been troubled by events. So they upped the ante and declared that 'herd protection' could only be guaranteed if 95 per cent of the 'herd' had been vaccinated. And that applies for all diseases for which a vaccine exists. For some nations, this means compelling all children to be vaccinated.

Undoubtedly the greatest absurdity of the propaganda on 'herd protection' is this: if 70 per cent of the victims were adults, not children, then how would vaccinating children protect their older siblings, let alone their mothers and fathers? After all, they'd already been vaccinated, and they were already 'protected'. Or were they?

Such outbreaks would suggest that vaccinations induce tolerance, rather than genuine immunity, to a disease. When an epidemic does occur, those people who have not been constantly topped up with boosters, are the most likely to succumb. And who do you suspect are the silent carriers of the disease? Here's a hint. In the epidemic that swept through Russia and the Newly Independent States, it was mainly mothers, not fathers, who came down with diphtheria.[57]

Many of them caught it from their vaccinated children, just as much of the adult population of Europe during the Second World War had caught it from their vaccinated children.

And as for the healthy, young, unvaccinated American GIs who had gone off to Europe to help fight the Nazi foe, only 2,500 out of as many as 3 million of them contracted the disease, and of those only 71 died.[48] Why was the rate, at 5.4 per 100,000 troops, so low? They were healthy, and as many as 80 per cent of those who had come from urban areas in the US had acquired lifelong immunity to the disease.[58]

The emperor's new clothes and the medical courtiers

Perhaps it began with the delusion that a vaccine had eradicated diphtheria. Perhaps it was the post-war hubris that technology could defeat all foes. Perhaps it was simply a noble desire to protect children. Whatever the reason, soon after World War II the germ of an idea began spreading like a contagion through western governments and drug companies: why not create vaccines to protect all children from all infectious diseases? Soon their 'experts', the medical courtiers, would jump on the bandwagon and begin singing the praises of the emperor's new clothes.

Tetanus

As we've seen, the diphtheria vaccine had been the first off the rank—and the courtiers proclaimed that that had been a total success—followed soon thereafter by the tetanus vaccine. Tetanus is not, of course, a contagious disease, but it can arise from penetrating wounds. Though the bacteria are present in human and animals faeces, it is only when the spores penetrate oxygen-deprived wounded tissues and begin to exude a strychnine-like toxin that they wreak havoc on our nervous systems: 'lockjaw' sums up the horror of it.

Wounded soldiers have always been prime candidates for contracting tetanus, particularly if their wounds are contaminated by debris from well manured soils, such as those of the Western Front in World War I.[59] For instance, for every 1,000 soldiers wounded on the fields of Spain and Portugal during the Peninsula War of 1808 to 1814, there had been 12.5 cases of tetanus; in the Crimean War, 2 cases.[60] The same rate of incidence had occurred during the American Civil War, but in that war tetanus had been particularly deadly: 89 per cent of those soldiers who contracted it had died from the disease.[61] Indeed, during that war, germs had claimed many a soldier's life: two-thirds of the 600,000 men who died during the war were killed by epidemics of infectious diseases that swept through the Union and Confederate armies.[62]

As the practice of resolving conflicts through war continued through the remainder of the 19th century, the prevalence of tetanus amongst wounded soldiers continued much as it had always been: amongst every 1,000 troops wounded on the well manured fields of Europe during the Franco-Prussian War in the early 1870s, there had been 3.5 cases of tetanus, and 90 per cent of those had died from it.[63] And yet on the barren African soils during the Boer War at the dawning of the new century, there had been only 0.28 cases in every 1,000 wounded soldiers.

During the 1890s, a tetanus antitoxin horse serum had been developed for passive 'immunisation' in the treatment of wounds. This vaccine had been widely used during the First World War, and was later touted as a godsend to wounded soldiers. Deaths from tetanus among wounded soldiers on the Allied side certainly did decline, from about 8 cases per 1,000 in 1914, to 1.4 per 1,000 during the following four years.[64] Hence, of the 520,000 wounded American soldiers, only 70 developed tetanus.[65] But amongst the wounded British soldiers, 2,595 had developed tetanus, 95 per cent of cases occurring on the Western Front.[63] And yet despite the anti-tetanus serum, 54 per cent of them had died of tetanus.

But what medical courtiers fail to tell us is that, as in every war, great strides had been made in surgical techniques and the treatment of wounds. During the Great War the occurrence of Clostridial infections (tetanus from *Clostridium tetani*, and gas gangrene from *Clostridium perfringens*) had been linked to the inadequate debridement of wounds (cleaning away damaged tissues and debris), and to early wound closure.[59] At the Inter-Allied Surgical Conference in Paris in 1917, delegates had established a new policy for the management of wounds: namely, debridement and delaying the suturing of large wounds. In other words, the best treatment for preventing tetanus is to thoroughly cleanse any wound and expose it to the air for at least four days, if not longer—which makes total sense since oxygen-hating Clostridial bacteria die when exposed to oxygen.

Moreover, from 1915, improved methods of transportation had facilitated the evacuation of wounded soldiers from the battlefields to hospitals so that their wounds could be properly treated.[63]

Hence, not only did tetanus decline, but so did gas gangrene: the latter from about 100 to 120 cases in every 1,000 wounded soldiers in 1914–1915, to about 10 cases per 1,000 wounded soldiers in 1918[63,66] —that's a drop of more than 90 per cent, and without a vaccine being used.

In addition, surgeons had begun using Dakin's hypochlorite solution for flushing wounds.[59] Hydrogen peroxide had also been extensively used from the early years of the 20th century till the 1950s for the same purpose. Such oxidising agents alone would have killed the oxygen-hating tetanus spores. Applying honey to wounds, a traditional folkloric practice in many parts of the world, particularly in Russia and China—and employed by Russian troops during the Great War—has the same effect. When diluted with bodily fluids in a wound, honey releases hydrogen peroxide.[67]

Nonetheless, the medical courtiers claimed that tetanus had been conquered by the tetanus antitoxin serum—they had no proof, just an empty claim. When World War II broke out, the lessons gleaned from the Great War about wound treatment and rapid evacuation of wounded soldiers to hospital facilities were readily put into practice. Doctors realised that the sooner a wound was debrided—and certainly within six hours—the better the chances of avoiding gas gangrene and tetanus. And of course, every soldier was inoculated with a newly-developed vaccine to produce 'active immunisation' in order to prevent tetanus developing in the first place.

Again, the great medical courtiers claimed that the reason why only 12 American soldiers out of 2,734,819 hospital admissions had contracted tetanus was because of the vaccine.[68] Five of those died;[69] which surely begs the question: if the vaccine was so successful, why did any soldier develop tetanus, let alone die from it? Another question also begs answering: why in the British Army was the death rate amongst vaccinated men not significantly lower than in unvaccinated men?[60]

As for gas gangrene, even the new wonder-drugs, pencillin and the sulphonamides, had failed to lower the incidence of deaths from it: the death rate was no different to the rate in the First World War, before the advent of antibiotics.[63] As British medical historian Dr Geoffrey Noon had noted, 'A quotation from a standard surgical textbook published after the Second World War, is apposite: "Gas gangrene, more than any other complication of wound infection, serves to point the moral that no ancillary methods will make amends for neglect of meticulous primary surgery." '[70] The same could be said for tetanus prevention.

Meanwhile, in the unvaccinated civilian population of Britain, the death rate from tetanus declined amongst males by 66 per cent between 1938 and 1957.[71] And in America, the death rate amongst unvaccinated young children dropped by 85 per cent between 1900 and 1940, and a further 8 per cent by 1950.[72] Which just goes to prove that cleanliness, not a hypodermic needle filled with a biochemical cocktail, is next to godliness.

Nevertheless, despite the overwhelming evidence that has been accruing since the 1940s in every vaccinated nation—at least 26 research papers have been published in peer-reviewed journals attesting to the fact that people who are fully vaccinated against tetanus can get still get the disease,[73–99] even when their antibody levels are 16 times the amount considered to be 'protective'[96]—the courtiers continue with their mantra that the emperor's new clothes are resplendent. And that a booster will make them more so.

As for mothers passing on to their children their own 'immunity', the World Health Organisation admits that, 'The number of reports from Asia and Africa describing the failure of tetanus toxoid to prevent neonatal tetanus in infants of immunised women has increased recently.'[100]

Now to put all this into perspective, from 40 to 50 (0.15 per million) Americans get tetanus every year, and 7 to 10 die from it.[101] And about 260 Americans are struck by lightning each year, and roughly 93 of them die from that.[102] Which means that you have roughly a six-times greater chance of being struck by lightning than of contracting tetanus, and about a 10-times greater chance of dying from being hit by lightning than from contracting tetanus.

To put this into the context of modern diseases, autism—which has been linked to the mercury compound, thiomersal (thimerosal in the US), in vaccines[103–110]—affects 1 in 150 children.[111] Which means that children have nearly a 45,000-times greater chance of becoming autistic than of contracting tetanus.

And given that Alzheimer's disease—which has been overwhelmingly linked to aluminium,[112–149] a toxic metal that occurs in many vaccines, including the tetanus toxoid—affects 1 in 8 Americans over the age of 55,[150] we can conclude that elderly Americans have at least a 830,000-times greater chance of getting Alzheimer's disease than tetanus.

Whooping cough

From the 1950s onwards, the tetanus toxoid for children would be accompanied by the biochemical cocktail of the vaccines against diphtheria and whooping cough: the DPT cocktail. And by the late 1960s, a vaccine to conquer measles mumps and rubella, all combined for convenience into one biochemical cocktail, the MMR vaccine, would be added to the list.

Admittedly, small outbreaks of whooping cough during the 1950s and '60s did blemish the emperor's finery, but the loyal courtiers blamed these on parents who had either failed to keep their children's inoculations up-to-date, or had refused point blank to have their children 'immunised'.

Then in the early 1970s something happened, something that government courtiers had not expected. And it wasn't the return of whooping cough epidemics, though that certainly precipitated the affair. It was the occasion of a Scotsman by the name of Gordon Stewart daring to break ranks and declare that the emperor has no clothes.

Stewart, then Emeritus Professor of Public Health at the University of Glasgow, had undertaken some epidemiological studies which revealed that during the 1975 whooping cough epidemic in Glasgow, nearly a third of the notified cases were fully vaccinated.[151] And where did he find the greatest prevalence of the disease? In the poorer districts of the city. 'The decline in recent years,' he reasoned, 'could be attributable to improvement in these conditions at least as much as to immunisation. [Hence] There is no epidemiological justification for continuing mass vaccination ... '.

Soon afterward, another Scotsman, Dr Robert Ditchburn from Shetland, would also break ranks with the medical courtiers. Ditchburn had good reason to observe the emperor up close. He had been a rural family doctor for years and had vaccinated 94 per cent of the children in the district. Only in 1974 did he stop using the whooping cough vaccine. Thus, when an epidemic swept through the island at the end of 1977, he could witness and document the effects of the disease on vaccinated and unvaccinated children.

And what an abysmal failure the vaccine was: 45 per cent of 144 children under the age of 16 developed whooping cough; 86 per cent of 3.5 to 5-year-olds who contracted the disease were fully vaccinated, as were 42 per cent of cases among the 6- to 10-year-olds and 50 per cent of cases among the 11- to 15 year-olds.[151,152] And as you would expect, of the 35 children born after he'd ceased giving the whooping cough vaccine, 46 per cent were naturally infected.

Overall, 54 per cent of all 'fully immunised' children had contracted the disease, as had 56 per cent of all unvaccinated children.[153] 'Heads I win, tails you lose,' sums up the charade. The vaccine was clearly a failure; the emperor was indeed naked. In his epitaph to the vaccine Ditchburn concluded: 'My findings ... do not support the routine use of pertussis immunisation in rural Shetland today.'

When the 1977–1979 epidemic finally subsided in Britain, 35 per cent of reported cases had occurred in fully vaccinated children aged between 1 and 5. But of the under-5s who had not been vaccinated, only 5 per cent had been recorded as having contracted the disease.[154] As Stewart noted, children who lived in deprived communities and those who had been vaccinated were the worst affected, many having to be hospitalised. Recall that Dr Hadwen had made the same observation about smallpox cases a century before.[17]

By 1983, 50 per cent of British parents were refusing to have their children inoculated with the vaccine. They, too, could see that the emperor was naked. Many had been swayed by the epitaph Professor Stewart wrote for the vaccine: 'In the United Kingdom and in many other countries, whooping cough (and measles) are no longer important as causes of death or severe illness except in a small minority of infants who are usually otherwise disadvantaged. In these circumstances, I cannot see how it is justifiable to promote mass vaccination of children everywhere against diseases which are generally mild, which confer lasting immunity, and which most children escape or overcome easily without being vaccinated.'[154]

But most of all, what clinched the decision for parents was Professor Stewart's revelation that in some children the vaccine had caused screaming attacks and convulsions, for others it had caused irreversible brain damage, and a few it had killed.[155,156] And his warning that for non-deprived children 'the risk of pertussis vaccine during the 1970–83 period exceeded those of whooping cough.'[157]

Britain's medical courtiers of course blamed the epidemic, which affected 200,000 people, on poor vaccination rates. But Britain was not the only nation to experience the failure of the vaccine. All nations, including those like the United States and the Netherlands with childhood vaccination rates as high as 96 per cent, experienced waves of epidemics beginning in the 1970s and their recurrence, on average, every four years to this very day.[158–176]

In the United States, for instance, between 1980 and 1986, 17,400 people contracted whooping cough, and 25 per cent of them were children aged from 1 to 4.[161] And United States health authorities prided themselves on the fact that 94 per cent of children were fully vaccinated by the time they started school.

Similarly in Australia, between 2003 and 2005, there were 25,000 reported cases of whooping cough, 5,200 of which were in children under the age of 15.[162] And Australian medical authorities proclaim that 86 per cent of children are fully vaccinated. A closer inspection of the Australian statistics reveals that 70 per cent of the 1- to 4-year-olds who contracted the disease were fully vaccinated, that 12 per cent were partially vaccinated, and that 61 per cent of the 4- to 9-year-old children were also fully vaccinated and 15 per cent were partially vaccinated. In other words, two-thirds of the children under the age of 9 who contracted the disease were either fully or partially vaccinated.

And there's plenty more evidence to prove the bleeding obvious: that the emperor is truly stark naked. In the 1993-94 epidemics that struck the US cities of Chicago and Cincinnati, for instance, 65 per cent of cases occurred in children under five-years-of-age.[161,164,165] According to the US Centers for Disease Control, 84 per cent of these children were fully or partially vaccinated. And in Cincinnati, nearly a third of children with whooping cough were hospitalised.

The hollow promise of using needle-dispensed white man's magic to eradicate whooping cough through 'herd protection', let alone halt outbreaks, in developing countries would also become evident. For example, in Cape Town, South Africa, a city where 95 per cent of children were fully vaccinated when a whooping cough epidemic struck in 1988–89, 33 per cent of pre-primary school children were affected.[166] And, as had happened in Cincinnati and Britain, a high number of vaccinated children had to be admitted to hospital.

In the West African nation of Gambia, there was an outbreak of measles and whooping cough during the early 1990s, even though childhood vaccination rates for both diseases were high.[167]

Swedish authorities were so disenchanted with their vaccine—after learning that 84 per cent of a sample of 620 children who had contracted the disease during epidemics in the mid-1970s were fully vaccinated—that they abandoned its use in 1979.[168]

Curiously, before the vaccination era, whooping cough—as with diphtheria, and measles and mumps, and all the other diseases for which a vaccine has been created—was remarkably rare in adults and rarely did it occur twice in the same person.[175,177] But now it is commonplace. Why would this be? Because not only does the whooping cough vaccine not confer lifelong immunity to the disease, but also, as Russian researchers had discovered during the diphtheria outbreaks in the early 1990s, because vaccinated children are the silent carriers of the disease.

This was exactly what Israeli researchers suspected when they investigated an outbreak of whooping cough in two day-care centres in 2000 and found that not only did 55 per cent of the 5- to 6-year old children, all of whom had received four shots of the DPT vaccine, have whooping cough, so did many of their siblings and parents.[176] The same had been apparent during a whooping cough outbreak in an isolated community in the Gascoyne region of Western Australia in late 1999, even though 96 per cent of children were fully vaccinated.[163]

Measles

Not surprisingly, the vaccines to conquer measles, mumps and rubella (German measles), combined for convenience into a single cocktail (MMR), have fared little better. Up until the 1960s, when the measles vaccine arrived on the scene, most children had contracted measles, mumps and rubella, and thereafter had lifelong immunity to these diseases.[178–183] Many parents had deliberately exposed their children to these endemic diseases—at 'measles parties', for example— knowing that contracting these diseases later in life could cause medical miseries; for example, meningitis, mastitis and inflammation of the testes from mumps. And when girls grew up and became mothers, they would pass on to their babies antibodies to the diseases to protect them during the first crucial year of life.

Moreover, most doctors knew how to treat these diseases. In a case of measles, for instance, the infected child was to be kept in a darkened room, out of draughts, and kept warm to ensure the measles rash became pronounced. They knew that should the rash disappear, the infection could turn inwards and affect the ears, eyes, lungs, heart, or brain. If that did happen, one technique employed was to make the child wear a vest that had been soaked in salty water. The skin would become irritated and the rash would soon appear. So long as no mischief was done—for instance, by quelling the child's fever with such antipyretic drugs as aspirin or paracetamol—then measles would run a benign course.[184] Of course, as with other diseases, impoverishment and malnourishment, by weakening a child's ability to fight off these diseases, could prove fatal.

By the 1950s, well before the programme to inject the measles vaccine into children's arms began, deaths from measles had plummeted; in Britain, for instance, by 99.4 per cent compared with the death rates in 1900,[185] and in the US by 99.7 per cent.[186,187] Nevertheless, governments and drug companies remained hell-bent on eradicating these diseases. Not once did they stop to consider that measles alone might serve some function in human health, that it might kick-start a child's immune system, that it might be a blessing or, as the physicians of India once believed, a visitation of the goddess.

Certainly in the 10 years following the advent of the measles vaccine in 1964, the prevalence of measles did decline in the United States, from about 400,000 cases each year during the 1950s to between 22,000 and 75,000 during the late 1960s and early 1970s.[187] Following each outbreak, scouts from state public health departments and the emperor's palace in Atlanta, Georgia, later to be known as the US Centers for Disease Control and Prevention, would be despatched to ascertain the reason for the vaccine's failure to protect.

In Jacksonville, Florida, for example, 28 kindergarten children had come down with the disease, even though 25 of them were vaccinated.[188] To make matters worse, there was little difference in the severity of the disease between the vaccinated and unvaccinated children.

Outbreaks continued during the 1970s, belying claims that measles was a 'vaccine-preventable disease'.[189–198] Even in schools where over 99 per cent of the children had been vaccinated, outbreaks still occurred; for example, in two schools in Erie County, New York in the spring of 1978.[198] Equally worrisome for the palace courtiers was the fact that from 84 to 94 per cent of the vaccinated children who contracted measles had sufficient antibodies to the disease to make them 'immune'. At least that was the courtiers' assumption. Moreover, there were negligible declines in the death rate from measles;[199] for example, 130 children had to be hospitalised and 6 of them died during the epidemic that swept through St Louis, Missouri, in 1971 to 1972, despite vaccination rates in school children being as high as 89 per cent.[194] Nevertheless, courtiers at the palace kept up the facade by using dubious statistical projections,[200] to spin the tale that 60 million doses of the vaccine in its first 10 years had saved 2,400 children's lives.[201]

Even though the United States had set the goal of eradicating measles by October 1982—indeed the palace courtiers could gloat that measles cases had reached an all time low of 1,497 cases in 1983[202]—outbreaks amongst vaccinated children continued to rise during the 1980s: for instance, 46 cases in Warren County, Pennsylvania in 1981/82, within two weeks of all children being vaccinated;[203] 16 cases among high school students in Illinois in 1983/84, all of whom were vaccinated.[204] There were also 1,806 cases among high school students in Corpus Christi, Texas, 99 per cent of whom were vaccinated, and of whom more than 95 per cent had antibodies to the measles virus;[205] 118 cases on a Blackfeet reservation in Montana, 82 per cent of whom were vaccinated; and 23 cases among school children in Browning, Montana, 98.7 per cent of whom were vaccinated.[206]

In fact, between 1985 and 1986 there had been over 253 measles outbreaks amongst the most vaccinated people on earth: 26 per cent of cases had occurred in pre-school age children, 14 per cent of whom were vaccinated; and 67 per cent of cases had occurred in 5- to 19-year-old school children, 60 per cent of whom were vaccinated.[207] During 1987 and 1988, measles outbreaks continued to occur amongst school age children, 98 per cent of whom were vaccinated,[208–210] averaging about 3,000 cases each year.[211]

But 1989 was the year measles epidemics erupted like a rash across the United States.[212] Within the first 26 weeks there had been 7,335 reported cases,[213] and by year's end the tally was 18,193 in 815 outbreaks.[211,214] Forty states were affected, and in particular the cities of Houston, Los Angeles and Chicago. According to the US Centers for Disease Control and Prevention, more than half of the cases occurred among appropriately vaccinated children aged 5 to 19; 30 per cent of cases occurred in children under 5; and the remainder of cases occurred in older adults who may or may not have been vaccinated.[213]

One instance of the vaccine's abysmal failure is that at a high school in Illinois where 68 measles cases occurred, yet 99.7 per cent of students at the school were vaccinated.[215]

All told, between 1989 and 1991 there had been 55,467 reported cases of measles, 11,251 hospital admissions, and 166 suspected measles-related deaths.[216] The total number of measles cases may well have been much higher, however, according to researchers who investigated the outbreaks in Wisconsin and Texas, because unlike unvaccinated children, 97 per cent of whom develop the typical measles rash, only about 15 per cent of vaccinated children who contract measles get the rash;[217,218] this is known as 'atypical measles'. Indeed, this had been identified in those who had been inoculated with the earlier killed-measles-virus vaccine, as well as the later live-attenuated-virus vaccine.[219] In other words, cases of measles are typically under-reported. Hence the vaccine's efficacy is overestimated.

Proof of under-reporting came in 1991, when researchers investigating a measles outbreak in New York City discovered that only 45 per cent of the 1,487 cases admitted to New York hospitals had been reported to public health authorities.[220]

The palace courtiers did at least acknowledge that measles was far harder to stamp out than they had previously thought.[213] Two researchers from the Mayo Clinic in Minnesota at least had the nous to conclude: 'The apparent paradox is that as measles immunisation rates rise to high levels in a population, measles becomes a disease of immunised persons. Because of the failure rate of the vaccine and the unique transmissibility of the measles virus, the currently available measles vaccine, used in a single-dose strategy, is unlikely to completely eliminate measles.'[221]

Realising that parents were unlikely to remain convinced about the splendour of the emperor's new clothes, the courtiers took a new tack: implement laws requiring all children to be inoculated twice with the failed MMR vaccine;[222] encourage health-care providers 'to take advantage of every opportunity' to vaccinate susceptible adolescents and adults; 'encourage persons in religious groups who do not seek health care to accept vaccination'; during an epidemic to make sure everyone at risk is inoculated; and, of course, continue to panic the population by stressing the 'seriousness of measles illness'.[223]

Since 1991 the number of reported cases of measles in the United States has certainly declined radically. When outbreaks do occur, they are often blamed on alien imports, on people who have come from or travelled through countries that have not caught America's obsession with defeating viruses through mandatory inoculations.

An outbreak in Indiana in 1991, for instance, was blamed on three measles-virus-carrying, albeit previously vaccinated New Zealand athletes.[223] State public health officials had gone to town to prevent an outbreak: the three athletes were quarantined for four days, 1,300 possible contacts were inoculated, and surveillance teams had been set up to record twice-daily reports from international athletic delegations. Come hell or high water, the efficacy of the double-dose MMR vaccine would not be put to the test. Nor would any imports tarnish America's reputation of having achieved 'herd protection'.

But it had already failed the test. Four healthcare workers at the Children's Hospital of Philadelphia had contracted measles from infected children in 1991.[224] Three of them had done the right thing and had had at least two doses of the measles vaccine, and all of them had levels of antibodies that courtiers would consider to indicate that they were 'immune' to the disease.

And the vaccine continues to fail the test to this very day. Reports from the Centers for Disease Control continue to identify cases of measles in people who have had two or even three doses of the MMR vaccine.[225–231]

The lengths to which courtiers will go when a viral foe threatens to expose the emperor's flanks is evident in their response to a measles outbreak in seven schools in Anchorage, Alaska in September 1998.[232] This had also been blamed on a foreign importation; in this instance, on a four-year-old visitor from Japan. Thirty-three people, mainly students, contracted the disease, reputedly from the child, even though 29 of them had had at least one inoculation against the disease, and one certainly had had two inoculations.

In response to the outbreak, Alaska's Department of Health and Social Services, issued an emergency decree that by mid-November 1998, all Anchorage school children must have received two doses of the vaccine. The order was subsequently expanded to require all students in Alaska to have two doses of the measles vaccine by early January 1999. The irony is that for the nation that purports to be 'the land of the free and the home of the brave', the decree smacked of the order issued by the German Reich 58 years earlier to inoculate its children against diphtheria.

Nonetheless, in March 2000, the United States proudly proclaimed that measles had been eradicated from the nation.[233] Thereafter, every case of measles, every outbreak, would be blamed on foreign importations.

But in every nation, whether richer or poorer, the measles vaccine from the outset has proved to be an abysmal failure.[234–277] Regardless of the percentage of the population that has been vaccinated—even when it is as high as 98, 99, or 100 per cent of the population,[237,240,248] and regardless of whether one or two shots of the vaccine are administered—outbreaks still continue to this very day. As two Canadian researchers concluded, 'Neither prior vaccination nor detectable secondary immune response [having specific antibodies to the measles virus] ensures protective immunity.'[239]

A classic case, not only of the failure of the vaccine to protect, but also of its dangers, occurred in Gambia.[250,251] In 1967, following a mass vaccination campaign in which 97 per cent of the population had been forced to be inoculated, the World Health Organisation proclaimed that measles had been eradicated from the nation. But in 1972 an epidemic erupted. And medical complications from the disease, and deaths, were significantly higher than they had ever been before.

As of 2004, the medical courtiers of over 50 per cent of the world's countries have managed to achieve childhood vaccination rates of more than 90 per cent.[278] But in 20 per cent of the world's nations, including Britain, France, Italy, Norway, China, New Zealand and South Africa, the courtiers have been battling to convince all parents that the emperor is clothed: vaccination rates are between 80 and 90 per cent. And doctors in the poorer nations aren't too convinced about white-man's magic either. Thus the idea of eradicating measles from the planet is pie in the sky.

Mumps

Perhaps the greatest joke the courtiers have spun is that mumps is a 'vaccine-preventable disease'. Introduced in the late 1960s and routinely used as the second 'M' of the MMR vaccine from the late 1970s, the vaccine started off with an apparently impressive record: in the first 18 years of its use the incidence of mumps in the United States declined by 98 per cent.

Foreshadowing subsequent epidemics, however, researchers had warned the courtiers that anti-mumps antibody levels in inoculated individuals were far lower than in those who had acquired natural immunity to the disease.[279]

Then in 1985 the lull broke. By the following year there were 7,790 reported cases in the United States. And in 1987, 12,848 cases had been recorded in 44 states.[280] The incidence had risen nearly five-fold in all age groups, and in the 15- to 19-year-olds there was over an eight-fold increase.

Outbreaks continued through the 1980s in highly vaccinated populations[281]— in Douglas County, Kansas, for instance, where 97.6 of the cases were fully vaccinated[282]—and on into the 1990s amongst school populations where 98 per cent of cases were fully vaccinated.[283–286]

The vaccine's appalling track record continued into the 21st century.[287–292] Even though 97 per cent of American elementary school children, and 98 per cent of middle school children, had been twice vaccinated against mumps, as had 84 per cent of 18- to 24-year-olds, an outbreak occurred in 2006, affecting 6,584 people in 11 states. Those most affected were the 18- to 24-year-olds, followed by the 5- to 17-year-olds. In Iowa alone, where the epidemic began, 94 per cent of the population of children and adolescents were vaccinated. The idea of 'herd immunity' had clearly been trashed.

Parents in Canada, Europe and Asia would have been as equally dismayed as their American counterparts at the vaccine's failure.[293–324] From the 1990s up until today, there have been mumps epidemics in highly vaccinated populations of people who never had a chance to acquire lifelong natural immunity to the disease. Affecting all age groups, but particularly adolescents and young adults, epidemics swept through Switzerland in 1993 (when the nation recorded its highest levels since records began in 1984,[295] and despite people having high levels of antibodies),[296] through Portugal in 1996–1997 (with 30,000 cases),[302] through Spain in 1997–1998 (with 6,915 cases, 93 per cent of whom were fully vaccinated),[300] through England and Wales in 2004–2005 (with 56,390 cases),[313] and through Poland in 2006 (with 15,115 cases).[322]

Two nations, the Czech Republic and Moldova, certainly had the opportunity to test the theory of 'herd immunity', since compulsory vaccinations had ensured that at least 95 per cent of their young populations had been vaccinated. But the Czech Republic was struck by a series of mumps epidemics, first in 1995–1996, affecting 11,680 people, then in 2003–2004, and again in 2005–2006.[318] And in Moldova in 2007–2008, there were 14,438 cases, the vast majority of whom had been inoculated with two doses of the vaccine.[319]

Rubella

As for rubella, it is a mild infectious disease causing a low-grade fever and typically a two-day rash. Before the vaccination era most children contracted the disease and hence acquired long-term immunity. Exposure to the freely circulating virus during epidemics would simply top up their immunity. In fact, the disease is so mild that 20 to 50 per cent of children get no symptoms at all, and thus the presence of a rubella infection can only be identified through blood tests.[325,326]

The only reason the rubella vaccine was introduced was to prevent women getting the virus while pregnant. In 1941, an Australian ophthalmologist, Dr Norman Gregg, had made the link between women having rubella while pregnant and subsequently giving birth to babies with a congenital syndrome of cataracts, deafness, and heart disorders. Mind you, catching many other diseases during pregnancy, particularly HIV, toxoplasmosis and cytomegalovirus infections, but also measles, mumps, chickenpox and even influenza, can cause congenital abnormalities in foetuses[327]—which is a good reason for girls to catch and acquire lifelong immunity to typical childhood infectious diseases, and for women to be healthy and have strong immune systems before they conceive.

In 1972, just as the rubella vaccine was being added to the medical armamentarium, the World Health Organisation estimated that as many as 10 to 15 per cent of women who contracted rubella during the first three months of pregnancy would give birth to a deformed child.[328] (As an indication of how the medical courtiers whip up public fear, nowadays they claim that the syndrome is likely to affect 80 per cent of babies if the mother is infected in the first eight weeks of pregnancy.[329]) But instead of finding out why 85 to 90 per cent of pregnant women who contracted rubella in the first 12 weeks of pregnancy did not give birth to deformed babies, rather than recognising that a diet containing high amounts of vitamin A and C could help prevent or reduce the severity of infectious diseases,[330] the thrust of medical prevention became focused on the new vaccine.

In the beginning, two different national approaches were adopted in the war on rubella. The United States, obsessed with 'herd immunity', decided on the potentially dangerous ethical concept in medical care of vaccinating one segment of society (young boys, as well as young girls), to prevent disease in a second segment of society (pregnant women) which in turn would prevent the disease in a third segment (foetuses). Canada, forever under the influence of its powerful neighbour, followed suit. Needless to say, the ethics of this approach, where boys gained no benefit whatsoever from a medical procedure inflicted on them, stirred up considerable controversy.[331-333] The same controversy would later emerge with the advent of the vaccine to tackle the human papilloma virus.[334,335] Other nations were less obsessed with the concept of 'herd immunity' and initially decided on vaccinating adolescent girls only. But during the 1980s and '90s, these nations adopted the American way of mass vacccination of children by adding the rubella vaccine to the measles and mumps vaccines (the MMR vaccine).

From the outset it was clear that the 'immunity' conferred by the attenuated virus in the rubella vaccine paled by comparison with the natural immunity gained through infection with the wild virus. Researchers had found that three to five years after being vaccinated, some children's antibody levels were undetectable, and that cell-mediated immunity was far stronger, and more persistent and stable in those who had acquired immunity from getting the disease.[336-338]

In 1979–80, eight years after Britain had begun vaccinating all 13-year-old school girls, researchers in Glasgow found that 11.5 per cent of females aged 13 to 21 had insufficient antibodies to protect them against rubella.[339] If ever there was proof that the rubella vaccine was a failure was the fact that 10 per cent of males in the same age group were also found to be susceptible to the virus … and they weren't even vaccinated. Ninety per cent of them had acquired natural immunity from being exposed to the freely circulating, wild rubella virus. The fact that there was no difference between vaccinated females and unvaccinated males prompted the researchers to comment: 'The rubella vaccination programme has clearly failed to reduce the number of susceptible women in this practice.'

Waning immunity in vaccinated adolescent females had also been identified by researchers in Canada, the United States, the Netherlands, Denmark, Switzerland and Finland.[340-354] Ten per cent of army recruits tested in a study in Canada, for instance, and 15 per cent of sixth-graders in a US study, had insufficient antibodies to protect them against rubella.[343,347] And according to a recent study in Finland, vaccine-induced 'immunity' dwindles so dramatically that by the age of 15, girls could well become infected with the very disease the vaccine was supposed to protect them against, especially when they're pregnant.[354] Indeed researchers in Switzerland suspected that the high percentage of Swiss women with antibodies, 15 years after they had been vaccinated, could be explained by them being reinfected by the wild virus, with no credit whatsoever being afforded to the rubella vaccine.[353]

So it should come as little surprise that rubella infections do occur in vaccinated individuals. One of the first researchers to discover the abysmal failure rate of the rubella vaccine was Australian virologist, Dr Beverley Allan. In 1972 she had monitored a group of male army recruits who were vaccinated, and who had produced antibodies to rubella, immediately prior to being sent to an army camp that typically had an annual outbreak of rubella. Four months later, when the outbreak did occur, 80 per cent of the vaccinated males contracted the disease.[355]

American researchers had also identified an 80 per cent failure rate of the vaccine during an epidemic in the late 1960s.[356] Studies have shown that during epidemics many vaccinated individuals do become infected with the rubella virus,[357–369] but from 50 to 80 per cent of them produce no clinical symptoms at all. In other words, only through blood tests can the infection be identified. According to Canadian researchers the actual number of rubella cases may well be 50 per cent higher that those reported;[370] hence, the claim that the incidence of rubella dropped dramatically after the advent of the vaccine is simply hype.

Moreover, far more vaccinated individuals become reinfected with the rubella virus, even after a second vaccination, than do people who have acquired natural immunity.[356,364,371] Because of this, and because of the failed immunity amongst vaccinated individuals and the continuing epidemics, the extents of which have clearly been under-reported, several researchers called into question the very concept of 'herd immunity' to the rubella virus.[331–333,372–375] Indeed, the very idea of vaccinating children had been predicated on the assumption that they were the major source of infection for pregnant women. But since the incidence of women giving birth to babies with congenital rubella syndrome is no greater in women who have several children compared with those with only one, this had been shown to be a flawed assumption.[376]

If the idea of vaccinating children was to prevent them infecting pregnant women, then how has it fared? If we are to believe the US Centers for Disease Control and Prevention, it has been a total success. In the year 2000 the emperor's palace in Atlanta, Georgia, announced that the United States was on the verge of eliminating both rubella and congenital rubella syndrome, and in 2004 it proclaimed that the goal had been achieved.[377,378]

Certainly many studies have shown that vaccinated women have developed subclinical rubella;[379–390] and that the foetuses of such women do become infected with the virus.[391–403] So what do many pregnant women do when they realise they've been infected with the virus? They opt for an abortion.

When a rubella epidemic struck the island of Oahu in Hawaii in 1977, for instance, 429 people, mainly women aged 20 to 24, were affected.[397] Twelve of them were pregnant, and 11 opted for an abortion; one, who contracted rubella in the second trimester of her pregnancy, decided to continue with the pregnancy, and she gave birth to a normal healthy baby.

Now it just so happens that neither the United States, nor Canada, nor most other nations monitor the number of pregnancies terminated because of rubella. Canadian authorities do at least acknowledge that the incidence of chronic rubella syndrome is vastly under-reported, and that the less severe cases of chronic rubella syndrome are not even being diagnosed, much less reported.[398–400] Undoubtedly therapeutic abortions do distort national statistics on the incidence of congenital rubella syndrome, and thereby create the illusion that the emperor's new clothes are immaculate.

Britain, Japan, and Israel, however, do record the number of pregnancies terminated because of exposure to, or infection with, the rubella virus. When a rubella epidemic struck Israel in 1972, for instance, Israel's Ministry of Health recorded as many as one-and-a-half times more abortions than in the previous three years—about 20 per cent of the abortions were due to a history of exposure to rubella in the first months of pregnancy.[401]

Similarly, Britain's Office of Population Censuses and Surveys identified that the number of abortions due to exposure to, or infection with, rubella between 1976 and 1978 was over 13 times higher than the number of babies born with congenital rubella syndrome.[402] In 1978 alone there were 830 abortions because pregnant women had contracted rubella.[403]

And when Japan was struck by a rubella epidemic in 1987—as it had done so every five years since 1976 despite the introduction of the rubella vaccine in 1977—Japanese authorities reported that 100 children were born with congenital rubella syndrome. But 2,500 women had decided to terminate their pregnancies.[405] Which means that the incidence of congenital rubella syndrome could be up to 25 times higher than the medical courtiers report.

In fact, in the late 1970s the Chief Medical Officer at the Department of Health and Social Security in Britain, Henry Yellowlees, contended that the incidence of congenital rubella syndrome (which at that time in Britain was assumed to be about 400 cases each year) was probably twice as high as recorded figures, even excluding abortions.[406]

Certainly the number of abortions due to rubella has dramatically declined in Britain in recent years.[407] But the incidence of congenital rubella syndrome is less easy to ascertain, the reason being that the syndrome can include delayed effects, including cataracts, autism and Type I diabetes.[408] Tellingly, the incidence of both autism and Type I diabetes in young children has skyrocketed in recent years, as have cases of atopic cataracts.[409–413] But because most young children are inoculated with the MMR vaccine and have vaccine-induced antibodies by the age of 15 months, no one can determine whether these, let alone deafness, are the result of congenital rubella syndrome or not.

To compound the mess, by vaccinating children the vaccinators shifted the incidence of rubella to older age groups, thereby creating a potential time bomb amongst the very people the vaccine had been purported to protect.[414] Thus, in the late 1960s, before the advent of the vaccine, only 23 per cent of rubella cases in the United States occurred in people over 15.[415] But by 1975, the figure was 62 per cent;[415] by 1990, 81 per cent;[416] and by 1997, 85 per cent.[417]

Further compounding the debacle was evidence from computer modelling that unless 60 per cent of the population was vaccinated with the MMR vaccine, then congenital rubella syndrome would increase.[418] To tackle this, the courtiers are now recommending that not only should all women of child-rearing age be vaccinated, but so too should menfolk. Hence, between 2007 and 2008, Brazil vaccinated 70 million males and females aged 20 to 39, Argentina vaccinated 6.5 million men aged 16 to 39, and Chile did the same to 1.3 million Chilean men aged 19-29.[419] And from Australia comes the recommendation that all men between 17 and 44 should be vaccinated with the vaccine.[420]

The absurdity of man-made 'immunity' is highlighted by an outbreak of rubella amongst an Amish community in the United States in 1991. Known for shunning modern lifestyles and maintaining their traditional healthy ways, the Amish have always refused to be vaccinated. During the epidemic, 20 per cent of those children affected had no symptoms save the typical rash, and not a single pregnant woman contracted rubella.[421] The reason is not hard to find. Their immunity, 17 years after an earlier epidemic, had protected them and their unborn babies, just as the 1991 epidemic would protect the next generation and *their* unborn babies.

But the final word on the MMR vaccine goes to doctors at the prestigious Cochrane Collaboration, a respected international organisation that conducts and publishes systematic reviews into the effectiveness of medical treatments. While acknowledging the decline in rubella worldwide, the Collaboration had identified 131 scientific articles on the efficacy of the MMR vaccine, and had reviewed 31 of them. Their conclusion was that not a single field study had identified the efficacy of the MMR vaccine.[422] Which is not surprising given that another study had noted that all vaccines have considerably less efficacy against mild disease than the published data would suggest; the reason being that highly biased observers will rate vaccines as being twice as effective as would less biased physicians.[423]

The polio scam

The disease that strikes the greatest fear into parents is polio. Images of withered limbs and iron lungs will stir many a parent to rush off and have their young child inoculated against the disease. But history reveals yet another sorry saga, one that is the undoubtedly the greatest vaccine scam of all.

Little is known about the disease before the 19th century, though some medical historians contend that the disease had afflicted ancient Egyptians, evident, so they claimed, in the withered limbs of people depicted on stelae. The first mention of acute paralysis in infants, as a disease entity, was by Michael Underwood, a London physician, in 1789.[424,425] The disease, he wrote, is characterised by 'debility of the lower extremities which gradually become more infirm, and after a few weeks are unable to support the body.' This syndrome he blamed on 'teething', 'foul bowels', or 'a fever'. No mention was made of the disease being contagious, nor did it pose a serious problem because it was so rare. Indeed, Underwood wrote that he had never seen a child die from the condition.

The culprit: poisons or germs?

As if a sign of the industrial revolutionary times, the first outbreak of infantile paralysis ever to be recorded happened in the early 1830s on Saint Helena, the island in the Atlantic Ocean, off Angola where Napoleon Bonaparte had been exiled.[426] Then, in 1835, an outbreak, affecting four young children, occurred in the English hamlet of Worksop, in Nottinghamshire.[427] The United States recorded its first outbreak, affecting 8 to 10 children, in Louisiana in 1841.[428] Norway was next in 1868 with 14 cases in Oslo, 5 of whom died; and Sweden had its first outbreak in the northern town of Umea in 1881, affecting 20 children. Sweden also had the world's first full-scale epidemic in 1887 in Stockholm, affecting 44 children, 3 of whom died; ominously, several of the cases were school age children rather than the typically affected under-fours.[429] France's first outbreak occurred in the village of Sainte-Foy-l'Argentière, near the city of Lyon, in 1885, affecting 13 young children.[430]

In the final decade of the 19th century the disease became more menacing. America's first epidemic struck Rutland County, Vermont in 1894, affecting 132 people, a quarter of whom were over the age of six: 18 people died and over 40 were left permanently paralysed in one or more limbs.[428,430–432] During the summer of 1907 'the crippler', as it later came to be called, struck many thousands of children, as well as adults, throughout the US's north-eastern states. New York City alone had over 2,700 cases. 'The crippler', and the ensuing public panic, returned in the summer of 1908, and it did so every summer thereafter for the next half-century, paralysing or killing nearly 400,000 Americans in total. The same was happening to populations throughout the industrialised world. But, tellingly, not in underdeveloped countries.

Was it contagious? And, more importantly, what was causing it? In 1840 a German orthopaedist, Jakob von Heine, had suspected that the disease was contagious. Other researchers, however, thought not. Dr Charles Caverly, who had investigated the epidemic that struck Massachusetts in 1908, believed the culprit to be a toxin, not a micro-organism, since there was no evidence of contagion.[432] Nevertheless, during the 1890s, Swedish paediatrician, Oskar Medin also came to suspect that the disease was contagious. Hence, for a long time infantile paralysis, which was beginning to strike down not only infants, but also children and some adults, was known as 'Heine-Medin disease'. Later, it was renamed 'poliomyelitis' after researchers in the 1840s had identified that the grey matter (*polios*, Greek) of the anterior horns of the spinal cord's motor neurons (*myela*, Greek) were inflamed (*itis*, Greek).

But it was Medin's student, Ivar Wickman who believed he had found confirmation of the contagious nature of the disease: its greatest prevalence occurred amongst children living near busy river ways and main roads; places, he reasoned, where travellers with mild symptoms of the disease could spread it to others.[429] And, of course, the only thing that is contagious is germs. Wickman had also noted that dogs, too, were being paralysed. The problem is, dogs do not get polio: only humans do.

Nevertheless, the time was ripe for searching for an infectious agent. After all, Louis Pasteur had only recently promulgated his germ theory of disease. So researchers began searching in earnest for the germy culprit. In 1908, two Austrian scientists, Karl Landsteiner and Erwin Popper, thought they had found it. They had extracted diseased tissues from the spinal cord of a nine-year-old boy who had died from infantile paralysis, minced up the tissues, filtered them to remove bacteria, made a suspension in water, and had then injected the noxious mix directly into the abdominal cavities of two rhesus monkeys. The diseased foreign proteins and toxins, human DNA, cellular debris and possibly a host of prions, micoplasmas and viruses made the two monkeys severely ill; one died and the other was left paralysed in the legs. After dissecting the monkeys' brains, the researchers found that the damage to their central nervous systems was similar to that found in victims of acute infantile paralysis.

Tellingly, when the monkeys were made to drink the vile brew they did not become paralysed; nor did those that acquired the disease after the abdominal injection pass the disease on to other monkeys.[433] As British-born human rights campaigner and investigative journalist Janine Roberts noted in her report on the polio vaccine scam, published in the *Ecologist* in May 2004, this evidence alone debunked the claims that polio was highly contagious. Nevertheless, the World Health Organisation still credits these two researchers with discovering the poliovirus.

Inspired by the crude experiment of the Austrian researchers, two US researchers, Simon Flexner and Paul Lewis of the Rockefeller Institute for Medical Research, conducted a similar experiment.[429] They injected a similarly noxious brew derived from the diseased spinal cord of a victim into the spinal cord of a rhesus monkey, allowed it to wreak its damage, then extracted some fluid from the monkey's inflamed spinal cord and injected this into another monkey's spinal cord, and so on through a series of monkeys. Again, unsurprisingly, all monkeys were left paralysed. But through twisted logic, Flexner and Lewis concluded that the culprit was an unidentified virus. It was not until the mid-1930s that electron microscopy enabled scientists to identify viruses, those packets of genetic material surrounded by a protein coat that are at least 50 times smaller than bacteria.

And so began the search for a vaccine to defeat the assumed viral foe. Not once did government health scientists stop to consider that toxins, as Dr Charles Caverly had suspected, may have been the culprit, that paralysis can be caused by various chemical nerve poisons. As Ralph Scobey, a New York poliomyelitis researcher, had written—in a statement prepared for the US House of Representatives Select Committee to Investigate the Use of Chemicals in Food Products, 1950-1952—there are over 170 diseases that cause polio-like signs and symptoms. Amongst them are those resulting from such nutritional deficiencies as beriberi (vitamin B1, or thiamine deficiency), pellagra (vitamin B3, or niacin deficiency), and scurvy (vitamin C, or ascorbic acid deficiency), as well as those from chemical poisoning.[434]

The Dutch physician Herman Boerhaave, for example, had in 1765 noted that if people inhaled the fumes of mercury they are 'rendered paralytic'.[435] Similarly, in 1924 the English scientist John Cooke had identified that inhaling the fumes of lead, arsenic or mercury, or drinking solutions of these poisons, often causes paralysis.[436] Further evidence of a link between infantile paralysis and toxins arrived in 1879 when French neurologist Alfred Vulpian found that lead poisoning in dogs caused not only paralysis of their extensor muscles, but also caused the same spinal cord lesions found in human victims of polio.[437] Indeed, Vulpian considered that what he had found was in fact poliomyelitis.

In 1881, the Russian researcher Popow had found that ingestion of arsenic could cause acute poliomyelitis.[438] And the Australian Dr Altman had noted that just prior to the first polio epidemic in Australia in 1897—in Port Lincoln, South Australia, which affected 18 children, none of whom died—phosphorus had been widely used in the district to kill an infestation of rabbits.[439] Indeed, an epidemic of paralysis had occurred in the spring of 1930 in Ohio, Kentucky, Alabama and Mississippi after people had drunk a commercial extract of Jamaican ginger contaminated with triorthocresyl phosphate.[440,441]

Many other reports have documented symptoms of polio in people who have been exposed to lead, arsenic, cyanide, and carbon monoxide.[442–446] And, as is typical of the so-called polio incubation period of seven to 10 days after the onset of fever, headaches, and vomiting, the symptoms of flaccid paralysis often occurred several days after exposure to the various chemical poisons. This had happened in Western Samoa in 1936, after people from 38 villages had been injected with an arsenical medication to treat an outbreak of the tropical skin and bone disease, yaws.[447]

But not once did government researchers consider this evidence. They ignored the fact that arsenic had been extensively used throughout the 19th century in paints and adhesive envelopes, in medicated soaps, in Fowler's solution—a remedy for numerous medical conditions including malaria and asthma—and as a fungicide in wallpaper. It is therefore not surprising that samples of Napoleon Bonaparte's hair, tested recently by Italian researchers, were found to contain levels of arsenic 100 times higher than would be found in people today.[448] And, in particular, the polio researchers ignored the fact that the mechanised spraying of an arsenic-based pesticide called Paris Green had been extensively used in all industrialised countries since 1868—the year of the first polio outbreak in Norway—to stop codling moth infestations destroying apple crops.

Nor did anyone connect the dots between the time when farmers began using the more deadly lead arsenate pesticide in Massachusetts in 1892 and the polio epidemic in the neighbouring state of Vermont two years later.[433,449] Nor between the three cotton mills in western Massachusetts that were extracting cottonseed oil, undoubtedly through the use of carbon tetrachloride, and the epidemic amongst people living in the river valleys downstream from the processing plants.[450]

As New York researcher Jim West has noted, 1907 was the year when the United States began high-volume production of carbon tetrachloride for use as a fumigant, herbicide, insecticide and cleaning solvent.[451–453] It was surely no coincidence that in the following year, small-scale polio epidemics erupted in Massachusetts. And, tellingly, 1915 was the year when high volume production of the neurotoxin chloral benzene began at two large chemical factories at Niagara Falls in upstate New York. The following year marked the first of America's major polio epidemics. This one swept through the north-eastern states, affecting 27,363 people and killing 7,179. In New York City alone, nearly 9,000 people were afflicted.

Government health authorities did not recognise the absurdity of claiming that a virus was causing the epidemics of human paralysis, when horses and chickens and pigs and dogs were also becoming paralysed.[454] After all, the medical 'experts' claimed that poliomyelitis was a peculiarly human affliction.

As more and more industrial poisons continued to be sprayed onto crops, flushed into rivers, and released into the air, the numbers of people affected by the epidemics of polio in the industrialised world kept rising.

Then in 1945, DDT and hexachlorobenzene (HCB) entered the arsenal in the war on germs. DDT was readily sprayed on everything, from crops and fabrics, people and dairy cows, and other animals, to whole cities, to kill off mosquitoes, flies and every other pest. Adding to the insanity was the belief that polio was spread by flies; hence DDT was considered the saviour, not the culprit. By 1954, 3.1 billion pounds of persistent pesticides had entered the human environment, which is the equivalent of a large cup of endocrine-disrupting, nerve-poisoning chemicals for every person then alive.[455]

In tandem with what American endocrinologist Morton Biskind had called 'the most intensive campaign of mass poisoning in known human history',[456] the incidence of polio skyrocketed. Biskind was one of the heroes of this saga for he, together with Ralph Scobey, had tried to alert the scientific community and the US House of Representatives to the human health dangers of pesticides and their link to polio.[457,458]

In the nine years leading up to the release of DDT, from 1937 until 1945, the US had had just under 87,000 polio cases.[459] That's an average of 9,600 a year. But in the nine years between the release of DDT in 1945 and 1954, the United States had suffered nearly 300,000 cases of polio. That's over 33,000 cases a year. The greatest epidemic of all occurred in 1952, when 57,897 people contracted polio, over 21,000 of whom had some degree of paralysis. Thus, once DDT entered the human environment, polio cases had skyrocketed by 345 per cent.

Adding to the damning evidence was the fact that during World War II Allied troops were in the habit of dousing themselves and their camps with DDT to exterminate lice, mosquitoes, bedbugs, cockroaches and fleas. And, of course, the incidence of polio among US troops abroad was far higher than among those at home.[460,461] As the United States Army's Surgeon General had reported: 'It became apparent during the years 1941–45 that men of military age, born and brought up in the United States during the 1920s and 1930s, were more susceptible to poliomyelitis than their fathers had been in 1917–18. This was unexpected.'[462] Also unexpected was the high death rate from polio.

Moreover, there had been unexpected polio epidemics amongst US, British and New Zealand troops in the hot climate of the Middle East.[463,464] And yet the population at large had been spared, just as the Philippine population had been spared the polio epidemic that had occurred among American troops stationed in Manila in 1936.[465]

Besides DDT there had been another load of toxins that was being added to children's bodies. These were the chemicals in vaccines: residues of formaldehyde used in killing the accompanying germ; the preservative thiomersal (a mercury-based compound); and aluminium sulphate (alum), used for stimulating an antibody response to the germ. Any toxicologist would have predicted problems arising from injecting these known neurotoxins into children's blood streams. But evidently, the medical courtiers either hadn't known or weren't interested.

Polio arising from vaccination soon came to be called 'provocation polio', and it has been well documented. In an article in the *Archives of Disease in Childhood*, in March 1950, a British doctor, JK Martin, gave details of 17 cases in which poliomyelitis followed within 28 days of children being inoculated: 8 cases followed inoculation with the alum-precipitated diphtheria toxoid; 5 had had the combined diphtheria and whooping cough vaccine; 2 had injections against diphtheria with a fluid toxoid alone; and 1 had had a whooping cough inoculation alone.[466] Meanwhile, two physicians, Bertram McCloskey in Australia and Dennis Geffen in Britain, had also identified 'provocation polio' in some children and found that paralysis was far more likely to have started in the limb in which the injection had been given.[467,468]

Alarmed by these findings, the British Ministry of Health arranged for two medical statisticians to investigate the risk between polio and vaccines. After examining all case histories of the under-fives who had been afflicted during the polio epidemic of 1949, they identified 410 cases where there was evidence of provocation polio.[469] 'We must conclude,' they wrote in the *British Medical Journal* of 1 July 1950, 'that in the 1949 epidemic of poliomyelitis in this country cases of paralysis were occurring which were associated with inoculation procedures carried out within the month preceding the recorded date of onset of the illness.'

As the editor of the *British Medical Journal* wrote: 'It may be that children with general malaise of incipient poliomyelitis are not taken to the clinic for inoculation, but it seems more likely that the effect of injection is to produce paralytic symptoms in a patient who might otherwise have exhibited few if any signs and symptoms of poliomyelitis infection.'[470] But as Lily Loat, Secretary of the National Anti-Vaccination League in Britain, had commented: 'Whether the inoculation caused the paralysis or whether it made the limb more susceptible to the poison of infantile paralysis hardly mattered if the inoculation was to blame.'[41]

There was further evidence that cast doubt on the germ theory of polio. Given that exposure to a micro-organism produces immunity, then why did some monkeys and humans get a second attack of poliomyelitis?[471–473] The viral theory of poliomyelitis became totally unhinged when researcher John Toomey, who chaired a committee of the American Academy of Pediatrics to investigate childhood acute diseases, confirmed earlier research that no matter how intimately laboratory monkeys were exposed to polio-infected monkeys, polio is not contagious.[474] Indeed, Toomey had doubted that the disease induced by injecting diseased human tissues into the brains and abdomens of laboratory monkeys was the same as human polio.

Casting further doubt on the need for a vaccine had been the findings of Frederick Klenner, an American physician who had pioneered the use of massive doses of vitamin C therapy for treating disease. He had discovered that by injecting 25 to 30 grams of vitamin C each day into adult polio sufferers, they overcame polio, becoming well within three days, and with no paralysis whatsoever.[475]

Furthermore, another American physician, Benjamin Sandler, who had investigated the link between diet and polio, had found that sugar leaches calcium from bones, muscles and nerves, and that the weakened nerves were readily attacked by polioviruses.[476] Tellingly, countries with the highest per capita sugar consumption had had the greatest incidence of polio. And when do children tend to eat sugary foods, such as sweets, ice cream and soft drinks? During the summer months, which was exactly the season of polio epidemics. Confirmation of Sandler's theory that sugar was another culprit for polio epidemics came in 1949. In the spring of that year, Sandler had aired his ideas on radio in North Carolina, and afterwards many people had shunned such foods, the result being that whereas there were 2,498 polio cases in North Carolina in 1948, there were only 229 cases in the summer of 1949.[477]

Despite all this evidence, and despite the fact that even during an epidemic 95 per cent of people who contract the designated virus get no symptoms whatsoever—which surely begs the questions: Why are 5 per cent vulnerable? Why do less than two percent of cases result in flaccid paralysis? And for that matter, why do only half of these result in permanent paralysis?[478]—the virus hunters remained obsessed with creating a vaccine. They even claimed that polio epidemics were the result of excessive cleanliness, of children no longer being exposed to the wild virus and thus not acquiring natural immunity. After all, US army doctors during World War II had found widespread immunity to the suspected poliovirus amongst people in the Middle East, Asia and Africa, and no evidence of infantile paralysis.[433] In Turkey, infantile paralysis was even known as 'the American disease'. If it were true that cleanliness was to blame for the polio epidemics, then why hadn't the courtiers claimed the same for smallpox, cholera, diphtheria and so on?

The quest for the saviour

Stirring the virus hunters into action had been public panic, engendered by the media and by the National Foundation for Infantile Research, together with the presidential push to conquer the disease. Franklin Delano Roosevelt (FDR) himself had been crippled by the disease in 1921, at the age of 39, while holidaying with his wife and children at the family retreat on Campobello, a small Canadian island across the bay of Fundy from Maine. Three days before the first appearance of signs of the disease that would leave him crippled in both legs, he had fallen from his yacht into the icy, and polluted, waters of the Bay of Fundy; and the day before, he had swum in these polluted waters. As Jim West has noted, there were many industries in the area—paint, clothing and hardware manufacturers, breweries, tanneries, ship builders, and oil refineries—many of which were undoubtedly dumping organochlorine wastes, as well as lead, arsenic and mercury into the bay.[479]

When FDR later became president, he inspired Americans to help conquer this foe, just as he had inspired them during the war years to conquer their human foes. Fund-raising began with the President's Birthday Balls. But the most successful campaign was that of the National Foundation for Infantile Paralysis, which he had founded in 1937. And though the Foundation promptly decided that there was no cure for the disease, its campaign rapidly became a media event to garner small coin contributions from the American public; hence it later came to be called the 'March of Dimes'.

Years later, Herbert Ratner, a public health official who would become a fierce critic of the polio immunisation programme, revealed that in order to keep the statistical incidence of polio elevated, and hence engender public panic and the concomitant flow of funds for research, the Foundation paid physicians $25 for each reported diagnosis of paralytic polio.[480]

Scientists and scientific institutions everywhere rapidly began jumping on the polio bandwagon. Fierce competition to find a vaccine had already tarnished such endeavours. Two US researchers, Drs Maurice Brodie from New York City and John Kolmer from Philadelphia, independently had created vaccines and tested them on nearly 20,000 children whose parents had 'volunteered' them for trials during 1934 and 1935. The result had been disastrous: many children contracted polio, 12 were paralysed and at least 3 died. But in the frenzy to find a vaccine, people soon forgot that disaster.

To create a polio vaccine researchers needed plenty of polioviruses. The problem was that the three strains of the poliovirus, discovered during the 1930s, were not always present in the diseased spinal cord of victims. As investigative journalist Janine Roberts has remarked, 'This should have stopped the vaccine trials dead.'[481] But it didn't, for two researchers had found a ready source of polioviruses in the excrement of paralysed children. They also discovered what later came to be called the Coxsackie virus, which also causes acute paralysis (but that inconvenient discovery was ignored in the stampede to create a polio vaccine).[482]

Another team of researchers, John Enders, Thomas Weller and Frederick Robbins, had found a way to grow these viruses, initially on the minced up tissues of aborted human foetuses, and later on the kidneys of monkeys, and for that feat they later received the Nobel Prize.[483] Years later, such cultures were discovered to harbour other virulent viruses, including the simian virus 40 (SV40), the simian cytomegalovirus (SCMV), and the simian immunodeficiency virus (SIV).

Thus, in the development of a polio vaccine, tens of thousands of monkeys were sacrificed in American laboratories. Jonas Salk, whose killed-virus vaccine was first off the rank, confessed to killing at least 17,000 rhesus monkeys in his research at the University of Pittsburgh.[433] Indeed he and his rival, Albert Sabin, had estimated that from a single monkey's kidney they could culture sufficient viruses to produce 6,000 doses; at three doses per child, that would mean roughly 47,000 monkeys would need to be sacrificed to vaccinate America's children.

After generating the living viruses on slices of monkey kidneys, Salk and his colleague, Julius Youngner (who incidentally received no kudos whatsoever for his part in the development of the vaccine), had killed them off with diluted formaldehyde and heat. At least, that's what they thought. The Salk vaccine was now ready for testing.

In 1954, in a trial of unprecedented size and scope, 440,000 second-grade school children in 44 American states, two Canadian provinces, and in the city of Helsinki, Finland, were injected with the vaccine. To ensure scientific rigour, epidemiologist Thomas Francis Jr., the official in charge of the trials, made sure that 210,000 first- and third-grade children were injected with a placebo; and that over a million children were observed as controls.

Salk had stipulated that children who received only one of the three injections were to be classified as 'not-inoculated'.[484] Ominously, that meant that adverse reactions to the initial dose would not be recorded.

Other worrisome signs were also emerging. In 1953, US researcher Albert Mitzer had warned that steeping the viruses in formaldehyde for nine days, as Salk had done, was insufficient time to kill all viruses.[485] After testing Salk's technique, the esteemed Swedish virologist Sven Gard had concluded that at least 12 weeks were needed. Even more alarming were the findings of Bernice Eddy, a researcher at the Laboratory of Biologics Control, a group at the US National Institutes of Health in Bethesda, Maryland.[486] She had been in charge of assessing the safety of Salk's vaccine and had discovered that monkeys, into whose brains and muscles she had injected Salk's vaccine, not only became paralysed, but also had live polioviruses in their spinal cords. Nevertheless, in the stampede to produce a vaccine, all this was ignored.

The National Foundation for Infantile Paralysis, which had paid for Salk's research and the mass trial, was so confident of the vaccine, it had ordered enough vaccine to inoculate nine million children.[487]

And so, on 12 April 1955, before an audience of 500 scientists and doctors and 150 reporters assembled in a makeshift newsroom in the Rackham Auditorium at the University of Michigan in Ann Arbor, and before 54,000 doctors watching the proceedings on closed-circuit television in theatres across the United States and Canada, and to people listening to radio broadcasts across America and, via *The Voice of America*, throughout the world, Dr Francis, announced that the Salk vaccine had proven to be totally 'safe, effective and potent'.

The news was greeted with jubilation. Across the nation church bells rang, air-raid sirens screamed, court-room proceedings were adjourned, and people stood for a minute's silence. Powerful symbolism was also afoot, for it was 10 years to the day since FDR, the most famous polio victim of all, had died; and it was 94 years to the day since the first salvoes had been fired against another enemy to announce the start of another war, the American Civil War.

Later that afternoon, William Workman, director of the Laboratory of Biologics Control convened a meeting of specialists to determine whether licences should be granted to five pharmaceutical companies for the manufacture of the vaccine. Despite the fact that the advisory committee had to assess 2,000 pages of information about the vaccine trial and the manufacturing procedures, it had agreed within two-and-a-half hours that the vaccine should be licensed. Today it takes at least one year to license a vaccine.[488] And William Workman, Bernice Eddy's boss, never said a word about her discovery that three of the six batches of vaccine, manufactured by Cutter Laboratories and submitted to her laboratory for assessment, had paralysed laboratory monkeys.[486]

Soon afterwards in Washington, DC, Oveta Culp Hobby, the US Secretary of Health, Education and Welfare, signed licences for the manufacture of the vaccine. Less than four hours later, Parke-Davis & Co, one of five drug companies under contract to the Foundation, made its first shipment of the vaccine.[487] Four days later, first- and second-graders in San Diego, California, became the first recipients of the vaccine.

The first shots in the war on polio

The jubilation was short-lived, however. Thirteen days after the war on polio had begun, after about a million children had been inoculated, the first casualties were announced: six cases of paralytic polio turned up in children who had received the vaccine manufactured by the Cutter Laboratories in Berkeley, California. The vaccines from Wyeth, Parke-Davis and Eli Lilly, three of the five manufacturers, were also implicated.[489] But it was the Cutter Laboratories that took the bad rap.

In the following days, health authorities discovered that of the 120,000 children who were inoculated with Cutter's vaccine, 40,000 had come down with mild symptoms of poliomyelitis, 51 were permanently paralysed—tellingly, in each case the paralysis began in the inoculated limb—and five had died.[488] Cutter's vaccine had also started an epidemic: 113 people in the inoculated children's families and communities were paralysed, and 5 had died. In his book, *The Cutter Incident, 50 Years Later*, paediatric immunologist Paul Offit, summed up the whole affair as '… one of the worst pharmaceutical disasters in U.S. history.'

The consensus was that the poliovirus had survived the formaldehyde treatment at the Cutter Laboratory, just as Albert Mitzer and Sven Gard had warned, and as Bernice Eddy had foreseen when she warned a friend: 'There's going to be a disaster. I know it.'[486]

The Cutter vaccine was immediately withdrawn, and on 7 May, the US Surgeon General called a halt to the vaccination programme, having been told by polio experts, to his surprise, that there were a variety of technical problems in the manufacture of the Salk vaccine, and that there could be no guarantees that the vaccine would be totally safe. But three weeks later, the vaccination programme was reinstated, thanks to the push by Jonas Salk and Thomas Francis to introduce 'improved' manufacturing procedures.

By late August that year, 150 million doses of the vaccine had been administered: half of the population under 40 had been injected with one dose, and one third had received three doses of the vaccine.

Was the vaccine an immediate success? No, it was an abysmal failure. Four months after the resumption of the programme, Boston recorded 2,000 cases of infantile paralysis, a seven-fold increase compared with the same time the previous year, and 130,000 children had been vaccinated.[490] The incidence of paralytic polio in Rhode Island and Wisconsin was five times higher than it had been at the same time the previous year, in Vermont three times higher, in Connecticut twice as high, and six other north-western states recorded incidences at least 50 per cent higher.

Not only was the Salk vaccine failing to protect children, it was even contributing to epidemics. Alarmed by the outbreaks, various state health authorities called a halt to their vaccination programmes. Newark, New Jersey, abandoned its programme in June 1955; Idaho followed suit on 1 July 1955 after a polio outbreak hospitalised 79 children and killed seven; and Utah did the same on 12 July.[490]

The vaccine's reputation fared little better during 1956. According to the *New York Times*, the national incidence of infantile paralysis during the first four months of the year had increased by 12 per cent over the rates during the same period in 1955.[491] Alarmed by the vaccine's track record in the United States, all European countries except Denmark called a halt to their vaccination programmes, just as Canada had done in July 1955. And by January 1957, 17 US states had followed suit.

A rose by any other name
Children certainly weren't being protected. But the medical courtiers were

determined to at least protect the US President, as well as Jonas Salk, the vaccine manufacturers, and themselves, from the humiliation of the vaccine being revealed as an outright failure. After all, the nation's reputation was at stake. Something had to be done.

And indeed it was. Taking a perverse interpretation of Shakespeare's famous lines—'What's in a name? that which we call a rose by any other name would smell as sweet'[492]—the courtiers began to rename polio to statistically create the illusion that polio was declining. The results of this charade would eventually go down in history as one of the most successful disappearing acts of all time.

First, they abandoned the World Health Organisation's definition of polio—the presence in a person of paralytic signs for 24 hours—and in its place adopted Salk's definition of polio, a definition he had used during his mass trial: the presence in a person of paralytic signs for at least 60 days. Because up to 98 per cent of people would recover within 60 days:[478] 'this nifty but dishonest administrative move,' wrote Australian research scientist Dr Viera Scheibner, 'excluded more than 90 per cent of polio cases from the definition of polio.'[493] That was undoubtedly an underestimate.

Second, all cases of polio that occurred within 30 days of inoculation were to be reclassified as 'pre-existing', just as Salk had done during the mass trial of his vaccine.[433]

By 1958, thanks to advances in microbiology, the courtiers alighted on a third ploy: shuffle as many cases of polio as possible into the categories of other diseases. Thus, where the victim suffered from inflammation of the membranes that protect the brain and spinal nerve cells and cause muscular weakness and pain—a syndrome that was previously diagnosed as 'non-paralytic poliomyelitis'—the disease was to be reclassified as 'aseptic meningitis' or 'viral meningitis'.[494]

And the fourth trick was to initially classify all cases of paralytic polio as 'acute flaccid paralysis'; and if no poliovirus could be found in the excrement of the patient, then the disease was definitely not to be classified as polio. It could be classified as Coxsackie virus infection, or as ECHO virus infection, both of which are clinically indistinguishable from paralytic poliomyelitis.[495] Or it could be classified as Guillain-Barré Syndrome, which some physicians suspect Franklin Delano Roosevelt had contracted.[496] Or it could be called myalgic encephalomyelitis (ME), a syndrome that first surfaced in 1954, and would later be named chronic fatigue syndrome.[497,498]

There was a final ploy the courtiers had hit upon to reduce the statistical incidence of polio. They redefined a 'polio epidemic': prior to 1955 it was 6 cases per 100,000 people, but after 1955 it was defined as 35 cases per 100,000.[499]

Unsurprisingly, the official statistics would show that the incidence of non-paralytic 'polio' had declined by 95 per cent between 1955 and 1960; and that paralytic polio had declined by 85 per cent.[459]

The person who had blown the whistle on the statistical manipulation was biostatistician Bernard Greenberg. A former Chairman of the Committee on

Evaluation and Standards for the American Public Health Association, he had informed colleagues at the 120th Annual Meeting of the Illinois Medical Society in May, 1960: 'My primary concern, my only concern, is the very misleading way that most of this data has been handled from a statistical point of view.'[500] And, further: 'A scientific examination of the data, and the manner in which the data were manipulated, will reveal that the true effectiveness of the present Salk vaccine is unknown and greatly overrated.'

The living virus lurking in the Salk vaccine

Worse was to come. Bernice Eddy, the researcher at the National Institutes of Health (NIH), who had already found problems with Salk's vaccine, had been inspired by the work of fellow researcher Sarah Stewart. The latter had discovered that viruses could cause cancer. That was the last thing their superiors at the NIH wanted to hear. So, without her boss's authorisation, Eddy went back to her laboratory to make further tests on the Salk vaccine. After injecting the monkey kidney tissues, upon which the polioviruses had been cultured, into 23 hamsters, she was horrified to discover that 20 of them grew large cancerous tumours.[501] By 1960, she knew that a virus, soon isolated by Ben Sweet and Maurice Hilleman (two scientists at the Merck research laboratories in Philadelphia), and dubbed SV40 because it was the 40th simian virus to be discovered, was the culprit, and that it had been far more resistant to being killed by formaldehyde than the poliovirus. She also discovered that it was capable of infecting recipients of the vaccine.[502,503]

Needless to say, Eddy's findings caused consternation amongst the medical courtiers. They certainly had cause for concern. Estimates were that from 10 to 30 per cent of Salk's vaccine had been contaminated with SV40, and they knew that about 98 million American children and adults—about 60 per cent of the American population—had been injected with the vaccine.[504] Several studies at the time had shown that SV40 caused brain tumours in experimental animals, and could cause cancer in human tissues.[505–508]

That meant that in the seven-year period from 1954 until 1961, as many as 30 million Americans, and up to 100 million people worldwide, were injected with a ticking time bomb from rhesus monkeys. As of 1968, the US had exported close to half a billion doses of the Salk vaccine. Britain alone imported 10 million doses.[501]

But according to Herbert Ratner, Director of Public Health in Oak Park, Illinois, editor of the *Bulletin of the American Association of Public Health Physicians*, and the man who chaired the meeting at which Greenberg had revealed the courtiers' statistical sleight of hand, 'The National Foundation for Infantile Paralysis and the US Public Health Service, who were recovering from previous troubles, were well aware how upset parents would be to discover that Salk anti-polio vaccinators, like a hoard of hungry mosquitoes, had descended on their children with African monkey viruses.'[501] Accordingly, government courtiers 'did what they could to suppress and minimise the discovery.' Even the National Cancer Institute soft-pedalled on the revelations to avoid publicity on the matter.

Although two of the four vaccine manufacturers, Merck and Parke-Davis, immediately recalled their polio vaccines, the courtiers at the US National Institutes of Health, as well as those in the departments of health in Britain and Canada, were more intent on saving reputations than children, and refused to recall the rest of the supply, fearing the public backlash would jeopardise the vaccination campaign.[509] Thus they knowingly allowed even more millions of people to be dosed with a cancer-causing virus. Tellingly, the US Public Health Service concealed that secret for 40 years.[510]

After a flurry of tests, the courtiers quickly concluded that there were no health risks from the Salk vaccine. The first public disclosure that the vaccine was contaminated with a monkey virus, and that Merck had withdrawn its vaccine, was buried on page 33 of the *New York Times* on 26 July 1961. When asked to comment, the US Public Health Service proclaimed that there was no evidence that the virus was dangerous.[511]

As for Bernice Eddy, because she had breached the official wall of silence by discussing her findings with other scientists, she, like many other whistle-blowers, was persecuted and demoted.

Out of Africa

The mood amongst physicians was rapidly turning sour. One writer in the 25 February 1961 edition of the *Journal of the American Medical Association*, aptly summed up the consensus: 'It is now generally recognised that much of the Salk vaccine used in the U.S. has been worthless.'[512] Such sentiments spurred the American Medical Association to exert pressure on the Federal Government to abandon the Salk vaccine and replace it with the Sabin vaccine. It was cheaper, it had been tested on tens of millions of children in Latvia, Estonia and Kazakhstan—albeit contaminated with SV40—and because it was taken by mouth on sugar cubes or as a liquid preparation, not injected, it was easier to administer. Because the vaccine contained a live but weakened poliovirus, the courtiers also believed it would more readily confer 'immunity' on recipients than the Salk vaccine. Data on the Salk vaccine showed that antibody levels two to four years after inoculation were so low that repeated, if not frequent, booster shots would be required to retain 'immunity.'[513] Moreover, Sabin's attenuated virus would remain in the intestinal tract of the recipient for at least six to eight weeks after the time of vaccination, and thus it would readily infect other members of the community—admittedly without their consent—but that was of no concern to the courtiers. At least it would ensure widespread 'immunity' to the weakened virus.

The courtiers were also confident in the safety of the oral vaccine, since researchers at the National Cancer Institute, in evaluating the carcinogenicity of SV40, had quickly concluded in 1963 that there were more dangers from Salk's injectable vaccine than from Sabin's oral vaccine.[514] Seven years after the horse had bolted, researchers conducted a follow-up study and found no evidence of deaths in newborn recipients of the Sabin vaccine.[515]

By 1963, the Sabin vaccine was off the starting blocks, with instructions to the three remaining manufacturers, Parke-Davis, Wyeth-Lederle, and Pfizer, to ensure that no SV40 was present in the vaccine. Merck had called a permanent halt to producing polio vaccine; in its letter to the US Surgeon General, it cited technical difficulties in removing all simian virus contaminants, 'which may be difficult if not impossible to detect at the present stage of technology.'[516]

That letter alone should have been sufficient warning to health officials that to continue with the vaccination programme was foolhardy. But policy was being made on the run, and the warning fell on deaf ears. To ensure no SV40 was present in any vaccine, regulations had been introduced in March 1961, stipulating that manufacturers were to test kidney cell cultures for at least 14 days to detect the presence of the virus. But according to scientists at the Division of Biologics Standards at the NIH, where Bernice Eddy had worked, at least five weeks were needed to detect SV40.[517] Curiously, the regulations did not stipulate that old seed stocks were to be discarded and started afresh, even though they undoubtedly carried SV40-contaminated poliovirus hybrids (recombinant mutants). In other words, the testing requirements to protect children from a cancer-causing virus were crude and unreliable, and had been based on poor science.

The US National Institutes of Health had also recommended to Sabin, and to Salk, that they switch from using the kidneys of rhesus monkeys to those of African green monkeys, which supposedly were not infected with SV40.

The change to using kidneys of African green monkeys was made quickly and quietly to ensure that the public would remain clueless to the fact that tens of millions of people had been infected with a cancer-causing virus. But, in the frenzy, no one had bothered to evaluate whether African green monkeys also carried viruses that could infect humans. That would later prove to have been a disastrous mistake.

What the courtiers also failed to see was that the live-virus vaccine was potentially more dangerous than Salk's vaccine. As was discovered later, the weakened viruses could revert to virulent strains—and hence give recipients paralytic polio; and through the shedding of the virus in their stools, those inoculated with it could spread it to other members of the community.[518] Ominously, the people who could least afford to be infected, either directly through inoculation, or indirectly by catching poliovirus from the recipient of the vaccine, were those with weak immune systems.

Concern about the Sabin vaccine harbouring unidentified and virulent viruses from African green monkeys spurred one of the two remaining Sabin vaccine manufacturers, Lederle, to request that studies be done on the vaccine. Together with the Bureau of Biologics, Lederle scientists found the simian cytomegalovirus (SCMV) in the kidneys of all 11 monkeys tested.[519] Yet again, the courtiers decided to suppress the information, as Australian-born virologist, John Martin, who had worked at the Bureau of Biologics during the 1970s, discovered. And so the story of SV40, like the virus itself and the 39 other simian viruses, remained hidden for another 20 years.

The Sabin vaccine's fall from grace

By the 1970s, the total number of paralytic polio cases had dropped to less than 25 per year, according to the US Centers for Disease Control and Prevention (CDC).[520] But in 1976, Jonas Salk, Sabin's arch-rival, testified before a Senate subcommittee that Albert Sabin's oral vaccine was the 'principal if not the sole cause' of all reported cases of paralytic polio in the United States since 1961. 'To avoid occurrence of such cases,' he warned, 'it would be necessary to discontinue the routine use of the live-polio vaccine.'[521] Over the years, each had accused the other of causing polio. And they were both right!

The CDC did at least acknowledge the dangers posed by the vaccine when it reported that all of the 21 cases that occurred during 1982–1983 were caused by the vaccine.[520]

There were hiccoughs with the vaccine overseas too. In Oman, for example, an epidemic of paralytic polio erupted six months after authorities had completed vaccinating 98 per cent of children. The highest incidence was in children under two-years-of-age, 87 per cent of whom had received three doses of the Sabin vaccine.[522]

In Romania, between 1984 and 1992, the risk of vaccine-associated paralytic polio was 14-times higher than in the United States, and 17 times higher than in other countries. Researchers were at a loss to explain why.[523] Moreover, doctors who examined Romanian children found that the chance of contracting paralytic polio was directly related to the number of antibiotic injections they had received: a single injection within one month of having received the Sabin vaccine raised the risk eight times; two injections, 27 times; 10 or more, 182 times.[524] This was nothing other than provocation polio.

Indeed, over 80 published studies on populations in 16 countries on all continents had shown that vaccine-associated paralytic polio was rife.[525]

Sabin's vaccine eventually fell from grace in 1994 when CDC researchers confirmed that the main cause of polio in the US was the vaccine.[526] Their recommendation was that the United States should switch back to the injectable, killed-poliovirus vaccine. But because production would take several years to get up and running, and because of heavy lobbying by the sole oral vaccine manufacturer, Lederle, the CDC would ordain an interim period when two shots of the Salk vaccine would be administered followed by two doses of the Sabin vaccine. Thus, in 2000 the Sabin vaccine became a mere footnote in the saga of medical history, though the effects of its Green monkey viral contaminants would continue.

Polio's great disappearing act

Certainly the medical courtiers had managed to pull off polio's great disappearing act. Thanks to the 'rose by any other name' ploy, Los Angeles County health authorities would note in 1967 how the statistics on non-paralytic polio had been swapped for those of viral meningitis. According to Christopher Kent, writer and later President of the Council on Chiropractic Practice, the report for 1967 stated:

'All cases [of polio] now reported as meningitis.'[527]

	Viral meningitis	Poliomyelitis
July 1955	50	273
July 1961	161	65
July 1963	151	31
September 1966	256	5

Nationally, non-paralytic polio's decline and demise, and viral meningitis's birth and reciprocal growth, are readily apparent in the following table presented by Gary Krasner, Director of the Coalition for Informed Choice, New York City:[528]

	Viral meningitis	Poliomyelitis
1951–1960	0	70,083
1961–1980	102,999	589
1983–1992	117,366	0

In 1997, the US Centers for Disease Control and Prevention did admit that 30,000 to 50,000 Americans contracted viral meningitis each year.[529] 'That's where all those 30,000–50,000 cases of polio disappeared after the introduction of mass vaccination,' declared Australian scientist Viera Scheibner.[493]

The aftermath

In 1954, a polio-like syndrome had surfaced, initially called 'myalgic encephalomyelitis' (ME) by British scientists. But because of pressure by their American counterparts, the name was changed by the 1980s to 'chronic fatigue syndrome' (CFS).[497,498] As British researcher Betty Dowsett would note, by emphasising a 'fatigue definition' of the syndrome, and the associated psychiatric inference in the term, the American courtiers managed to distract attention from serious research into the viral aspects and clinical features of the syndrome.[530] After all, some researchers had noted that the syndrome was indistinguishable from non-paralytic polio, once known as 'abortive polio', or 'atypical polio', and, in particular, the chronic phase known as 'post-polio syndrome'.[531–534] It had simply been rebadged.

More to the point, there were suspicions that ME/CFS was caused by any combination of the 69 strains of enteroviruses that are genetically related to the three strains of poliovirus. These include the Coxsackie viruses and ECHO viruses. At least 69 epidemics of the syndrome have been recorded since 1934.[534] But, as Dr Richard Bruno, American clinical psychophysiologist, expert in post-polio sequelae, and Director of the Post-Polio Institute, International Centre for Post-Polio Education and Research and Fatigue Management Programs at New Jersey's Englewood Hospital and Medical Center, explains, '… something unexpected, frightening and unrecognised happened after the polio vaccine was distributed: the number of cases of CFS/ME went through the roof.'[535] The reason?

'It appears that the vaccine that eliminated polio had an unintended consequence,' Bruno continues.[535] 'The elimination of the three types of poliovirus left a vacuum that had to be filled. Just as a flock of dominant and aggressive blue jays blocks less aggressive robins from roosting in your back yard, poliovirus are the bluejays of enteroviruses, the viruses that live and grow in your intestines. When poliovirus "blue jays" disappeared from your intestines thanks to the vaccine, other enteroviruses "robins" took over the poliovirus' old intestinal breeding ground and filled the vacuum. With the polioviruses gone other enteroviruses were able to multiply, spill into the bloodstream and enter the spinal cord and brain.' In other words, by changing our intestinal microflora, the Salk vaccine, and particularly the oral Sabin vaccine, indirectly caused ME/CFS.[536]

Given that about one million Americans suffer from ME/CFS, as do about 200,000 Britons, 90,000 Canadians, 65,000 Australians and 12,000 New Zealanders, and that a quarter of them are severely incapacitated, we can begin to understand the enormous consequences of the polio vaccination campaign.

But one researcher believes that ME/CFS, as well as many other diseases of epidemic proportions, including autism and attention-deficit-hyperactivity disorder in children, as well as cancer, fibromyalgia, and a host of neurological disorders, are the direct result of Sabin's polio vaccine. Dr John Martin, the Australian virologist who had worked at the Bureau of Biologics during the 1970s, and then went on to become Professor of Pathology at the University of Southern California School of Medicine, and to establish the privately-funded Center for Complex Infectious Diseases in Rosemead, California, had taken a keen interest in the simian cytomegalovirus (SCMV). His interest had been whetted after discovering that SCMV was a green monkey contaminant in the Sabin polio vaccine, and that the medical courtiers had suppressed that information, not only from the public, but also from the scientific community. Using a recently developed, sophisticated analytic technique called the polymerase chain reaction (PCR) that enables scientists to identify gene sequences, he had identified DNA fragments of SCMV in many people suffering from ME/CFS.[537,538] Normally our immune system reacts to a viral infection with an inflammatory response, but curiously the viruses he extracted and cultured from brain biopsies, the cerebrospinal fluid, and the blood of people with ME/CFS, had somehow managed to evade that immune response.[539,540]

Equally disturbing was his discovery that fragments of these immune-eluding viruses readily combined with fragments of bacterial DNA (which he dubbed viteria), with DNA fragments of other viruses, and with DNA fragments of our own genes, potentially including our own oncogenes (cancer-causing genes). And they can capture, amplify and mutate cellular genes without our immune system being any the wiser. Thus he coined the term 'stealth viruses'.[541]

To prove the point, Martin injected cats with stealth viruses taken from people suffering from ME/CFS. The cats ended up with encephalopathy (brain dysfunction).[542] And when an epidemic of encephalopathy struck people in the

Mohave Valley, Arizona, in 1996, they too showed the tell-tale signs of a stealth virus.[543] Further proof of the epidemic's stealth-viral origin emerged in the case of a young boy from the Valley who was so severely affected that doctors expected him to die within months. He recovered after being prescribed an antiviral drug.[544]

In essence, the polio vaccine has been responsible for creating new and potentially virulent life forms called 'stealth viruses', which, as Martin has portrayed them, are 'nature's biological weapons programme'. Except that they were spawned in human laboratories.

Unsurprisingly, the courtiers were furious, for Martin had dared to reveal that the emperor's naked body was not only appallingly grubby, but also a festering mess. Despite repeatedly urging the CDC to investigate the issues, his efforts have come to nought. His proposals for funding to investigate the risks, submitted in 1978, and again in 1995, were rejected, and several abstracts submitted to CDC meetings were also rejected. He has even been denied the right to test patients for stealth viruses. The courtiers' message is clear: if you break the code of silence and impugn the excellence of the emperor's new clothes, then you will be ostracised, if not pilloried.

And whatever became of SV40? Well, if the courtiers had heeded the warnings from researchers in the 1960s—that, when injected into hamsters, SV40 caused ependymomas, a rare form of brain cancer; that it caused chromosomal aberrations in human kidney cell cultures; and that, when injected into human cells, it produced tumours—then they may have foreseen that sooner or later some of the recipients of the Salk vaccine, or their children, would end up with various cancers.[505–508]

If they had but trawled through the details of all epidemiological studies on the impact of SV40, they would have found, as did a group of Canadian and Italian biostatisticians,[545] that according to an Australian study, children who had been inoculated with the Salk vaccine had a 40 per cent greater risk of developing cancer within 10 years of the shots than those who hadn't been inoculated, and for children over the age of one, the risk was 69 per cent higher.[546] According to the Connecticut Tumor Registry, children born between 1956 and 1962 had twice the risk of central nervous system tumours compared with other children, and that 66 per cent of medulloblastomas, a variety of brain cancer, contained SV40.[547] According to a group of researchers at the Boston Medical Center, not only was there an increased incidence of ependymomas in children born between 1956 and 1962, but the children of mothers inoculated during these years had two-and-a-half times the risk of getting cancer; and if their mothers had been inoculated during the first four months of their pregnancy, then the risk was 13 times greater than expected, and if inoculated in the first three months of pregnancy, then the risk of cancer was more than 15 times greater.[548]

The courtiers' game of make-believe should have been over in 1988, when a team of US physicians and scientists, using the newly developed polymerase chain reaction, found that half the children they examined who had choroid plexus papilloma (a form of brain cancer), and all but one of the 11 children with ependymomas, had the DNA-footprints of SV40 in their tumours.[549] Several years later, the same researchers found that 14 of 17 children with choroid plexus papillomas and ependymomas had the SV40 footprints.[550]

Then in 1993 more bad news arrived. Italian researchers had found that when SV40 was injected into hamsters it caused mesothelioma, a lung cancer normally associated with exposure to asbestos.[551] One of the researchers, molecular pathologist Michele Carbone, now working at Chicago's Loyola University Medical Center, followed his hunch and he and his colleagues, using the polymerase chain reaction, examined the lung tissues of patients with mesothelioma. What they found was astounding, particularly since the disease was blamed entirely on asbestos: 60 per cent of cases had the tell-tale DNA footprints of SV40.[552]

Was SV40 the reason why mesothelioma first emerged during the 1950s? And was that the reason why cases of mesothelioma in Turkey, which didn't start its polio vaccination programme until the 1970s, and in Finland, which never used SV40-contaminated vaccine, showed no evidence of SV40?[553,554] Given that 80 per cent of cases of mesothelioma in the western world develop in individuals who have been exposed to excessive levels of asbestos, and yet only a fraction of people thus exposed will go on to develop mesothelioma, is SV40 the hidden factor, a co-carcinogen?[555] Carbone and his fellow research scientists certainly believe so.[556–559]

Two years later, Carbone and his colleagues would detect SV40 in 60 per cent of osteosarcomas, a type of bone cancer.[560]

By 1996, dozens of scientists had reported finding SV40 in a wide variety of brain and bone cancers, in mesothelioma, and in non-Hodgkin's lymphoma. But the courtiers were sceptical. Between 1997 and 2003, more than 25 peer-reviewed studies were published on the link between SV40 and mesothelioma, and 16 other studies had been published on the connection between SV40 and brain and bone cancers, non-Hodgkin's lymphoma, and other cancers, including kidney tumours.[510,556–572] And by 2003, the link between SV40 and these cancers had been identified in 18 developed countries. But the courtiers remained sceptical, at least publicly.

On the issue of brain cancers, for instance, researchers from Italy, France, and China had found SV40 footprints in a high percentage of all types of brain cancers. The Italian team headed by Professor Mauro Tognon, at the University of Ferrara's School of Medicine, found that SV40 was present in 83 per cent of choroid plexus papillomas, 75 per cent of ependymomas, 47 per cent of astrocytomas, and 37 per cent of glioblastomas.[567,568] The French team at the International Agency for Research on Cancer, in Lyons, had found SV40 in all brain tumour types, including 56 per cent of ependymomas in children, 38 per cent of choroid plexus papillomas, and 29 per cent of medulloblastomas.[569] And a Chinese team at the Department of Neurosurgery at Xijing Hospital in Xi'an had found SV40 in each of the common brain tumours, including all cases of ependymomas and choroid plexus papillomas, 90 per cent of pituitary adenomas, 73 per cent of astrocytomas, 50 per cent of glioblastomas, and 33 per cent of medulloblastomas.[570] Ominously, the Italian team had discovered that SV40 was present in 8 per cent of normal brain tissue.[568]

SV40 had even been detected in 45 per cent of sperm specimens and 23 per cent of blood samples collected from healthy adults.[571,572]

Revelations

One question arising from all this is, how does SV40 cause cancer? According to research scientists, the answer is that the simian virus 40 acts like a hit-and-run driver, wreaking havoc as it goes.[573] Its power lies in one of its proteins, which binds to and inactivates our body's own tumour-suppressing proteins, particularly a protein known as 'the guardian of the genome,' or less poetically 'p53'.[574] This is probably the reason why cancers that contain SV40 are less likely to be responsive to chemotherapy and radiation therapy.[575] To make matters worse, SV40 also causes cellular aberrations in immune system cells, as is readily apparent in its link to lymphomas.

But the big question is, how did SV40 end up in children who were born long after Salk's SV40-contaminated vaccine was removed from vaccination programmes? Many researchers suspect that the virus can be passed from a mother to her unborn child, that it can be sexually transmitted, and that it can be transmitted through blood transfusions.[568,572,576,577] Undoubtedly a person's health also plays a huge part, because researchers at Baylor College of Medicine in Houston, Texas, noted that six per cent of hospitalised children, many of whom were immune-compromised, had antibodies to SV40.[576]

Mysteriously, American researchers had noted that some mothers of children who had brain tumours containing SV40 had no evidence themselves of antibodies to the virus.[578,579] A case in point is that of Alexander Horwin, a young American boy who contracted a malignant brain tumour, medulloblastoma, eight months after having received the oral polio vaccine.[575] He died five months later, four months shy of his third birthday. Neither his parents, nor his placenta, carried any sign of SV40; but according to four independent laboratories, SV40 footprints were apparent in his tumour. Believing that their son's cancer was caused by the polio vaccine, Michael and Raphaele Horwin, from a beachside suburb in Los Angeles, would go on to establish the SV40 Foundation, to help other parents of children with cancer, and to alert the public and the US Congress to the issues surrounding SV40 and the polio vaccine.

But that mystery may have been solved, not by a scientist, but by a lawyer. Over the years, Philadelphia-based lawyer Stanley Kops had represented allegedly vaccine-damaged plaintiffs in litigation against the US Government and vaccine manufacturers. He had read and heard a lot about manufacturing procedures. And he wasn't impressed. He was particularly irked by statements made by representatives of Lederle, the leading US manufacturer of oral vaccines since 1963, and the sole manufacturer from 1978 until 2000; the company prided itself on the fact that it had distributed 650 million doses of the vaccine in the United States since 1963. At an international conference in early January, 1997, entitled 'Simian

Virus 40: A Possible Human Polyoma Virus Workshop', organised by the US Department of Health and Human Services, and attended by officials from the FDA and the CDC, as well as scientists from around the world, a representative of Lederle had assured the assembly that Lederle's oral polio vaccine was SV40-free, and that their testing had proved it so.[580] Kops knew it wasn't true.

So, three years later, after reading through numerous scientific articles on SV40, Kops blew the whistle amongst the science community, and in the process undoubtedly set a precedent for being the only lawyer to have an article published in a peer-reviewed medical journal.[581] He warned readers of the November/December 2000 edition of *Anticancer Research* that all scientific literature and research on SV40 up until that time had been based on the assumption that SV40 had been removed from all oral polio vaccines since 1963. But he knew that the evidence suggested otherwise. Even though manufacturers were required by law from 25 March 1961, to ensure there were no extraneous microbial contaminants at each stage of the manufacturing process, documents subpoenaed from Lederle during litigation involving its oral polio vaccine failed to reveal that the original Sabin SV40-contaminated poliovirus seeds had been removed from manufacturing procedures, or that procedures for neutralising and testing the vaccine lots cultured from these seeds had been carried out. Tellingly, neither Lederle nor the FDA could produce documented evidence that all the poliovirus seeds were tested and that they all passed the mandated standards.[582]

Kops didn't pull his punches when he testified three years later, in September 2003, before the US House of Representatives Subcommittee on Human Rights and Wellness of the Committee on Government Reform, on the subject of 'The SV40 Virus: Has Tainted Polio Vaccine Caused an Increase in Cancer?'. Coincidentally, the topic was the result of efforts by Michael and Raphaele Horwin to persuade the Chairman of the Committee, Congressman Dan Burton, to investigate the relationship between SV40 and public health.

In his damning testimony Kops reeled off a litany of allegations against Lederle:[583] that it knew that 10 per cent of the green monkeys it used were infected with SV40; that from 1963 until 1980 it cultured the master seeds of two of the three strains of poliovirus on rhesus monkey kidneys, not those of green monkeys; that it knew that 50 to 60 per cent of the rhesus monkeys it used were infected with SV40; that from the 1980 until 2000 it cultured vaccines on monkeys previously used in experiments; and that it had continually failed to follow the mandated requirements for testing its vaccine.

A year earlier, in July 2002, Kops had presented the same issues in a presentation at an Institute of Medicine (IOM) meeting on 'SV40 Contamination of Polio Vaccine and Cancer' in Washington, DC. The Institute had been so concerned that the regulatory agency, the FDA, had made no response to Kop's allegations that its report in October of that year stated: 'The committee urges that the FDA or other agencies address these claims to try to resolve the uncertainty regarding the possibility of exposure to SV40 after 1963.'[584]

And the response of the FDA to the IOM's request? Deathly silence.

But Lederle was not the only drug company to have made an SV40-contaminated polio vaccine. An international team of scientists had undertaken the task of testing the quality of 13 oral vaccines manufactured around the world. Alarmingly, they found that a major eastern European manufacturer had made an SV40-contaminated vaccine from the early 1960s until about 1978, and had distributed it not only to eastern Europe and the USSR, but also to Africa and Asia.[585]

The big question arising from this is, could the simian virus 40 be transmitted via SV40-contaminated oral polio vaccine? The answer had arrived in 1962, when two American researchers discovered that SV40, as with the poliovirus, could be found in the faeces of recipients of the oral vaccine for up to five weeks after taking the vaccine.[586] The faecal-oral route could account for any contagion.

Meanwhile, Herbert Ratner, the public health official who had been a fierce critic of the polio vaccination programme, re-entered the scene. He had retrieved some old vials of Salk vaccine from 1955 that he had kept in his refrigerator, and he presented them to Michele Carbone and his fellow scientists to run some tests. What they found was alarming. There was not just one strain of SV40 virus, but two: the second was much slower growing and hence would have escaped detection by the mandated protocols.[587] They would have needed at least 21 days culture, not 14 days as was the mandated safety protocol, to have been detected. And what was even more alarming was that the original flawed testing protocols were the only safety tests required right up until 2000. The more sophisticated PCR tests had never been made a requirement.

Notwithstanding all this evidence, the courtiers of the US Public Health Service, from its regional castles to the grand palace in Atlanta, Georgia, could not, and would not, accept any of it. They quibbled about the reliability of the PCR tests, and, in particular, they refused to accept any connection between SV40 and cancer. However, they did at least accept that SV40 came from contaminated polio vaccines.

Thus in 2004, the National Cancer Institute, citing two studies that had shown that antibodies to SV40 were no higher in people with non-Hodgkin's lymphoma than in controls, stated: 'Studies investigating the possible connection between SV40 and human cancer have been inconclusive.'[588]

To state otherwise would have meant admitting to a hideous error. And worse, at least for the courtiers, it would have undermined the whole vaccination programme that purported to prevent disease, not cause it. And so they fell back on the old political ploy of casting doubt about an inconvenient truth. It had been used before, and it would be used again later.

The Legacy

Imagine this: You're in charge of assessing the safety of medicines for children. You're presented with a list of recipes that the manufacturer claims will prevent a variety of infectious diseases when injected into children's bodies. You find that each one contains a veritable cocktail of chemicals, so you check the material safety data sheets on each. Unfortunately, there is virtually no information about the long-term, low-dose toxicity of any ingredient. But material safety data sheets and other toxicological data do list the acute, higher-dose toxicity of each: formalehyde, mercury and aluminium compounds (although thiomersal, an ethyl mercury preservative, was supposedly removed from most vaccines, it is still present in both the infant and adult influenza vaccines),[589] sulphate and phosphate compounds, phenol, 2-phenoxyethanol, borax, glutaraldehyde, polysorbate 20/80, polyethylene 9–10 nonyl phenol, sorbitol, aspartame, beta-propiolactone, benzethonium chloride, monosodium glutamate (MSG), and so on. In fact, there are about 40 chemical compounds you need to check off.

You find that many of the ingredients, at least in high doses, are neurotoxic, mutagenic or carcinogenic; some are toxic to the gastrointestinal system, the respiratory system, the reproductive system, the cardiovascular system, the blood and the liver; and others interfere with a child's development. Unfortunately, you have no information whatsoever about the synergistic effects of all these chemicals together, about how they interact.

Next, you assess the safety of injecting into a child the various antifungal and antibiotic agents, antioxidants, amino acids and other culture nutrients. Add to this the foreign proteins and DNA, and possibly micoplasmas and prions, from a host of viruses, bacteria, and animals upon which the medicines have been cultured: organ tissues and blood from monkeys, cow hearts, calf serum, chicken embryos and eggs, duck eggs, pig blood, sheep blood, horse blood, dog kidneys, rabbit brains, and aborted human foetuses; large foreign proteins from egg albumen, casein (milk protein); and gelatin from calves, cattle skins, de-mineralised cattle bones, or pork skin.

The manufacturer has run some short-term tests on various animals, as well as on healthy human adult volunteers. Curiously, the manufacturer hasn't bothered to evaluate whether or not the proposed vaccine has the potential to cause cancer, genetic mutations or infertility (see Chapter 3, 'Clinical tests'). The limited tests reveal that there were no adverse effects; and that antibodies to the infectious germs were produced.

Now it's decision time. What do you do, particularly knowing that children as young as two months of age will be injected with them (in fact, for Hepatitis B shots, at birth)? And that a child will receive over 60 doses of combinations of these substances. Do you approve them, as our medical courtiers have done?

Or do you refuse, knowing that the US Vaccine Adverse Events Reporting System (VAERS), part of an agency established in 1986 to compensate American victims of vaccines, receives approximately 11,000–12,000 reports of adverse reactions to vaccines every year, of which about 15 per cent prove to be serious—meaning they require hospitalisation, are life-threatening, lead to permanent disability or are fatal—and that from 100 to 200 people die.[590] And that's only the tip of the iceberg, because the CDC and the FDA estimate that only 1 to 10 per cent of reactions are reported.[591,592]

And if you did approve the vaccines, how do you think you'd feel when you realised they were being linked to some of the following diseases and syndromes?: convulsions and seizures; sudden infant death syndrome (SIDS or cot death); developmental problems, attention deficit/hyperactivity disorder, and social violence; epilepsy, paralysis, cerebral palsy, mental retardation, autism and other neurological disorders; allergies, asthma, and anaphylaxis; leukaemia, lymphoma, brain tumours, and other cancers; Crohn's disease, multiple sclerosis, Guillain-Barré syndrome, amyotrophic lateral sclerosis (Lou Gerig's disease), systemic lupus erythematosus, Type I diabetes, and other autoimmune diseases.[23,589,593–596] And that's just to name a few.

How would you feel knowing you contributed to the 'approved vaccines'? You'd probably go into denial, which is a normal human defence mechanism to shocking news. So is anger. Perhaps you'd muddy the waters by setting up experiments to prove you were right all along. Maybe you'd even disparage or demote those who dared to break ranks. So imagine how doctors must feel, knowing that they may have done far more harm than good, particularly to their youngest patients.

On top of that, how would you deal with the knowledge that a child with a compromised immune system should never be vaccinated? And yet, according to the Medical Advisory Committee of the Immune Deficiency Foundation, in Towson, Maryland, most immune deficiencies cannot be diagnosed until a child is one year old.[597] The insanity of vaccinating children before they are one is obvious.

The charade, the subterfuge and the propaganda

The courtiers, of course, went far further than denial, or denigrating and demoting whistle-blowers and renegade scientists. They used every trick in the book. In summing up the charade, the subterfuge and the propaganda employed, Paul King and Gary Goldman, two American research scientists writing in *Medical Veritas*, a journal that seeks the truth in medical science, said it perfectly: 'The propaganda dispensed by Public health care and vaccine apologists is, at best, a weak attempt to rationalize the healthcare establishment's positions using all the tools of doublespeak or, as George Orwell called it in his book *1984*, "newspeak", to: (a) mislead, (b) distort reality, (c) pretend to communicate, (d) make the bad seem good, (e) avoid and/or shift responsibility, (f) make the negative appear positive, (g) create a false verbal map of the world, and (h) create dissonance between reality and what their narrative said or did not say.'[595]

And these researchers continue, detailing the subterfuge employed: 'Such propaganda often relies on half-truths and/or superficially logical, but foundationally flawed, phrasing. However, this propaganda is fundamentally flawed and based on pseudo-science or non-reviewable statistical studies of medical records, where, contrary to ethical science, the study design, data selection/rejection criteria, exact approach used to evaluate the data, and/or the original data itself are kept confidential making independent evaluation/verification of the published findings impossible.'[595]

But cancer registries don't lie. In the United States, for instance, the incidence of childhood cancer has continued to rise since the 1930s, as it has in other developed countries.[596,605–606] Between 1935 and 1979, in the state of Connecticut, for instance, there was a three-fold increase in the incidence of cancer in the under-five-year-olds.[598] Other age groups fared little better. Particularly significant in the under-fives was a rise in the incidence of neuroblastoma, a tumour of the central nervous system. And neuroblastomas are linked to SV40 from polio vaccines.[607]

Meanwhile, in the state of Minnesota, cancer incidence in under-15-year-olds increased by 1 per cent each year from 1970 to 1989.[603] The greatest increase was in tumours of the central nervous system, which increased by 2.7 per cent each year. During the same time period, the national incidence of osteosarcoma (bone cancer), astrocytoma (a form of brain cancer), and rhabdomyosarcoma (soft tissue cancer) in the under-15s increased by 2 per cent per annum.[601] These cancers have also been linked to SV40 from polio vaccines.[560,567,568,608] The greatest rise was in children under three. And for children in their first year of life, the greatest increase was in cases of neuroblastoma and retinoblastoma (cancer of the eye's retina), both of which are linked to SV40.[607,609]

Tellingly, the abrupt rise in childhood leukaemia, cancers of the central nervous system, and infant neuroblastomas, began in the mid-1980s, soon after the MMR vaccine had been added to the medical armamentarium.[605,606]

In Australia—a nation that has played deputy dog to the United States in many things since World War II, including using the same FDA-approved medicines—the national incidence of childhood cancer during the 1980s was 34 per cent higher than in the United Kingdom.[610]

The medical courtiers have no answers to what has caused the rise in childhood cancer, but they contend that it's definitely not vaccines.

The incidence of autism shows the same rising trend. First identified in the 1940s, it has continued to rise ever since the advent of mass childhood vaccination programmes. During the 1960s, it was estimated that 1 in every 2,000 children had the condition.[611,612] By the mid-1970s it was 1 in 250 children.[613,614] Today, autism affects 1 in every 150 US children, and 1 in 160 Australian children.[615,616] If the less severe forms of autism, such as Asperger's Syndrome, are included in what is now called the Autistic Spectrum, then about 1 in 100 children are affected.

The medical courtiers have no answers to what causes autism. But they claim that it's definitely not vaccines.

Whistle-blowers

Despite the courtiers' propaganda, many people with autistic children, as well as many members of the medical profession, are unconvinced.[589,595,596,617] A case in point is that of Dr Jon Poling, a neurologist from Athens in the US state of Georgia, whose daughter Hannah developed regressive autism soon after receiving a series of vaccines in 2002 at the age of 18 months. Medical professionals eventually conceded that vaccinations had caused Hannah's regressive autism. As a result, the US Department of Health and Human Services eventually paid compensation to the family. The message from the US Government was clear: for the first time it had conceded that children can develop regressive autism following vaccinations.

As Dr Jon Poling and his wife Terry wrote in the *New York Times* in April 2008, in response to misstatements made in a previous letter to the newspaper by Paul A. Offit, Chief of Infectious Diseases at the Children's Hospital of Philadelphia, Professor of Pediatrics at the University of Pennsylvania School of Medicine, and chief US propagandist for vaccinations:[619] 'Our daughter, Hannah, developed normally until receiving nine vaccines at once. She immediately developed a fever and encephalopathy, deteriorating into what was diagnosed, based on the Diagnostic and Statistical Manual of Mental Disorders, or D.S.M. IV, as autism.'[596]

In response to Offit's claim that a pre-existing medical condition contributed to Hannah Poling's autism[618]—and definitely not vaccines—the Polings continued: 'Dr Offit's assertion that "even five vaccines at once would not place an unusually high burden on a child's immune system" is theory and risky practice for a toddler's developing brain. No one knows if Hannah's mitochondrial dysfunction existed before receiving vaccines. Dr Offit's claim that Hannah had "already weakened cells" is unfounded.'[596]

Ever the vaccine propagandist, Dr Offit repeated his inaccurate statements in a May 2008 edition of *The New England Journal of Medicine*.[619] To alert medical professionals to the issues, and to correct Offit publicly for the second time, Dr Poling wrote a letter to the same journal, published three months later.[620]

Not once have the courtiers at the CDC, FDA, NIH, the American Medical Association, or the American Academy of Pediatrics thought to compare the data on the prevalence of autism, let alone any other medical condition, in vaccinated and non-vaccinated children.

Given that the American Academy of Pediatrics admits that 1 in 6 American children are diagnosed with a developmental and/or behavioural problem, it may well be that more than 20 per cent of American children have some vaccine-induced deficit.[621] No wonder the courtiers would prefer to muddy the waters than investigate the issues.

But evidence for harm is emerging. A recent Canadian study, for example, examined the prevalence of asthma in more than 11,500 children in Manitoba.[622] Those children whose first shot of the DPT vaccine had been delayed by at least two months had half the risk of developing asthma than those who had their first shot at the recommended two-months-of-age. And delaying all three DPT shots by more than two months reduced the risk of having life-long asthma by 60 per cent.

Conversely, some vaccines administered two months after a child is born seem to be more dangerous than if given at birth. J. Barthelow Classen, a former researcher at the US National Institutes of Health, and founder and CEO of

Classen Immunotherapies in Baltimore, Maryland, found that vaccinating a baby with Hepatitis B shots at birth—supposedly for newborn 'prostitutes and intravenous drug users'—is far less likely to result in insulin-dependent diabetes than starting at least three or more weeks after birth.[623–625] And the Haemophilus influenza type b (Hib) vaccine seems to do the exactly the same.[626] Of course, the more shots a child receives, the greater the risk of developing juvenile diabetes.

Thus, when medical courtiers in New Zealand undertook an intensive campaign in 1988 to inoculate children at six weeks of age with the Hepatitis B vaccine, the incidence of Type I diabetes increased by 60 per cent during the following three years.[627] And Finland's incidence of juvenile diabetes increased 147 per cent in the under-five-year-olds after three new vaccines were introduced during the 1970s; and, during the 1980s, when the MMR and Hib vaccines were introduced, the incidence in the 5- to 9-year-olds increased by 40 per cent.[623]

Since 1985, sharp rises of early onset diabetes have also been recorded in the under-fives in both the United States and Britain—the incidence in Britain soaring by 11 per cent each year between 1985 and 1995.[628,629] And the rising incidence corresponded with the advent of the Hib and HBV (Hepatitis B virus) vaccines.

The courtiers had of course added another line to former US Secretary of Defense, Donald Rumsfeld's immortal lines on knowing and not knowing. Theirs is: 'There are some things we know we don't want to know.' But some physicians did get to know what the courtiers preferred they didn't know.

During the late 1960s, the impact of vaccines, and particularly the DPT vaccine, on Aboriginal health had prompted two prominent members of Australia's medical profession to break ranks. At the time, Archie Kalokerinos had just become Medical Superintendent of Collarenebri Hospital, in rural New South Wales, 840 kilometers (500 miles) north-west of Sydney. He was a firm supporter of vaccines. But he was appalled to find an extraordinarily high rate of infant mortality among Aboriginal babies.[630] He soon came to realise that many Aboriginal infants became ill after receiving routine vaccines. Some became extremely ill, and many died. In some Aboriginal communities every second baby died after being vaccinated. Hence the title of his book, *Every Second Child*.[631]

He noted that illness or death was more likely to occur in infants who were ill at the time of receiving a vaccine, or in infants who had recently been ill, or in those who were incubating an infection (and there is no way that physicians can clinically detect disease in its incubation period). But by giving babies an intramuscular or intravenous injection of a high dose of vitamin C, he could reverse the reaction and lives would be saved.

This wonderful news about preventing sudden infant death syndrome, or SIDS, was greeted with extreme hostility by Australia's medical courtiers. But as Kalokerinos explains, 'This forced me to look into the question of vaccination further, and the further I looked into it the more shocked I became. I found that the whole vaccine business was indeed a gigantic hoax. Most doctors are convinced that they are useful, but if you look at the proper statistics and study the instance of these diseases you will realise that this is not so.'[632]

Then in 1969 the Australasian College of Biomedical Science appointed Melbourne pathologist Glen Dettman to head a research team to investigate the claims made by Archie Kalokerinos, that children were dying because of subclinical scurvy (vitamin C deficiency) brought on by impoverished diets and infections, and by the added burden of vaccines. Indeed, viral infections alone have been shown to reduce vitamin C levels by 50 per cent.[633] Vaccines, Kalokerinos reasoned, were simply an affront to their already weakened immune systems.

Dettman was soon convinced of the veracity of Kalokerinos's findings, and joined forces with him, publishing articles on the myth that vaccines conquered various diseases, and trying to convince the courtiers of the dangers of vaccinating sick children.[25,634–637] But their efforts were all in vain, for the medical courtiers clung to the opposite belief: that sick children must be vaccinated to protect them.

Nevertheless, through their efforts the Aboriginal infant mortality rate in Kalokerino's health district dropped to zero.

Then, as chance would have it, a politician, one of Kalokerinos's ex-patients, asked him to investigate why the Aboriginal infant death rate in the Northern Territory had suddenly doubled in 1975, and was set to double again by the following year. There was no obvious explanation. Then Kalokerinos was stuck by an epiphany: to improve Aboriginal health, the authorities had stepped up their vaccination campaign. In other words they were vaccinating sick children. He went off to investigate. What he witnessed horrified him. Health authorities had stormed into Aboriginal communities, rounding up children even though their mothers may have refused permission for their children to be vaccinated, even chasing fleeing children on foot or in Land Rovers and then forcibly vaccinating them. A few weeks later, the vaccination merry-go-round would begin again as the children were forcibly given booster shots. As Kalokerinos remarked, 'It is a wonder that any kid survived really, not that the death rate had just doubled. It is a wonder that anyone survived.'[632]

Years later, Kalokerinos would state about his experiences: 'Deliberate attempts have been made to allow (Aboriginal) infants under my care to die. The real authorities don't want these infants to live. The real intention on the part of the authorities is genocide.'[638]

Kalokerinos's appraisal of international organisations that promote vaccinations is no less savage: 'My final conclusion after forty years or more in this business is that the unofficial policy of the World Health Organisation and the unofficial policy of "Save the Children's Fund" and almost all those organisations is one of murder and genocide. They want to make it appear as if they are saving these kids, but in actual fact they don't. I am talking of those at the very top. Beneath that level is another level of doctors and health workers, like myself, who don't really understand what they are doing. But I cannot see any other possible explanation, it is murder and it is genocide.'[632]

Because of the overwhelming evidence for harm, many doctors who dare to think have broken ranks. Almost a century ago, Dr Walter R. Hadwen had done just that. He was the physician who had witnessed the devastating effects of the smallpox vaccine upon Britain's population during the late 19th century; the man who had persuaded the townsfolk of Gloucester not to get vaccinated against smallpox during the epidemic of 1895–1896, who watched as the whole child population, only 4 per cent of which was vaccinated, passed through the epidemic unscathed; who recorded that of the 2,000 people who did contract smallpox, two-thirds of them had indeed been vaccinated; and who had identified the culprit—leaking sewers near drinking water pipes.[639]

After winning a legal case of alleged manslaughter brought by the medical courtiers, and before a packed audience in Queen's Hall, London, on Friday 6 February 1925 Hadwen declared: 'I once believed in Jenner; I once believed in Pasteur. I believed in vaccination. I believed in vivisection. But I changed my views as the result of hard thinking.'[640]

The importance of infections

If doctors had done the hard thinking, then they might have come to understand that viral and bacterial infections, even parasitic infections, in childhood are essential for human health.

For example, in *Immunology Today* in an article entitled 'Give us this day our daily germs', two British medical microbiologists, Professor Graham Rook and Laura Brunet, have suggested that our use of vaccinations and antibiotics, our fear of germs, and our obsession with hygiene, are depriving our children of the very germs that play a role in the correct maturation of their immune systems.[641]

In other words, we are born with the hardware of an immune system that is primed to deal constantly with environmental germs, but its correct functioning depends on the information fed into its software after birth. But because the fine cytokine balance and fine-tuning of T-cell regulation have never been kick-started by persistent exposure to viruses, bacteria and parasites, our immune systems have never learned to switch off. This 'hygiene hypothesis of atopy' (allergy), the two medical microbiologists contend, may explain the soaring prevalence of asthma, allergies and autoimmune diseases throughout the developed world.

Though the importance of acute illnesses for human health, and their treatment, will be dealt with in Volume 2, suffice it to say here that there is overwhelming evidence that children from farming communities, where they are exposed to farmyard germs; from Rudolf Steiner schools, where treatment with vaccines, antibiotics, and antipyretics (drugs that reduce fever) is discouraged; from large families, and those from small families who go to playschool during their first year of life, and hence are exposed to numerous germs from other children; that all these children have far less eczema, hayfever and asthma, than other children.[642–645]

And there is clear evidence that girls who catch mumps early in childhood are far less likely to develop ovarian cancer later in life.[646–649]

Measles alone, according to many studies, prevents or reduces the tendency to develop skin allergies and sensitivity to house dust mites, hayfever and asthma, malaria in tropical climes, autoimmune diseases, various degenerative diseases of the bones, juvenile rheumatoid arthritis (Still's disease), various tumours, psoriasis, Parkinson's disease, and even epilepsy.[650–666]

Children exposed to the tuberculosis bacillus or Hepatitis A virus earlier in their lives also have less asthma and allergies than other children.[667,668] The same applies to those who are infected with parasitic worms (helminths: tape worm, fluke worms and nematodes)[669] British researchers suspect that hookworms, caught only through walking barefoot on contaminated soil, may help people overcome Crohn's disease (an intestinal autoimmune disease).[670] Indeed, Japanese researchers have found that intractable epileptic seizures disappear within two weeks after a child has had not only measles but also mumps, rotavirus colitis, or exanthema subitum (roseola rash).[671]

In other words, being healthy, but nevertheless being exposed to unhygienic living conditions early in life, is evidently a recipe for health. And the earlier the exposure to germs, the better.

Moreover, catching a cold, or the flu, or some other viral infections, may prevent cancer and even destroy cancer cells.[672–6]

According to a group of researchers at the University of Newcastle, in New South Wales, Australia, a wild-type, common cold-producing virus, Coxsackievirus A21, has powerful anti-tumour activity against malignant melanomas, multiple myeloma, prostate cancer and breast cancer.[672–676] And the ECHO virus (an intestinal infection that although potentially life threatening in babies, usually produces minimal symptoms in adults) apparently targets and destroys human ovarian cancer cells.[677]

Groups of American and Canadian researchers have recently found that infection with reovirus (which may elicit no symptoms at all) also destroys cancer cells, in particular breast cancer and prostate cancer cells.[678–681] Scottish and American researchers found that the same applies to the herpes simplex virus.[682,683] And according to researchers in the US and Japan, the flu virus apparently triggers our immune systems to target and kill off cancerous cells;[684–691] as does the human respiratory syncytial virus, and the human cytomegalavirus.[692,693]

Hidden footnotes to the vaccination saga

This investigation of vaccines would not be complete without mention of two diseases, the origins of which still lurk in the shadows: AIDS and the Gulf War Syndrome.

AIDS

Seven years and a day after the WHO proclaimed that it had wiped smallpox from the face of the Earth, *The Times* of London ran a front page story stating that the epidemic of AIDS sweeping through Central Africa may have been triggered by the WHO's final assault on the smallpox virus.[694] Using a 'modified version' of the vaccine, the WHO had inoculated nearly 100 million people in seven Central Africa states, as well as in Brazil. During the 13-year campaign, which ended in 1980, 14,000 Haitians working for the UN in Zaire had also been inoculated. And in which countries did the AIDS epidemic suddenly appear, as if out of nowhere, in about 1978? In the very countries the WHO had just vaccinated.

As the WHO adviser who tipped off *The Times* stated: 'I thought it was just a coincidence until we studied the latest findings about the reactions which can be caused by Vaccinia [the cowpox virus]. Now I believe the smallpox vaccine theory is the explanation for the explosion of AIDS.'

Furthermore, *The Times* reported that according to the Walter Reed Army Medical Center in Washington, DC, a previously healthy 19-year-old US Army recruit, who had received the vaccine during routine 'immunisations' against possible biological warfare agents, had also contracted AIDS, and soon thereafter had died.

But the American media remained stony silent, proving that politics, not newsworthiness, was at play.

To allay fears and dumb-down the public, the medical courtiers had contrived the following racist fantasy: HIV/AIDS had been transmitted through a bite from a jungle-dwelling African green monkey to some person in Central Africa.[695] That person's body had transformed the green monkey simian immunodeficiency virus (SIV)—which incidentally was also present in the polio vaccine—into human immunodeficiency virus (HIV), and then that person had transmitted the new virus through sexual intercourse (homosexual or heterosexual) to another person, and so on. And because African males are a promiscuous lot, the infection had rapidly spread through rural communities into city dwellers, and then exploded into such plague proportions that to date 15 million Africans have died of AIDS and about 25 million are infected with HIV.[696]

Some courtiers had come up with variations on the mode of transmission. They included such racist hypotheses as contracting the disease through sex with a green monkey; parents allowing their children to play with dead monkeys as toys, and hence becoming infected; or adults inoculating themselves with monkey blood around their pubic region and thighs to induce sexual fervour.[697,698]

During the 1990s, the courtiers decided to change the hypothesised animal vector from a green monkey to a chimpanzee. But in their scurry to announce such fantasies, the courtiers never thought to investigate whether AIDS was rife amongst the very people who hunt monkeys and chimpanzees, the Pygmies. In fact, AIDS is notable for its absence amongst these people.[699] Moreover, the virus thought to be the culprit, SIV, was found to have no effect whatsoever on green monkeys, nor did it genetically resemble HIV.[700,701]

The courtiers couldn't even agree on when AIDS first arose. Some thought it was during the 1930s, some claimed it emerged during the late 1950s, and Jonas Salk contended that it arose in Africa 900 years ago—which begs the question:

given that African peoples have always travelled the world, and that at least 100 million had been forcibly transported as slaves to the New World, why wasn't the rest of the world affected with AIDS long ago?

The courtiers have an even more fantastical explanation for how AIDS suddenly erupted throughout gay communities in the United States. The story goes like this: Some of the 14,000 Haitian men who had been working in Africa when the disease erupted there had carried the virus back to their home country, and then transmitted it to American homosexual and bisexual men who frequented the island for sex. The gay American holiday makers had, in turn, taken the virus back to the United States. And because they, too, are a promiscuous lot, had rapidly spread it amongst gay communities.

Come hell or high water, the courtiers could not afford to have the public discover that AIDS in the US had been caused by a vaccine trial approved by the National Institutes of Health. The trial of a new Hepatitis B vaccine had been conducted by Professor Wolf Szmuness, an epidemiologist from the Columbia University School of Public Health and New York City's Blood Center. In 1978, he had selected over 1,000 healthy, young, highly promiscuous, homosexual and bisexual men from New York City, and had inoculated them with the vaccine. A year later he had vaccinated another 3,400 gay men from New York City. Then in 1980, he selected similar cohorts of thousands of gay men from the cities of San Francisco, Los Angeles, Chicago, St Louis, and Denver and inoculated them.

The first hint that something was amiss had become apparent by March 1981. Amongst young gay men in New York City there had been at least eight cases of a rare form of cancer, Kaposi's sarcoma, and it was far more aggressive than was typical.[702] About the same time, researchers from the CDC noted that cases of both Kaposi's sarcoma and a rare lung infection, *Pneumocystis carinii* pneumonia, were coming to light amongst the gay communities of New York and California.[703,704] What researchers were looking at were the first cases of people with AIDS.

CDC investigators noted that 6 of the first 10 cases of AIDS in San Francisco were part of the 6,800 gay men who participated in Szmuness's Hepatitis B trial.[705] Taking a representative sample of the trial cohort, they found that HIV infection had risen from just over 4 per cent of the group during the period 1978 to 1980, to 67 per cent in 1984, and 73 per cent by 1985. Clearly most had been infected by the hepatitis vaccine. Of the 31 members of the representative sample, 10 had developed AIDS or AIDS-related conditions by 1981. And of the whole cohort of human experimental guinea pigs, 166 of them had AIDS by 1984. By 1985, the number had increased to 262.

As for the 4,400 gay men who participated in Szmuness's Hepatitis B trial in New York City, five years later 48 per cent of them were infected with HIV.[706]

Meanwhile, other CDC investigators had noted outbreaks of AIDS in the same cities in which Szmuness trialled the Hepatitis B vaccine. In fact, the CDC acknowledged that those cities accounted for 80 per cent of all AIDS cases in the United States.[707] In New York City and San Francisco alone, the number of AIDS cases per million was 10 times higher than that for the entire nation.

This marked the beginning of America's AIDS epidemic. Seventeen years after the trials in New York and San Francisco, 57 per cent of the gay men who had received the Hepatitis B shots were dead: 95 per cent of them from AIDS.[708]

Contrary to the courtiers' racist propaganda that AIDS came out of Africa,[709] it is clear that AIDS emerged from American laboratories that manufactured the lethal Hepatitis B vaccine, and from laboratories that supplied the smallpox vaccine to the WHO Smallpox Eradication Programme in Central Africa.

Was HIV deliberately or accidentally made? Many Black Americans believe it's the former. In a survey conducted in 1990, 35 per cent of Black American church members believed AIDS is a form of genocide; 1 in 10 believed HIV was deliberately created to infect black people, and an additional 2 out of 10 thought it might be so.[710]

Black Americans certainly had good reason to suspect sinister motives on the part of the US Government. Since the 1930s, the US Government and its agencies had conducted many experiments on its unsuspecting citizens. For example, the US Public Health Service had conducted a 40-year experiment on poor, illiterate, syphilis-infected, black sharecroppers in Tuskagee, Alabama.[711] Government researchers had withheld medication for, and knowledge about, the men's medical condition, all in the name of investigating how syphilis impacted on the men and their families.

Black Americans may have also noted that the prevalence of AIDS in the United States, which during the 1980s was a disease primarily of white, gay men, had by 2008 become a disease primarily of minority groups, the virus's prevalence being particularly high in women and children of Black, Hispanic , and Native American ethnicity.[710] According to two British investigative journalists, these ethnic groups have twice the rate of HIV infections compared with American Whites, and account for 80 per cent of children and 90 per cent of infants with AIDs.[712]

Moreover, the number of sub-Saharan Africans living with HIV/AIDS accounts for two-thirds of all cases in the world today.[713] As a New York Department of Health official had forewarned the *New York Times* in April 1992, 'AIDs in future generations may be primarily a disease of black people.'[710]

Some researchers suspect sinister motives lie behind the creation of the virus. In their books, *The Extremely Unfortunate Skull Valley Incident*, and *AIDS: The Crime Beyond Belief*, Donald W. Scott—editor of *The Journal of Degenerative Diseases*, co-founder of the Common Cause Medical Research Foundation in Ontario, Canada, and Adjunct Professor at the Institute for Molecular Medicine at Huntington Beach, California—and his son William have documented many of the government dealings that led up to the release of the HIV.[714,715] Similarly, British investigative journalists Robert Harris and Jeremy Paxman have documented in their book, *A Higher Form of Killing*, the international story of the development of chemical and biological warfare, and its ties to medical research; and have looked particularly at the US Army's objective of developing ethnic weapons.[712] Alan Cantwell, a New

York dermatologist who took a particular interest in the origins of HIV, has written several books on the subject.[716–719] Investigative journalist Harry V. Martin has also revealed evidence that the AIDS virus was tested on expendable people.[720] And Leonard G. Horowitz, an American public health authority, explains in his book, *Emerging Viruses: AIDS and Ebola*, how a small group of virologists working for major military-medical contractors, and under the auspices of the US National Cancer Institute and the WHO, had for years conducted dangerous experiments with viruses that ravage the human immune system.[721]

As long ago as 1966, scientists as esteemed as Australia's Frank Macfarlane Burnet had warned molecular biologists against tampering with life, that there were limits beyond which there were grave dangers.[722] But no one took any notice of such warnings, the reason being that politics, money and egos were at play. Author and editor Jonathon Vankin summed up the situation perfectly: 'Public comprehension of science is scant, depending entirely on third-party interpreters, "experts" who have agendas of their own. Not only is general scientific knowledge therefore minimal, more importantly few people understand how science works. We think we're getting objective truth when what we're seeing is a political acerbically personal process involving billions of dollars, reputations and egos, and belief systems that censor large slices of fact and theory.'[723]

Thus politics, money and egos, together with a belief system that life is a toy to be played with, was the reason why Dr Donald MacArthur, US Deputy Director of Defense Research and Engineering, requested in 1968 that a US Congress Appropriations Committee fund a research programme into engineering new micro-organisms … and the funds were granted.[724] It is also why a committee at the WHO recommended the following: 'An attempt should be made to ascertain whether viruses can in fact exert selective effects on immune function, e.g. by depressing 7S versus 19S antibody, or by affecting T cell function as opposed to B cell function. The possibility should also be looked into that the immune response to the virus may itself be impaired if the infecting virus damages more or less selectively the cells responding to the viral antigens.'[725] In other words, the World Health Organisation recommended that an AIDS-causing virus be created and tested.

By playing God, the science of molecular biology was certainly toying with potentially catastrophic dangers. Thus, during the 1980s, when scientists began to examine the genetic structure of HIV, they discovered that it was nothing like a monkey virus. Both Robert Strecker, a Californian pathologist, and J. Grote, an AIDS researcher in London stated that the virus appeared to be a recombinant virus, a cross between a sheep and a bovine virus called *bovine visna* virus.[726,727] In a letter to the *Journal of the Royal Society of Medicine*, Dr Grote wrote that the bovine visna virus was a known contaminant of foetal calf serum.[727] Foetal calf serum just happens to be one of the cell cultures used in the manufacture of vaccines. So perhaps the virus was accidentally created through contaminated Hepatitis B vaccines and smallpox vaccines.

Incidentally, Robert Strecker tried to alert the medical profession to his findings, but not one medical journal would publish his evidence. Undeterred, he created a video, *The Strecker Memorandum*, to at least alert the public.[726]

Whether deliberate or accidental, the courtiers could never admit that HIV had been spread by vaccines. To do so would have been to hammer the greatest nail into the coffin of vaccination campaigns.

The Gulf War Syndrome

Nor could the courtiers admit that Gulf War syndrome was caused by an experimental vaccine. In his book, *Vaccine A: The Covert Government Experiment That's Killing Our Soldiers*, investigative journalist Gary Matsumoto unearthed shocking evidence that the US Department of Defense and the British Ministry of Defence approved an experimental vaccine to protect armed forces personnel against anthrax.[728] The justification for using the vaccine was that Saddam Hussein might deploy chemical weapons against coalition forces after the UN decision had been made to drive Iraqi forces out of Kuwait, which Iraq had invaded and annexed on August 2, 1990.

Time was of the essence, and the licensed vaccines took up to eight months to produce 'immunity' to anthrax.[729] The defence establishments in the United States and Britain needed a vaccine that worked quickly. So US military doctors added an unlicensed adjuvant (a chemical that stimulates the body to produce antibodies) to the vaccine. This adjuvant was squalene, an oil-based substance found in olive oil. When squalene is injected into the bloodstream it had been shown in peer-reviewed scientific literature to be capable of causing incurable, if not fatal, diseases.[730]

By the time the United Nations sanctioned a coalition of military forces from 34 nations to drive Hussein's troops out of Kuwait, 41 per cent of US combat soldiers and 57–75 per cent of UK combat soldiers had been inoculated against anthrax, though not all with the experimental vaccine.[731]

About a year after hostilities ended, reports began to emerge about a strange malady that afflicted many military veterans from America, Britain, Australia and Canada.[732] Symptoms included chronic fatigue, dizziness and headaches, loss of balance, short-term memory loss, muscle and joint pains, shortness of breath, skin rashes, diarrhoea, dyspepsia and indigestion, weight loss, hair loss, sore gums, fibromyalgia, terminal tumours, and a host of autoimmune diseases including multiple sclerosis, systemic lupus erythematosus, amyotrophic lateral sclerosis (Lou Gerig's disease), Guillain-Barré syndrome, inflammatory arthritis, endocarditis, thyroiditis, polyarteritis nodosa, and collagen vascular disease.

The victorious coalition forces suffered only 190 combat deaths and, sadly, 379 deaths by accidents or 'friendly' fire; the US suffered only 148 combat deaths, though a quarter of these were by 'friendly' fire.[733] But however successful the armed conflict had been in its strategic aims and limited loss of life, the aftermath was horrendous. Of the 700,000 American servicemen and women who participated in the war, over a third of them (183,000) have been declared permanently disabled by the US Department of Veteran Affairs.[731]

Moreover, according to a US survey, Gulf War veterans are at least twice as likely to have children with birth defects compared to veterans who were never deployed to the Gulf, and who therefore never received the anthrax vaccine.[734] Of course, the courtiers could never accept that a vaccine caused such human misery. They blamed the syndrome on denatured uranium, on a US Army engineering battalion inadvertently releasing a plume of nerve agent from an Iraqi chemical munitions stockpile at Khamisiyah, on the extensive use of pesticides by English-speaking troops, and even on the stresses of war.[735]

The courtiers were clearly clutching at straws, for they'd overlooked the fact that many army personnel who had never departed their home shores were also suffering from the syndrome. Moreover, soldiers from most countries in the anti-Iraq coalition did not suffer from the malady, nor did Arab soldiers or civilians on either side of the conflict, nor did any journalist, 'embedded' or not, get sick.[732]

The generals and officials at the US Department of Defense even hid from Congress and public scrutiny the fact that by continuing to use the vaccine, long after the First Gulf War, over 20,000 military personnel between 1998 and 2000 had been hospitalised immediately after receiving the squalene-containing anthrax vaccine.[736] According to *The Newport Daily News* in Virginia, military officials misled Congress and the public by claiming that fewer than 100 people had been hospitalised or become seriously ill after receiving the shot; and they failed to report three cases of amyotrophic lateral sclerosis.[736]

Though researchers at Tulane University had repeatedly identified antibodies to squalene in military personnel who were suffering from symptoms of Gulf War syndrome,[737] and even though those same researchers had later found that 47 per cent of military recipients inoculated after 1997 with the anthrax vaccine had antibodies to squalene—squalene is still present in the anthrax vaccine, as well as many influenza vaccines—and that recipients of other vaccines had no antibodies whatsoever to squalene,[738] the US Department of Defense, in 2009, proudly published a study that claimed it had found no relationship between squalene antibodies and symptoms. The Defense Department researchers concluded: 'We found no association between squalene antibody and chronic multisystem disease. The etiology of Gulf War syndrome remains unknown, but should not include squalene antibody status.'[739] This is an abstruse way of saying, 'Let's drown the subject.'

Perhaps the wisest words, and most prescient, on the dangers of vaccines had been uttered by Nicholas Wade, a British-born science reporter, who is now an author of several books, and writes for the 'Science Times' section of the *New York Times*. In an article entitled 'The boat that never rocks', published in *Science* magazine in 1972, he wrote: 'There can be few graver opportunities for man-made disaster than the mass immunization campaigns that are now routine in many countries.'[740]

PART TWO

BLINKERED SCIENCE AND THE VITAL FORCE

Chapter 6

How Do We Know?

> *Our scientific power has outrun our spiritual power.*
> *We have guided missiles and misguided men.*
> Dr Martin Luther King Jr, American clergyman and civil rights activist
> (1929–1968).

Where are we going?—A summary

Throughout Part One we have examined the popular spin that our collective health has never been better. And we found that despite the band-aid solution it has never been worse. We also identified the harm modern medicine is inflicting on untold numbers of people—the collateral damage from the war on disease—and some of the reasons for it.

Now it's time to get down to the root of the problem; to fathom out the reason why modern medicine is failing to halt the onslaught of modern diseases. As we've seen, our culture not only conveniently ignores the root cause of poverty, drug-taking, crime, terror and everything else it wages war on, it also has a blind spot for the root cause of disease. Needless to say, it's also clueless to the root cause of health.

Here in Part Two, we'll first examine the philosophical roots of our modern mindset about life, the universe, and everything, including health and disease. Then we'll identify what medical science deleted from the equation: the vital force (see Chapters 8, 9, and 10). Indeed Western culture is the only culture that has no vitalistic approach to life, health and disease. Next we'll add the vital force back into the equation and revisit health and disease (see Chapter 11). And finally, in Part Three, we'll identify the root cause of modern diseases: many of our technologies and our disconnected lifestyles.

Science

Our beliefs about the world and life in general, and about health and disease in particular, have been powerfully shaped by modern science. Our culture prides itself on being scientific, and even refers to our time as the 'Scientific Age'. Thanks to the discoveries of science we have created our technological world and our chemical armouries in the fight against disease. And when push comes to shove, science is considered by most people to be the final arbiter of truth. Until something is 'scientifically proven' it's only 'anecdotal': someone's story.

The proof of the efficacy and safety of traditional medicines, for example, is considered to be established only through scientific research. Traditional usage is considered to be insufficient evidence; it's only someone's story, not objective fact. Hence, traditional knowledge is considered inferior to scientific validation and is not to be trusted. Traditional insights into the workings of our minds are also dismissed in favour of the revelations from the pseudoscientific disciplines of psychology and psychiatry and the science of neurology. When scientific evidence conflicts with traditional knowledge, science inevitably wins.

But what does 'science' mean?

Two modes of consciousness, two kinds of knowledge

The word 'science' derives from the Latin *scire*, to know. Therefore science is the pursuit of knowledge. 'Knowledge', however, has two meanings. One deals with facts and information about things out in the world. The other involves the experiences of the observer—experiences that may include intuition or gut instincts, dreams, aches and pains, and the whole gamut of human emotion and consciousness, as well as sensory experience.

For the past 2,500 years, the Western approach to knowledge has been fixed on one aspect of knowledge: the intellectual pursuit of finding the truth about things, about defining reality, about asking the 'what' and the 'why' of things. As Aristotle had once written in reference to his country folk, '… men do not think they know a thing till they have grasped the "why" of it'.[1]

Incidentally, throughout this book we're following in that great Western traditional by asking the 'what' and the 'why' about health and disease. It's not until Volume 2 that Eastern and indigenous peoples' tradition will be incorporated, and the 'how' about improving our health will be presented.

The Western focus on the intellectual aspect of knowledge began with the debates between the Athenian philosophers, Plato and Aristotle.[1-10] They were trying to solve the age-old intellectual problem of 'what' we can know for certain about the world, since there appears to be a gap between appearance and reality, between our awareness of the world and the world itself.

If you doubt there is a gap between appearance and reality, watch how the lines between them are blurred as you cringe during the blood-curdling scenes of a horror film even though you know they're only flickering images on a screen. A more powerful example of the gap is portrayed in the movie *The Matrix*.[11] The characters trapped inside the matrix experience a world of illusions and phantoms, a virtual reality. They believe it is real, and for them it feels real. But the ultimate reality lies outside the matrix.

The gap between appearance and reality is also a central feature in the legal system. In any court proceedings, whether before a jury in a criminal trial to determine the guilt or innocence of a defendant, or before a judge in a civil court to determine the liability of the accused, the judge or jury has to weigh up the hard evidence and the various perspectives presented in the testimonies of witnesses to render an impartial verdict. This requires bridging the gap through deductive reasoning in order to infer the guilt or innocence, or legal liability, of the accused.

Echoes of the gap are also found in the poetry and literature of Europe. In *The Tempest*, for instance, Shakespeare wrote: 'We are such stuff as dreams are made on, and our little life is rounded with a sleep.'[12]

Both Plato and Aristotle believed that our subjective experience of the world, which is gained through our senses, does not equate to the world itself.[1-10] Both accepted that they had to solve the conundrum of the gap between people's experience 'in here' and the world 'out there'. Not until they had resolved the problem could they begin asking why the world works the way it does and thereby start building the foundations for a systematic body of knowledge.

Indian and Chinese sages had also been aware of the apparent gap between appearance and reality.[13,14] Like Plato, they considered the material world, the world of maya, to be images or shadows of an ever-changing cosmos that flicker across our minds. Unlike Plato, however, they denied that there was any permanent or essential nature of things in the world.

For them, all things are continuously flowing and changing and perpetually being transformed. We experience the dynamic and cyclic interplay of these changes as movements between polar forces or opposites. That, by the way, is one of the attributes of the vital force that will be examined in Chapter 9. The Greek philosopher Heraclitus taught that any pair of opposing forces acts as a single unity.[15,16] Chinese philosophers similarly recognised the interplay of these forces that both oppose and complement each other, just as the sunny side of a mountain (yang) soon becomes the shady side (yin), and the next morning becomes the sunny side again, and so on in a never-ending cycle.[14]

Where Plato and Aristotle were obsessed with finding the true nature of things—known to the Greeks as *physis*, from which we derive the word 'physics'—the founders and sages of Buddhism and Taoism, as with the earlier Hindu philosophers, were focused on 'how' we experience the world. Human experience, specifically human consciousness, was their central focus. By claiming that we create our world through our beliefs, they would challenge our commonsense perspective that there is an enormous difference between what we imagine and what is real. Thus they would challenge one of the central tenets of western thinking today: that reality is 'out there'.

The Eastern path therefore led to the other aspect of knowledge: intuitive insight or mystical knowledge, which is implied in the Greek word, *gnosis*, from which we derive the word 'knowledge'. By focusing on human experience they swept aside the apparent gap between appearance and reality that Plato and Aristotle were grappling with. For the Eastern mystics, as with all schools of mysticism, including those of indigenous cultures, there is no split between perceptions and material reality, between material and spiritual realms, between mind and body, between life and death, between animate and inanimate, between 'in here' and 'out there'. For them there is quite simply no dualism. As we'll see later, some of the 20th century quantum physicists came to much the same conclusion.

From the Eastern perspective all things are aspects and manifestations of an ultimate reality. In other words, the divinity or ultimate being of beings pervades everything. In Hindu mythology, for example, the ultimate reality is portrayed as Brahman, the divine actor and magician who becomes the world. And in the end the world becomes Brahman. The divinity is the glue that connects everything, including our experiences, to everything else. The Hindu net of Indra, a garment covered in mirrors, is a marvellous image that exemplifies this idea. Each mirror reflects every other mirror in an endless process of reflections.

Because the Eastern religious philosophies, and indigenous cultures worldwide, took a mystical approach to knowledge there was no need to quest after truth or to storm the gates of heaven. Their focus was, and still is, on experiencing union with the ultimate source of being. Unlike the mainstream of the Judaeo-Christian and Islamic religions, which held that the ultimate source is a personal God who, though He created the world, is outside the world in some transcendent realm, the Eastern and indigenous traditions perceived the ultimate source to pervade everything, to be both immanent and numinous.

Plato's solution to the problem of the gap was not dissimilar to that of Eastern cultures, though his was an intellectual rather than an experiential solution. The problem he and Aristotle both faced was that Greece's Eleatic school of thought had relegated the divinity or Divine Principle to a transcendent realm outside the world of matter, men and gods.[7,8] Plato argued that the ultimate reality can be known through our minds, through awareness, reasoning and intuition.[9,10] He would argue that we intuitively know the archetypal essence of things, of maleness or femaleness, for example, of fear or love, of beauty and ugliness, of good and bad, of time and of space. Our senses, he reasoned, simply fill in the gaps about particular things of the mundane world.

Despite his efforts to resolve the issue by making our minds the link between the transcendent and material realms, Plato simply perpetuated the split between appearance and reality.

Aristotle's solution was to reject any idea of a connection between the non-material, transcendent world and the material world.[2] Instead he opted for the notion of reality residing in the material world 'out there' which can be known through our senses, through observation.

These two Greek philosophers had therefore set Western civilisation on two different paths to knowledge: the Platonic, ideational or rationalist path, which focused on aesthetics, metaphysics, ethics, justice and politics; and the Aristotelian, sensate or empirical path, which led to the exploration of the material world.

The waxing and waning of knowledge

At various times over the past 2,500 years, the Platonic and Aristotelian paths have diverged and converged, narrowed and broadened. The sociologist Pitirim Sorokin noted that when a culture experiences a convergence and a mingling of the two paths it flourishes, not only in its technology but also in its flexibility towards, and its creativity in, all human endeavours.[17,18] Such a culture is distinguished by its idealistic values.

Greece, for example, experienced such a convergence during the 5th and 4th centuries BC. The philosophical, mathematical, medical, architectural and artistic ideas of such geniuses as Aristotle and Plato, Pythagorus, Hippocrates, Pheidias, Euripides and Aeschylus, among others, still impact on our modern civilisation. And, as we'll see, nearly 2,000 years later a similar convergence occurred in Europe and centred on Italy: the Renaissance. Even during the 20th century, there was a similar brief moment of idealistic resurgence among the young people of the counter-culture that arose during the 1960s, as the American psychologist Carl Rogers had noted.[19]

The mingling of the two paths continued to influence Greece, and the Roman Republic; though by the beginning of the Christian era, both paths were rapidly moving apart and each became narrower in perspective. After the collapse of the Roman Empire in the 4th century AD, the ideational, Platonic path suddenly broadened when the Christian Church took the helm.

One of the functions of myths and religion, according to the American scholar of comparative religion, Joseph Campbell, is to help us understand and give meaning to the nature of the world, and to explain why the world is the way it is.[20] Whether enacted through rituals or daily activities, religion also provides a cultural framework, a cosmology, from which we can experience a sense of connection to the world, and a sense of place and even awe in the apparent chaos of the universe. Even the roots of our language reveal this meaning: the word 'religion' derives from the Latin *re-ligare* meaning to 're-connect' or 'tie back'.

The myths of all cultures reveal how important the experience of being connected is to our wellbeing. We are told of the human connection to the air and the sky, to the world of plants and animals, the seasons, day and night, birth and death. Some stories warn us of the dangers of being disconnected, not only from the world and other people, but also from ourselves and from the stages of life's journey.

Religion also has a sociological function, since it provides us with ethical guidelines, and a pedagogical function through teaching us how to live a human life under any circumstance.

But when religion jumps into bed with politics, the upshot is likely to be rigid control of the populace. And that's exactly what happened after the Christian Church came to power in Europe.

For 1,000 years, from the 4th to the 14th centuries AD, truth was dictated by Church dogma. If the Church considered that the ideas and gleanings of the earlier

Greek geniuses clashed with the Church's dogma, the Church won. Fortunately for the Church, though Aristotle had proposed a philosophical approach to investigating the nature of the world, he was far more smitten with contemplating ideas about the human soul and God's perfection.

And so the Church selectively used Aristotle's ideas to perpetuate its stranglehold on knowledge. Its most powerful weapon against the heresy of challenging institutionalised truths was the Inquisition. Galileo Gallilei, for instance, was forced under threat of torture to recant his confirmation of Copernicus's discovery that the sun was the centre of the known universe in favour of the Church's tenet of a geocentric universe. Because the cogs of institutionalised power invariably grind slowly, it was not until 1992, four hundred years later, that the Catholic Church absolved Galileo of heresy.

During this rigid ideational era, medieval scholars followed Aristotle's ideal and Plato's obsession by focusing their attention on the importance of God, on the human soul, and on ethical matters, to understand the purposes underlying natural phenomena. The power to predict and control nature were of lesser concern to them.

Although Italy was the seat of the Church's power, it was also the place where an emerging cultural movement began charging along the sensate path towards the Church's ideational rut—perhaps proving that only in the darkest places do we see the brightest lights. The convergence of these two paths produced the intellectual and artistic flowering of the Renaissance, which culminated in Italy during the 16th century and influenced much of Western Europe. The ideas, works and discoveries of this era's geniuses, from Leonardo Da Vinci to Shakespeare, from Galileo to Descartes, still resonate through our modern culture.

The dream of a certain Descartes

On the 10th of November, 1619, after a night of dreaming, a 23-year-old French soldier and philosopher, René Decartes sent the ball rolling down the sensate, empirical path. Arguably, Plato would have been proud of Descartes, for he had tapped into his inner knowledge through a series of dreams.[21] In the days following his revelation, Descartes set down the philosophical, scientific and mathematical foundations for a new way of thinking about the world that would form the basis for the entire structure of modern Western knowledge.

The starting point of Descartes' new method for discovering the truth about the natural world was to attack his own beliefs with radical doubt.[22] He doubted traditional knowledge; he doubted his own sensory experiences. He even doubted the existence of his body. Finally, after he'd whittled away at his beliefs, he arrived at the one thing he had no doubt about: his thoughts about doubting.

This was encapsulated in his celebrated statement: *cogito ergo sum*, 'I think therefore I am'.[23] Perhaps closer to the mark is *dubito ergo sum*, 'I doubt therefore I am'. Thus the only certainty Descartes admitted to was his mind, his conscious experience, and, with it, his own existence.

But there was something else Descartes had assumed was certain, and that was the existence of God. God, he reasoned, had created the realm of mind, and specifically its reasoning ability, to understand His other creation, the world of matter. Thus with a leap of faith Descartes had bridged the gap. At least, that's what he thought.

And his method for arriving at the truth about natural phenomena? Exactly the same method he had used to discover the certainty of his own existence: to use the human mind to split, to cleave, to pare down and reduce things to their smallest constituent parts. For the mental realm, to analyse complex thoughts and problems; today we'd call this left-brain or analytic thinking: it's the essence of logic. And, for the worldly realm, to reduce it down and examine its smallest bits.

Thus, only by establishing the truth about each of the smallest components of our thoughts and observations, so Descartes reasoned, could we build an argument through deductive reasoning to establish the truth about the whole. And indeed this is the way theories are born.

In other words, Descartes sent modern science down the path of believing that the only way humankind could build up a body of scientific knowledge based upon absolute certainty was to engage in analysis and reductionism, and to have God in the middle.

Life seen through the prism of science

Today, this analytic and reductionist approach permeates the life sciences, though God has been left out of the equation. The fundamental basis of life, according to modern biology, is molecules. The assumption is that all organisms, including human beings, are nothing more than tremendously complex and organised chemical factories. The blueprint for life, so biologists tell us, is to be found in the genetic material that each life-form inherits from its parents. Each organism has its own unique code that commands all the chemical processes that determine its physical make-up, development, growth and reproduction.

But what about the influences of the environment, or psychological processes on our biochemistry or genetic codes? What impact, for that matter, do the chemical processes in one part of our bodies have on the chemistry of other parts of our bodies or, more generally, on our genes? The answer is: no one knows.

Though the brilliance of the reductionist approach to discovering things is that researchers can peer at microscopic bits of our bodies and use specific molecular tools to ask precise questions, that microcosm is also the place of its failing. Put simply, it cannot see the forest for the trees. It doesn't just have a blind spot, it is blind to the whole panorama. Medical researchers cannot watch the whole body operating in its entirety, let alone observe the impact of the sun, the moon, our foods or thoughts on the molecular processes under examination.

As Canadian geneticist David Suzuki noted in reference to the interdependence of molecular and genetic phenomena with other aspects of our bodies: 'Just like the blind men, each of them [researchers] can at once be entirely correct about a piece of the system and mistaken about the appearance of the whole beast'.[24]

Certainly, analysis is a powerful tool when we want to get to the bottom of a problem. I've used it here in this chapter to try and get to the crux of modern medicine's problems. But analysis alone leads only to bits of knowledge. What is also required is synthesis: putting it all back together again to give an overall view. Or, to paraphrase one of the German psychologists who founded the school of Gestalt psychology: the whole is more than merely the sum of its parts.[25]

A slice of Bacon

Modern science is also fixated on experimentation. Indeed this is at the heart of the scientific method. This began with the ideas of the English philosopher Francis Bacon, a contemporary of Descartes. Rather than simply observing nature, as Descartes had espoused, Bacon was obsessed with the idea of manipulating nature in order to understand each facet of it. Then, through inductive reasoning, he argued, we could apply those findings generally to the whole field under investigation.[18,26]

Bacon would have argued, for example, that if a drug is proven to have a safe anti-inflammatory effect on a group of healthy volunteers, then you could generalise, and expect the same would apply to the whole population, including the sick. The problem is, it doesn't mean that at all. Inductive reasoning can never prove certainty.[27] At best, it can suggest a probability that something will occur.

Nevertheless, thanks to Bacon, the age-old duo of 'observation and experience' (sensate and ideational knowledge) was replaced by the lone ranger of 'observation and experiment' (sensate only).

Bacon's fanaticism also changed the direction that science had previously taken. The ancient quest of science had been wisdom, understanding the natural order of things and helping people to live in harmony with nature. This had been evident in the way ancient cultures, including Greece, had integrated science, mathematics, religion and arts into a unified system. Suddenly, a new direction was being charted, one that sought control and domination of nature.

Though echoes of this are to be found in the Bible—in man having dominion over the creatures of the Earth[28]—Bacon set the juggernaut rolling. His legacy is readily apparent today in the manipulation and exploitation of everything on the planet. Its worst manifestations are seen in the rush to genetically manipulate plants and animals and, through patent laws, to own life-forms.

Science's failings

By combining Descartes' reductionist and analytic ideas with Bacon's beliefs about the need for the experimentation with and manipulation of nature, science began to build up an enormous amount of information about parts of the world. Hence the need for specialists.

Today, medical science abounds with specialists, experts who know the minutest details of their chosen component of the human body, but who are oblivious to the multitude of factors that impact on the bits they know so well. And, while General Practice is clamouring to be identified as a 'speciality' on its own, that is more out of a desire to be given more weight amongst the medical fraternity than anything else.

Another of Descartes' ideas, and one that has continued to haunt Western science, is the split between mind and matter, often referred to as dualism. Because the existence of mind was more certain—at least in Descartes' mind—than matter, he concluded that the two were separate and fundamentally different, though both were creations of God.

Descartes' adherence to doubt had clearly lapsed for he had borrowed the Christian idea that only humans had a mind or soul. The human body, animals, plants, and everything else in the material world, so Descartes reasoned, are nothing but machines that work like clocks according to mechanical laws. Though Isaac Newton would later expand on this mechanistic view of things, Descartes believed that everything in nature can be explained in terms of the arrangement and movement of its parts. He even compared a sick man with an ill-made clock, and a healthy man with a well-made clock.[18,29]

Galileo, another contemporary of Descartes, was more enamoured with matter than mind, and so contended that science should study only the essential properties of things—such as shapes, numbers and movement—that could be measured and quantified.[18,30] The subjectively assessed properties of colour, taste, touch, smell and sound were to be excluded from the domain of science.

The emphasis on mathematics, originating from Descartes' ideas, expanded upon by Galileo when he combined scientific experimentation with mathematics, was incorporated by Isaac Newton into a complete mathematical formulation of the mechanistic view of nature, which, despite the findings of quantum physics, is still the basis for other sciences.

Today, God has been left out of the equation, at least for science. Science explains everything, including spiritual and psychological phenomena, in materialistic terms; for the latter, as biochemical processes, nothing more, nothing less. This approach to knowledge can be referred to as materialistic monism.[17]

But in our everyday language, Descartes' mind/body split remains. The co-existence of Cartesian dualism with science's materialistic monism has led to endless confusion about the relationship between mind and brain, and between the roles of priest and psychiatrist, doctor and psychologist. It also caused headaches for the founders of quantum physics who recognised that the observer of atomic phenomena also influences the observations.[31-34]

During the 20th century this trend to dismiss all but the supposedly objective, verifiable, and quantifiable events, has meant that science ignores all subjective human experiences. If you can't measure the size or weight or movement of a thought, then clearly thoughts will be excluded from scientific investigation. Ironically, Descartes' thoughts and dreams, which founded the whole of modern science, are also excluded from the domain of science.

Today the language of science is dominated by numbers, since all physical phenomena have been reduced to exact mathematical relationships. Our health is measured in figures, in lung-function print-outs, in cardiographs and blood assays. Our psyches are measured in terms of quantifiable stimuli and responses. Our lives are measured in long lists of nitrogenous base-pairs that constitute our individual genomes. And the social quality of our lives is measured as digits of GDP (gross domestic product).

But like the dates on a tombstone, these figures ignore what it is to be human. It's the dash or gap in between the birth and the death dates, between the digits, where it all happens, where we live our lives. The things that medical science ignores are the very essence of what it means to be human: thoughts, feelings, motives, intentions, values and ethical sensibilities, relationships, aesthetics, consciousness, soul and spirit.

To compound science's difficulties in getting to the root cause of modern diseases, is its relationship with commerce. Commerce has been the driving force of politics ever since the 1970s, when Western governments became seduced by the ideology of economic rationalism. It's not surprising, therefore, that once science had jumped into bed with commerce, a profit-driven agenda emerged; and that its institutional power would surge by becoming the final arbiter of truth today, just as the Church had been the repository of truth during the Dark Ages.

It's equally unsurprising that disease should become an industry; the cancer industry, for example. And that the focus of medicine should be on treating, rather than preventing, disease, an approach known to traditional Chinese physicians as stem treatment. Maybe this is why medicine has pinned its hopes for cures on stem-cell treatment.

The challenge

Though the materialist paradigm still dominates most sciences, it is being challenged, at least at the theoretical level. The first challenge emerged from the most reductionist of all sciences: physics, in the guise of quantum physics.

As several of the founders of quantum physics—including Neils Bohr, Werner Heisenberg and Julius Oppenheimer—noted, the properties and interactions of subatomic particles, of which all matter is made, prove that the cosmos, including the observer of any aspect of it, is one inseparable reality.[33,35-38] This idea parallels those expressed by mystics of all traditions: that the cosmos is a unified whole, both spiritual and material, that is constantly moving, alive and organic.[35]

Moreover, quantum physics has also revealed that the belief in the certainty of scientific knowledge—which Descartes kick-started, and which still lies at the heart of our current world-view—is an illusion. The Eastern sages would have agreed with quantum physicists that there is no absolute truth in science. All our theories and concepts about how things work are limited and approximate only. This discovery, however, has yet to penetrate the life sciences.

The second major challenge has emerged from chaos theory. And from where did this theory arise? From the science that continuously struggles to make predictions: meteorology. We all know that weather forecasts are often wrong. The reason for this, according to chaos theory, is that there are too many factors that influence weather patterns, and too many events occurring everywhere all at the same time, for anyone to cull, let alone observe, all this information to make an accurate long-term prediction.[39] The 'butterfly effect' illustrates the point. When a butterfly on one side of the world flutters its wings, it can set off a train of events that eventually causes a tornado on the other side of the world.

The same theme of the interconnectedness and interdependence of all things was also held by mystics and Eastern philosophers. Chaos theory therefore suggests that science's predictive ability is tenuous at best, and illusory at worst. Chaos theory has also revealed that although enormous numbers of components and events occur in any system, there is nevertheless a dynamic order in the apparent chaos. In other words, patterns and cycles of movement emerge, patterns that the Chinese referred to as yin and yang.

The third major challenge comes from some scientists who question some of the very principles that underlie the material world, particularly living organisms. One assumption of the current world-view is that complex systems, such as living organisms and even weather patterns, are merely complicated versions of simple systems. But theoretical biologist Robert Rosen and theoretical physicist Paul Davies question whether the simple systems that have been investigated, and upon which the physical laws are based, are not a very restricted area of nature, and, indeed, whether there are simple systems anyway.[40,41] As Paul Davies asks of living processes: 'How can individual atoms, moving strictly in accordance with the causal laws of physics, responding only to local forces that happen to be produced by neighbouring atoms, nevertheless act collectively in a purposeful, organised and co-operative fashion over length scales vastly in excess of intermolecular distances?'[42]

Moreover, the principle of entropy, of the increasingly disordered energies in a 'closed system' that are posited in the second law of thermodynamics, appear to be defied in life—at least, for the duration of an individual's life—if not throughout the universe. In other words, unlike machines, we're not falling apart. Admittedly, living organisms are not 'closed systems' and hence strictly do not defy the rigid formalism of the second law of thermodynamics. Nevertheless, from the moment the universe came into being—the Big Bang, according to cosmologists—complete and utter chaos (maximum entropy) seems to have been replaced by increasing dynamic order. We certainly experience a world that is continuously and spontaneously evolving and generating dynamic order. And everywhere we look we find life constantly renewing itself.

Why science is not scientific enough

From our position today we may be inclined to think that science holds the key to the truth about health and disease. After all, it's a powerful force to contend with, let alone disagree with. In many ways, particularly in its institutionalised power, in its position as the arbiter of truth, in the very truths it clings to, and in its intellectual hubris, science today mirrors the Church in its heyday.

But just as we may look back on yesterday's truths as quaint or strange, much of what is held to be true today may, in hindsight, be seen as a mistake. Somebody once remarked to the eminent philosopher, Ludwig Wittgenstein, how stupid Mediaeval Europeans must have been prior to Copernicus, to believe that the sun circled the Earth.[43] He is reputed to have replied, 'I agree. But I do wonder what it would have looked like if the sun had been circling the Earth.' The very point is that it would have looked exactly the same.

As you can appreciate, on the slippery road to knowledge, yesterday's heresy often becomes today's truth, and—as is already evident with the claimed curative powers for many drugs—tomorrow's hideous error.

Modern science certainly excels in analysis and reductionism, in quantification, in left-brain thinking, in construing things as being mechanisms that are isolated from everything else. In its techniques of discovery it tends to be aggressive and invasive. In its technological applications it is dominant and powerful. In essence, modern science and its artful twin, technology, are archetypically male or yang.

The duo of modern science and technology has created everything our culture prides itself on—computers and cars, missiles and skyscrapers, drugs and heart-lung machines. It's the reason why President John Kennedy's promise to put a man on the moon by the end of the 1960s was fulfilled.

But science's myopia blinds it to the whole panorama of life, to the consciousness that resides not only in humans but also in animals and plants, and everything else in the universe. It is blind to the uniqueness of each individual, to right-brain thinking, to the intuitive, the gentle, the receptive, the inclusive, the synthetic, the interconnected; the archetypically female or yin.

And that explains why President Richard Nixon's promise of finding a cure for cancer by the end of the 1970s failed. And why modern medicine is failing to halt the onslaught of other modern diseases.

In other words, in its consideration of the whole gamut of life, including health and disease, science is not scientific enough.

Chapter 7

Two Ways to View Health and Disease

It is difficult to get a man to understand something when his salary depends upon his not understanding it.
Upton Sinclair, Pulitzer Prize-winning American author (1878–1968).

A modern perspective

Think about the last time you experienced pain or discomfort. Did you think, 'Wow, I feel great'? Of course not. You probably felt lousy, even awful. You may still be suffering. Perhaps you don't sleep as well as you did, or you're breathless when you walk, or your bowel or bladder habits have gone haywire, or you're depressed or anxious. None of the symptoms of illness is pleasant.

But just because we feel bad or are suffering doesn't necessarily mean our bodies or minds have gone wrong. They could be doing the right thing. They could be trying to clean out and repair their own tissues. They could be warning us to slow down or change our ways. They could even be trying to keep us going despite our wayward lifestyles and abusive habits.

But that's not how we think, nor what we're taught. We assume things have gone wrong because we feel ill. Thus we confuse feeling 'bad' with things going 'wrong'.

One of the reasons for this muddle of meanings is to be found in the origins of the word 'ill' and its association with ethical issues about right and wrong. 'Ill' derives from the Old Norse word *illr*, meaning 'evil'. That 'evil' is 'live' spelt backwards is perhaps not coincidental. Perhaps linguistic wisdom is telling us that evil is anti-life.

But our culture went one step further. Dominated by the Christian religion for the past 1,500 years, mainstream European culture lumped evil and the work of the Devil together, thus showing that only the letter 'D' separates the Devil from his deeds. And because the Devil wages war against God, God-fearing followers of the faith have a moral imperative to do the right thing by opposing anything construed as evil, be it events, bodily functions and processes, or behaviour. That as many as nine million 'witches' were hanged, drowned, or burned at the stake between the 12th and 17th centuries AD,[1] reveals how deadly such righteous opposition to 'evil' can be.

If the Church's beliefs about moral conflicts—between God and the Devil, good and evil, right and wrong, truth and heresy—are applied to health and disease, we can readily appreciate why our culture came to view illness not only as both evil and wrong, but also as another thing to fight.

The other reason we've learned to equate illness with malfunction is because that's what our doctors tell us. And where did their ideas come from? From the maelstrom of power, money, academia and science that is today's beast of institutionalised medicine.

This beast views disease as a disorder of function or structure. As a pathology, an impairment, a malfunction. Disease is the body going wrong. In the case of psychopathology, it's the mind going wrong. Whichever way you look at it, disease is construed as both bad and wrong.

We've progressed, at least to the extent that illnesses are no longer blamed on the Devil. Instead, our modern sleuths search through the smallest nooks and crannies of the material world for an explanation of disease. And somewhere in the beehive of chemical processes, genes, and germs they hunt down the culprits.

So today we can blame our illnesses on an attack of demon germs, or on the curse of rogue chemical processes, or, in more recent times, on being possessed by defective ancestral genes. For many diseases, however, the explanation remains elusive.

Regardless of whether *the* causes, *a* cause or *no* cause at all is found, the same mediaeval mindset of opposing evil persists. Drugs that counter or oppose our bodies' processes abound, and germs are annihilated with anti-microbials. Undoubtedly next in line will be weapons to obliterate wicked genes.

As for health, modern medicine flounders, for its focus is on disease, on diagnosing disease, on identifying the microscopic processes of disease, and on treating disease. From its point of view, health is simply the absence of disease and is confirmed, again, by biochemical markers that reveal no impairment is present. Descartes' words about disease being a malfunctioning of the human machine still echo through the corridors of modern medicine.

A vitalistic approach

Now to a profoundly different way of looking at health and disease: the holistic perspective. If you can grasp the basics of this approach, not only will you begin to marvel at our natural healing abilities, you'll also appreciate why working with, rather than against, the vital force, is essential for health. By working with life you'll also be acknowledging its sacredness, an attitude that is missing from the modern mechanistic view of life.

The term 'holistic' was first coined by South African philosopher, lawyer and political leader Jan Christian Smuts in 1926, in reference to nature's tendency to produce 'wholes' (life-forms) from the ordered groupings of smaller units (cells, tissues and organs).[2] The idea is implied in the writings of British physicist Paul

Davies, and in the observations of the founders of quantum physics, as well as in chaos theory.

The basic concept of wholeness, however, extends far back into the early history of medicine. As evidence of the fertile ground of the word's origins, 'whole' derives from the Indo-European word *kailo*, meaning 'whole' or 'intact', as do the words 'health', 'hale', 'hail', 'hallow', 'holy' and 'heal'.[2] There's no escaping the importance of wholeness when we're dealing with health.

Central to the holistic approach is the concept of the vital force. It forms the foundation of all systems of medicine. Except, that is, for modern medicine. So, what is the vital force?

According to the *Oxford English Dictionary* it is 'an immaterial force or principle which is present in living beings or organisms, and by which they are animated and their functions maintained'.[3] In other words, the lexicographers of the *Oxford English Dictionary* chose to define the vital force as an explanation for why life works the way it does. Remember Aristotle's observation, that people do not think they understand something until they fathom the 'why' of it?

By this definition, modern biologists, unsurprisingly, would deny the existence of a vital force. Their argument is: if it's not made of matter then it doesn't exist. For them, life is animated by purely physical and chemical processes, not by some ghost in the machine.

For the physicians of ancient civilisations, however, the vital force was a description, not an explanation. It was a description borne of observation and experience, not just observation and experiment. For them, the vital force was a manifestation of the divinity that imbues life, the universe, and everything with order and stability. To grasp this idea, imagine that the divinity is the grand computer programme that runs the entire universe. It's also the material hardware of which the universe is made, and the mind behind the whole shebang.

Whereas modern biologists scrutinise the hardware of life—the biochemical molecules and cellular structures—in order to understand why life works or malfunctions as it does, their ancient counterparts tried to understand the interplay between the programme and the hardware; not just in life, but everywhere.

One aspect of the dynamics of the vital force—and it is central to our discussion about health—was identified by the ancient Greeks as the *vis medicatrix naturae*, the body's natural ability to heal itself. Again, this was not an explanation derived from observation and experiment, but a description of living organisms, borne of observation and experience.

Ancient seers had identified at least three principles that operate together in the grand scheme of things: the principles of unity, energy and intelligence. Hence they are aspects of the vital force. To understand and, later, apply these principles, we'll examine each one separately.

Chapter 8

The Vital Force 1: Stuck in the Whole

There are more things in heaven and earth, Horatio,
than are dreamt of in your philosophy.
Shakespeare. *Hamlet*, Act 1, scene 5, line 166.

Where are we going?—a preview

In this and the following two chapters we'll examine the attributes of the vital force. As we've seen, modern medicine denies the existence of the vital force. Natural therapists do use the term, though only to describe the body's natural ability to heal itself. The vital force is not limited to the human body, however, for it encompasses all bodies, all minds, all life forms, all environments; indeed, the whole universe.

Nor is the vital force simply an intellectual construct. At its core is an attitude, a mode of perception borne of both observation and experience, of gnosis, of intuition; of that slab of knowledge to which modern science is blind. And it is a mode of perception many of us have never experienced because of the impact of science, and particularly medical science, on our beliefs.

So here you may well be encountering new territory, a world view that may seem quaint. This territory has been the playground of many a culture—including our own long ago—and this world view has also been adopted by many of those at the forefront of modern science, including many quantum physicists,[1–5] some biologists such as Rupert Sheldrake and Robert Rosen,[6,7] and British anthropologist and philosopher Gregory Bateson.[8,9]

If you can grasp the ideas presented here, you'll be on your way to changing your attitudes about life, the universe and everything. And just by doing that, you'll be well on your way to improving your health. And that's because health is ultimately about relationships: relationships between you and your body and mind, between you and your breathing and drinks and foods, and between you and your loved ones and your community, your environment, and the world.

The universal glue

The principle of unity or cohesion simply means that all parts are related to each other and also to the whole. In other words, we're all stuck together by a universal glue.

For the mystics of India, who rapturously probed the mind of the divinity through their altered states of consciousness, the cosmic glue is love. The theme of love as the great connector also reverberates through the works of the Romantic poets, particularly in those of Keats, Shelley, Byron, and also Wordsworth while he was young. And of course many a songwriter today waxes lyrical about love and its many splendid connections.

Other cultures, both civilised and primitive, were satisfied with simply experiencing the interconnectedness and interdependence of everything. For them, the divinity (for many Chinese, the Tao) is not simply present in the world but inherent in its substance.

The important point is that ancient sages and initiates in mystical rites, as well as many a poet, consciously experienced the unity of all things. Such an experience was important for their psychological, social and spiritual health. Rather than feeling themselves to be separate entities who resided in an alien world, they knew that the macrocosm was mirrored in the microcosm, that the human mind was an aspect of the cosmic mind, that each person was the macrocosm in miniature. As the Hermetic sages of the Hellenist Egyptian tradition had stated, 'As above, so below', or more correctly, 'That which is below corresponds to that which is above, and that which is above corresponds to that which is below'.[10]

If we leave God out of the equation, as the ancient Chinese sages had, we can still understand and perhaps consciously experience the interconnectedness and interdependence of everything in the material world.

We know, for instance, that atoms are timeless, and are constantly being circulated and recycled. In the great circle of life, all living things only borrow them for a short while. According to medical writer Deepak Chopra, 98 per cent of our bodies' atoms weren't part of us a year ago, and won't be with us in a year from today.[11] Within a month, atoms of carbon, hydrogen, oxygen and nitrogen—which pass freely back and forth through the 75–100 trillion cells of our bodies, including those of our apparently solid skeletons—will have returned to the environment via urine, faeces, sweat, breath and the sloughing of skin. Indeed our skin renews itself every month. For the slow moving atoms, such as calcium and iron, their journey through our bodies may take a year.

Hence some of our atoms today may, a few weeks ago, have been atoms of apples and carrots, or oceans and forests. The atoms of the air we now breathe, and the water we drink, may have travelled through countless human bodies, dung beetles, wombats, slime moulds and river red gums. And they once circulated through the world of our ancient ancestors and before them the dinosaurs. Ultimately, atoms are the stuff of stars.

We also recognise life's interdependence. In the food chain, animals and insects depend directly or indirectly on plants and algae. As the lungs of the Earth, they also supply atmospheric oxygen. Plant life in turn depends upon millions of different micro-organisms in the soil and water to help them convert inorganic minerals into organic materials. Many micro-organisms, particularly the much-maligned bacteria, are the planet's garbage eaters, converting dead matter back into inorganic material. And, ultimately, all life is powered by sunlight.

Then there's social cohesion, a major ingredient of human life and health. Alienation, loneliness, poverty, crime and suicide are symptoms of a society where the glue is coming unstuck. And the worst form of social disintegration is war.

Acausal connections

For ancient sages, everything was connected and interdependent, not only through causal connections where one thing leads to another, but also through acausal connections. They had identified that the humdrum chains of causal events were often disrupted by coincidences, serendipities or ill fortune. So what are acausal connections? They are those spontaneous and ever-present connections that are outside the known laws of cause and effect.

Until about the 18th century, acausal connections were considered of equal importance with causality in influencing people's lives, including their illnesses and health. They were also considered to impact on the world at large. Acausal connections (sometimes called non-local connections) were first noted by Hippocrates as 'one common flow, one common breathing, where all things are in sympathy'.[12] Everything hangs together, not by mechanical causes but by hidden 'affinities'.

This theme is echoed in the Pythagorean concept of the Harmony of the Spheres, a concept that was revived by the Elizabethans, and existed in the teachings of Neo-Platonists and Renaissance philosophers. It is apparent in the ancient idea that the finger of 'fate' determines our destinies. It is implied in the German concept of *Zeitgeist*, which can be understood as the spirit, mood and ideas of an era whose time has come. Because astrology deals with our connections with the planets and stars, this ancient science also acknowledges acausal connections. And it's also at the heart of traditional systems of medicine.

Foucault's pendulum
Despite modern science's assertion that only causal connections exist in our humdrum, day-to-day, macroscopic world, it is obvious that many events confound this dogma. One that strikes at the heart of science's belief about the material world is the enigma of inertia. According to Newton's First Law of Motion, inertia is the tendency of a body to preserve its state of rest or its uniform motion in any given direction. The book in your hand remains there because of inertia.

In 1851, the French physicist Jean Foucault set up an experiment to test inertia.[13] He demonstrated that a huge pendulum he had set swinging in a church in Paris, strangely did not continue to oscillate in the same direction, at least relative to the Earth, as would be expected from Newton's First Law. Instead, the oscillations of his pendulum slowly rotated, completing a turn every 24 hours, thereby demonstrating the Earth's rotation.

Curiously, Foucault's pendulum continued to oscillate relative to the distant stars, and not between two fixed points in the church where it was suspended. This experiment demonstrated that inertia is produced by the mass of the universe, not by the Earth, nor by the Sun. Einstein later postulated—but he did not venture to give a causal explanation—that the phenomenon is another manifestation of gravity, due not to the stars as such but to their rotation.

But how the rotation of the universe, how the rotation of 300 billion stars in our own galaxy and those in the 100 billion galaxies in the observable universe, how they could affect Foucault's pendulum or the resting state of the book in your hand is, as philosopher Arthur Koestler, exclaimed in *The Roots of Coincidence*, anybody's guess.[13]

The Hundredth Monkey Phenomenon

Nor does science offer a causal explanation for the Hundredth Monkey Phenomenon that scientists had identified in the behaviour of monkeys. It began with a scientific study of Japanese monkeys living in the wild on various Japanese islands, and on the mainland at Takasakiyama.[14,15] Scientists were providing the monkeys with sweet potatoes dropped in the sand.

Then, one day in 1952, scientists on the island of Koshimo noticed that a young female monkey began washing her sandy sweet potatoes in a nearby stream.[16] Soon the trick for removing the dirt was learned by other monkeys in the troop. By 1958, the innovative behaviour had spread to monkeys in other troops, though no one knows how many.[17] Let's suppose it was 99.

Then suddenly in the autumn of 1958, as if some critical mass in monkey consciousness occurred when the 'hundredth monkey' caught on to the idea, all the monkeys on Koshimo began washing their gritty sweet potatoes. And so did the monkeys on all the other islands. And on the mainland.[18]

Common acausal connections

Strange as these phenomena may at first seem, acausal connections are far more common than many of us may realise. For the Swiss psychologist Carl Jung, they are identified in the 'synchronicity' of events.[19] For the philosopher Arthur Koestler they are 'confluential events'.[13] Sceptics would call them serendipity, luck, or chance. Non-believers would emphasise their random nature by qualifying the noun: 'pure' luck, 'blind' chance—the blind chance of random mutations together with natural selection is, after all, the basis of the theory of evolution. Many of us would recognise them as meaningful coincidences.

From time to time, all of us experience such connections: in dreams perhaps, or from hunches and gut instincts, or maybe from observing strange behaviour in an animal. Some of us may even interpret them as 'signs', just as people in primitive societies had.

Causal and acausal connections, and health

The impact of causal and acausal connections form the foundation of the humoral systems of medicine. These systems are based on identifying the qualities of, and relationships between, the humours: elements and seasons, foods, colours, tastes, smells, activities, emotions, types of diseases, functions of the body, and so on. This approach to patterns of events was employed by all cultures, including Western culture, until the advent of the chemistry's periodic table. Today, however, the language of chemistry is employed to explain most biological phenomena.

For the ancient Chinese philosophers, both causal and acausal connections were apparent in the 'concordances' or 'patterns' of events that 'correspond' with the five elements they had identified in nature: fire, earth, metal, water and wood (see Table 1, and Figure 1).

In traditional Chinese medicine, the metal element, for example, corresponds with the season of autumn, the direction of west, the planet Venus, the number nine and the colour white. It is also associated with an aromatic taste, the smell of rotting flesh, and dryness. In bodily structures, the metal element is linked to the skin, the body hair, and mucus secretions. It also corresponds with the functions of the nose and lungs, and the small intestines. And with the emotions of sadness and courage, grief and loss.

For most people, including Western-trained doctors, this undoubtedly would be seen as a tangled web of irrelevancies to anyone's health. Perhaps the only relationship that could be found would be the causal link between autumn and lung or nasal congestion, for it is a time when allergens, particularly from grasses, float on the air. But science has never identified any causal connection, barring crying, between respiratory congestion and grief. And yet, Chinese medicine does successfully treat some types of respiratory congestion with counselling, as well as with herbs and acupuncture, to deal with past losses or grief.

The Chinese use of concordances can also be applied to psychological and even social health. Relationships, for example, both with yourself and with others, correspond with the earth element. If you're lacking in self-esteem or feeling lonely, your fire element, which nurtures your earth element, may need stoking. This can be achieved by eating small amounts of bitter-tasting foods and herbs, getting some fun into your life, and laughing, even if it's only at yourself. The weakness of the earth element may also be caused by an excess of the wood element. Excessive anger, or sour-tasting foods, or even windy weather, may be the culprit.

Though the Chinese humoral system is too complex to incorporate into this book, for it also relies on pulse and tongue diagnoses, these examples should help you to appreciate that Chinese physicians—in the hospitals of China, even to this day—fully recognise the impact that emotions, foods, climate and so on have on human health.

The Greek and Indian humoral systems of medicine also work with patterns of events, both causal and acausal. The Greek system, known as Unani Medicine, or Unani Tibb—which is still used today, primarily in Pakistan—incorporates the elements, or humours, of fire, water, earth and air into the human temperaments of choleric, phlegmatic, melancholic and sanguine, respectively (see Table 2, and Figure 2).

Ayurveda, the Indian humoral system, which is an integral part of India's medical system today, amalgamates the five elements recognised by the ancient Indian culture into three main types of human constitution: Vata (ether and air), Pitta (fire), and Kapha (earth and water) (see Table 3, and Figure 3). In Volume 2 of this work, you will see how to apply these concepts to your foods and lifestyle.

Astrology, the ancient science of investigating and interpreting the influence of the stars on us, relative to both our time of birth and the present time, also recognises acausal connections and incorporates them into a humoral system (see Table 4, and Figure 4).

Of the 12 constellation signs, three correspond with the fire element (Aries, Leo and Sagittarius) three with the earth element (Taurus, Virgo and Capricorn), three with the air element (Gemini, Libra and Aquarius), and three with the water element (Cancer, Scorpio and Pisces). These four humours—fire, earth, air and water—form the foundation of the Greek system of medicine.

Each of these humours has, as in the Indian system, one of three qualities: the cardinal or Pitta qualities of fire (Aries, Cancer, Libra and Capricorn), the fixed or Kapha qualities of earth (Taurus, Leo, Scorpio and Aquarius), and the mutable or Vata qualities of air (Gemini, Virgo, Sagittarius and Pisces).

Indeed, the quadripartite humours of Greece and the triadic humours of Indian medicine may well have originated in the world's oldest civilisation, Sumer, in the land that is present-day Iraq.

Of the fire signs, for example, Aries consists of a double dose of fire; Leo has qualities of both fire and earth; and Sagittarius has qualities of fire that is tempered by the moving qualities of air.

Needless to say, science disparages astrology, accusing its adherents of hocus pocus. But the fact remains that Foucault's pendulum was somehow influenced by the mass of the distant twinkling stars. The ancient Sumerians and Chaldeans who developed the science of astrology simply plotted the effects of the mass of the universe at specific times on the corresponding patterns of energy here on Earth. Thus, they acknowledged the cosmic space-time continuum that Albert Einstein would mathematically describe 6,000 years later in his special theory of relativity.

Table 1: Concordances of Humours in Traditional Chinese Medicine

	Wood	Fire	Earth	Metal	Water
Season	Spring	Summer	Late summer	Autumn	Winter
Climate	Windy	Hot	Damp	Dry	Cold
Energy	Generative	Expansive	Stabilising	Contracting	Conserving
Development	Germination	Growth	Transformation	Harvest	Storage
Stages of life	Birth	Youth	Adulthood	Old age	Death
Direction	East	South	Centre	West	North
Planet	Jupiter	Mars	Saturn	Venus	Mercury
Colour	Green/dark blue	Red	Yellow	White	Black
Solid organs	Liver	Heart	Spleen	Lungs	Kidneys
Hollow organs	Bladder	Large intestines	Gall bladder	Small intestines	Stomach
Body part	Ligaments	Blood vessels	Flesh/fat/muscles	Skin/body hair	Bones/scalp hair
Sensory organ	Eyes	Tongue	Mouth	Nose	Ears
Sense	Sight	Speech	Taste/touch	Smell	Hearing
Body fluid	Tears	Sweat	Saliva	Mucus	Urine
Taste	Sour	Bitter	Sweet	Spicy	Salty
Smell	Rancid	Scorched	Fragrant	Rotten	Putrid
Emotion	Anger	Joy	Anxiety/sympathy	Grief	Fear
Sounds	Shouting	Laughing	Singing	Wailing	Groaning
Attributes	Creative	Focused	Contemplative	Courageous	Wilful
Negative	Depressive	Manic/erratic	Obsessive	Anguished	Fearful
Aggravated by	Over-use of eyes/ wind	Over-walking/ heat	Over-sitting/ humidity	Over-lying down/ dryness	Over-standing/ cold
Movement	Upward and outward	Rising	Circular	Contracting	Downward

Table 2: Concordances of Humours in Greek Medicine

	Air	Fire	Earth	Water
Season	Spring	Summer	Autumn	Winter
Climate	Moist/warm	Warm/dry	Dry/cool	Cool/moist
Energy	Floating/moving/ forever changing	Energetic/purifying/ intense/destructive	Nurturing/ stabilising	Flowing/cleansing
Development	Germination	Growth/blooming	Consolidation	Decay
Stages of life	Childhood	Youth	Middle age	Old age/birth
Direction	East	South	West	North
Celestial body	Jupiter/Mercury	Sun/Mars	Saturn/Earth	Venus/Moon
Nature	Light/thin/porous/ variable/fickle	Light/bright	Dense/heavy/hard/ rough	Soft/smooth/ shape-changing
Colour	Red	Yellow	Black	White
Temperament	Sanguine	Choleric	Melancholic	Phlegmatic
Humour	Blood	Yellow bile	Black bile	Phlegm
Bodily organs	Heart/ blood vessels	Liver/gall bladder/	Spleen/brain/ bones/hair	Lungs/sex organs/muscles kidneys/bowels/ mucosa
Function	Respiration	Digestion	Bodily structure	Nutrition
Sensory organ	Ears	Eyes/nose	Skin	Tongue
Sense	Hearing	Sight/smell	Touch	Taste
Excretion	Saliva	Sweat/tears	Faeces	Urine
Tastes	Salty	Bitter/acrid/pungent	Sour/astringent	Sweet/oily
Emotion	Spontaneity/joy	Determination/ anger	Contemplation/ fear/worry/grief	Calmness/ indifference
Tendencies	Thinking	Activities/behaviour	Physical sensations	Emotions
Feelings	Quick to arouse/ quick to dissipate	Quick to arouse/ long-lasting	Slow to arouse/ long-lasting	Slow to arouse/ quick to dissipate
Introversion/ extroversion	Extroverted	Extroverted	Introverted	Introverted
In balance	Adaptable/ friendly/creative/ imaginative	Intense/ strong-willed/ fearless/self-reliant	Stable/loyal/loving/ compassionate/ reliable/logical/ trustworthy	Patient/caring/ faithful
Out of balance	Hyperactive/ agitated/unreliable/ inconsistent/ fearful/depressed	Impetuous/ headstrong/wilful/ hateful/vindictive/ destructive	Morose/aloof/ indecisive/highly suspicious/critical/ unforgiving/ depressed	Greedy/selfish/ slothful/apathetic/ unreliable
Likes	Change and excitement	Being in control/being an achiever/goal-oriented	Order and perfection/ fairness/solitude/ security	Peace and harmony/ and to be accepted
Aggravated by	Wind	Heat	Dryness	Cold
Movement	To and fro	Rising	Spreading	Downward

Table 3: Concordances of Humours in Ayurveda

	Ether/Air	Fire	Water/Earth
Season	Autumn	Summer	Winter and spring
Climate	Windy/dry/cool	Hot and dry	Cold and wet
Energy	Light/dry/motile/rough/cool/subtle/clear/dispersing/erratic	Hot/dry/light/motile/intense/liquid/oily/fast	Liquid/cold/heavy/sticky/oily/dense/cloudy/smooth/soft/slow
Development	Conception, life force, and death	Transformation and harvest	Germination, growth, and decay
Stages of life	Maturity and old age	Young adulthood	Childhood
Direction	West	South	East/north
Planet	Mercury/Saturn/Venus (secondary)	Sun/Mars/Jupiter (secondary)	Jupiter/Moon/Saturn (secondary)
Colour	Brown/black	Yellow/orange/red	White/blue/green
Humour	Vata	Pitta	Kapha
Seat of humour	Colon/hips/thighs/ears/bones/large/intestine/pelvic cavity/skin	Small intestine/stomach/sweat glands/blood/fat/eyes/skin	Chest/throat/head/sinuses/nose/mouth/stomach/joints/plasma/mucus
Bodily organ	Brain and lungs	Intestines	Kidneys and heart
Function	Movements/breathing/circulation/nerves/skin/elimination	Digestion/metabolism	Structure of fluid balance/muscles/fat/bone/sinew
Sensory organ	Ears/skin	Eyes	Tongue/nose
Sense	Hearing/touch	Sight	Taste/smell
Taste	Bitter/pungent (air and fire)/ astringent (air and earth)	Pungent (fire and air)/ sour (fire and earth)/ salty (fire and water)	Sweet/salty (water and fire)/sour (earth and fire)/astringent (earth and air)
Emotional tendencies	Wavering/fearful/anxious/fearful/insecure	Determined/angry/irritable/contentious/jealous	Calm/content/attached/steady/loyal/sentimental/greedy
In balance	Energetic/adaptable/flexible/enthusiastic/spontaneous/an initiator and communicator	Intelligent/clear/friendly/Discriminating/independent/courageous/a leader	Calm/peaceful/stable/loyal/consistent/compassionate/patient/devoted/nurturing
Out of balance	Indecisive/unreliable/hyperactive/agitated/disruptive/anxious	Wilful/impulsive/ambitious/aggressive/critical/proud/vain/manipulating/angry	Controlling/attached/greedy/seeks security, comfort and luxury
Very disturbed	Secretive/fearful/servile/depressed/self-destructive/suicidal	Hateful/destructive/vindictive/dangerous to others	Dull/apathetic/slothful/insensitive/a hoarder
Likes	Excitement and change	Power and control	Peace and harmony
Aggravated by	Foods: dried, bitter, hot spicy, astringent. Irregularity in daily activities/windy weather.	Foods: hot spicy, sour, dried, excess salty. Excessive stimulation/hot weather.	Foods: oily, heavy, sweet, sour, salty, astringent. Lack of stimulation/damp, cold weather.
Improved by	Foods: sweet, sour, salty, mild spicy. Regularity in daily activities.	Foods: bitter, sweet, astringent. Purity in lifestyle.	Foods: bitter, hot spicy. Stimulating activities.
Movement	Scattering/dispersing	Rising	Falling

Table 4: Concordances of Humours in Astrology

	Air	Fire	Earth	Water
Season	Spring	Summer	Autumn	Winter
Climate	Windy/warm/wet	Hot/dry	Cold/dry	Cold/wet
Energy	Flexible/communicative	Energetic/assertive	Practical/restrained	Emotional/intuitive
Positive (yang): active, self-expressive, spontaneous	Libra Aquarius Gemini	Aries Leo Sagittarius		
Negative (yin): self-repressed, passive			Capricorn Taurus Virgo	Cancer Scorpio Pisces
Nature	Light	Ardent	Heavy	Soft
Celestial bodies:	Libra, Aquarius, Gemini:	Aries, Leo, Sagittarius:	Capricorn, Taurus, Virgo:	Cancer, Scorpio, Pisces:
Day ruler	Saturn	Sun	Venus	Venus
Night ruler	Mercury	Jupiter	Moon	Mars
Participating ruler	Jupiter	Saturn	Mars	Moon
Direction	East	South	West	North
Qualities: Cardinal (Enterprising) Kapha-like qualities	Libra	Aries	Capricorn	Cancer
Fixed (Immovable) Pitta-like qualities	Aquarius	Leo	Taurus	Scorpio
Mutable (Adaptable) Vata-like qualities	Gemini	Sagittarius	Virgo	Pisces
Jungian types	Thinking	Feeling	Sensation	Intuition
Body parts	Libra: kidneys/lumbar region Aquarius: calves/ankles Gemini: lung/chest	Aries: head Leo: heart Sagittarius: hips/thighs	Capricorn: knees Taurus: throat/neck Virgo: abdomen/intestines	Cancer: breasts/stomach Scorpio: genitals/bladder Pisces: feet
Colour	Libra: green Aquarius: turquoise Gemini: yellow	Aries: red Leo: ruby Sagittarius: royal blue/deep purple	Capricorn: grey/dark green Taurus: pale pink/green/blue Virgo: navy/chocolate	Cancer: silver/metallic blue Scorpio: maroon/blood red Pisces: white/silvery green
Tastes	Libra: warm/sweet/mildly aromatic Aquarius: salty/astringent Gemini: mildly astringent/cold/aromatic	Aries: pungent/astringent Leo: pungent/rich/sweet Sagittarius: sweet/aromatic	Capricorn: cold/sour/astringent/stodgy Taurus: sweet/spicy/rich Virgo: cold/mildy astringent/simple	Cancer: watery/milky/insipid Scorpio: intense/bitter Pisces: alcohol/watery foods
Attributes	Libra: enterprising/urge for harmony/easy going/romantic Aquarius: idealistic/detached/steadfast/unconventional Gemini: mentally active/communicative/spontaneous/adaptable	Aries: quick-witted/courageous/fearless/impatient/passionate Leo: energetic/Intense/assertive/generous/conceited/confident Sagittarius: self-expressive/assertive/energetic/ optimistic	Capricorn: passive/self-restrained/rational/prudent Taurus: restrained/passive/intense/sensual Virgo: analytical/urge for perfection/practical/logical	Cancer: emotional/intuitive/sensitive/loyal/protective Scorpio: emotional/intuitive/intense/perceptive/passionate Pisces: intuitive/adaptable/nebulous attitude/emotional

References:

Mayo J. *Teach Yourself Astrology*, English University Press Ltd, London, UK, 1973.

Lad V. Ayurveda: *The Science of Self-Healing, A Practical Guide*, Lotus Press, Wilmot, Wisconsin, USA, 1984.

Frawley D, and Lad V. *The Yoga of Herbs: An Ayurvedic Guide to Herbal Medicine*, Lotus Press, Twin Lakes, Wisconsin, USA, 1986.

Frawley D. Ayurvedic *Healing: A Comprehensive Guide*, Passage Press, Salt Lake City, Utah, USA, 1989.

Tobyn G. *Culpeper's Medicine: A Practice of Western Holistic Medicine*, Element Books Ltd, Shaftesbury, Dorset, UK, 1997.

Eastwood BS. "Galen on the Elements of Olfactory Sensation", Journal: *Rheinisches Museum fuer Philologie*, 1981; 124: 268-289.
[Online, accessed 24th January, 2010].
URL:http://www.rhm.uni-koeln.de/124/Eastwood.pdf

Aquinas T. *Commentary on Aristotle's De Senso et Sensato*, K White (translator), Catholic University Press of America, 2005.
[Online, accessed 24th January, 2010].
URL:http://dhspriory.org/thomas/SensuSensato.htm

Kapchuk TJ. *Chinese Medicine: The Web That Has No Weaver*, Rider and Company, London, UK, 1987.

Kratky KW. *Comparative and Integrative Medicine. II: Health Geometry and Life Spiral*, Institute of Experimental Physics, University of Vienna, Austria, 2002.
[Online, accessed 24th January, 2010].
URL:http://www.energie-institut.com/service/forschung/2002%20Kratky%20II%20Health% 20Geometry.pdf

Figure 1: Chinese Medicine- Five phases (Wu Xing)

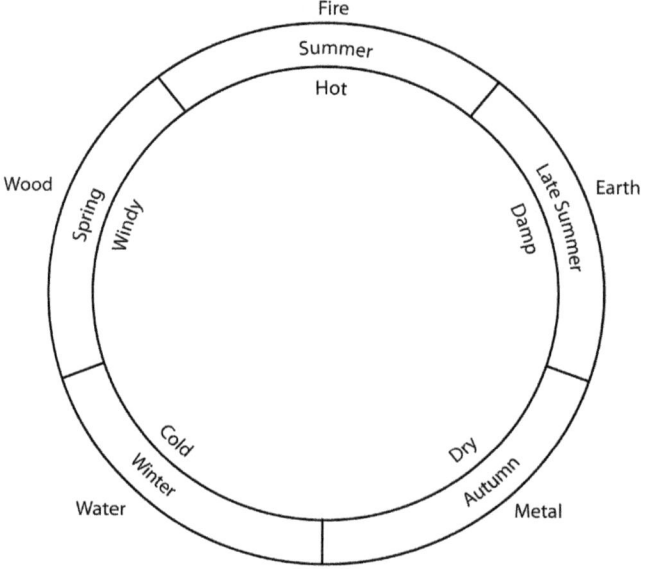

Figure 2: Greek Medicine- Four elements and humours

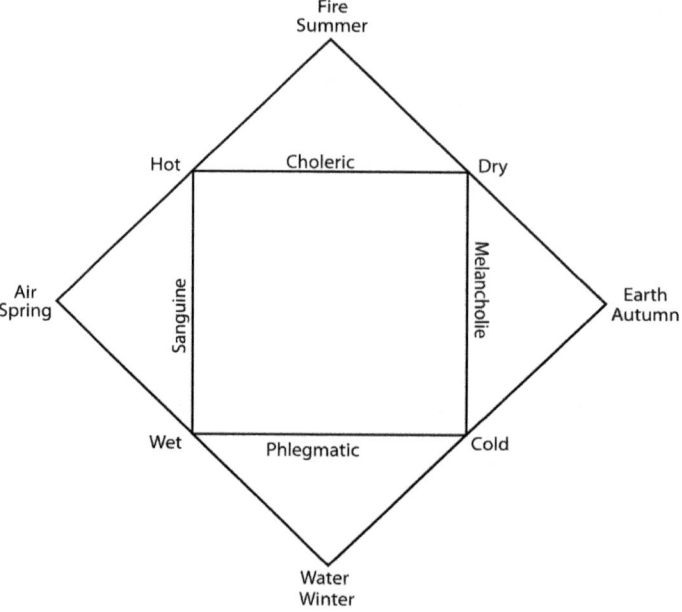

Figure 3: Ayurveda- Five elements and three humours (doshas)

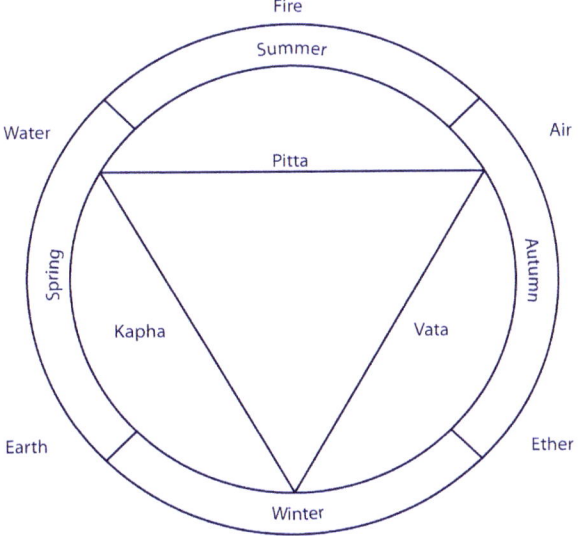

Figure 4: Astrology- Four elements twelve signs and three qualities

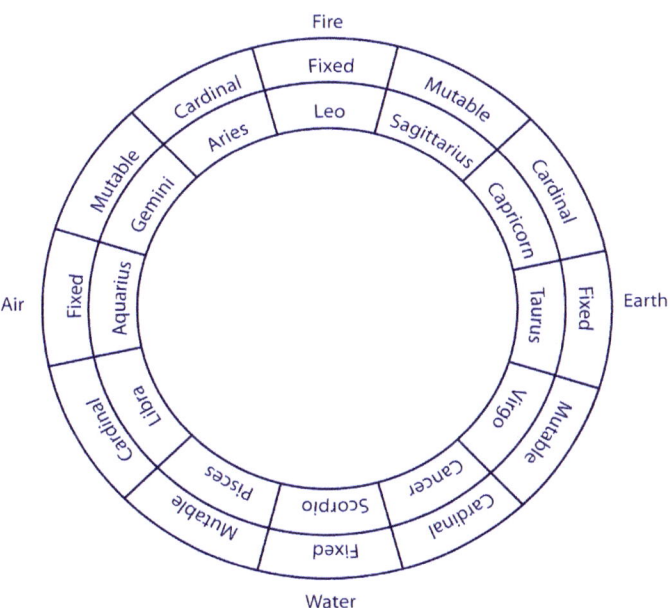

What modern science says about connections

So far we've explored the unity of everything, and the significance of acausal connections in our lives. But what does science have to say about this? In medical science, nothing. In physics, however, a lot. Although it is the most reductionist of all sciences, physics has cut to the core of both the cosmic and microcosmic levels of the universe.

In Chapter 6 we briefly touched on the challenge to science posed by several of the founders of quantum physics—that the properties and interactions of subatomic particles prove that the cosmos, including the observer of any aspect of it, is one inseparable reality. But what did they discover about causality?

Let's start with our 'Middle Earth' reality. At the heart of our view of the day-to-day world in which we live, even of the microscopic world of bacteria and viruses at which scientists peer, are our concepts of time and space, matter and objects, velocity and energy, and cause and effect. We experience events occurring at a certain place and at a certain time.

Time, at least for us in our culture, seems to move forward. (Some cultures do experience time as standing still, and believe that we are moving backwards into the future, watching past events recede). We feel objects to be solid, and we see the effects of the deterministic law of cause and effect, where this leads to that, everywhere we look. Even chaos theory—remember the butterfly effect?—is based on an understanding of the incredibly complex and tangled web of cascading causes and effects.

Einstein had, of course, changed scientific conceptions about time and space at the cosmic level, when he theorised that time and space were woven together in a four dimensional, space-time continuum. But no one was prepared for what quantum physicists discovered in the subatomic world. As in the *Alice's Adventures in Wonderland*, everything is not as it seems.

Like Peeping Toms at a keyhole, the founders of quantum physics watched the footprints of subatomic events in a shadow world that they could only make sense of by using mathematical formulations.[20,21] Down there—in here—the objective world of space and time, matter and causation, has no meaning. Matter turns out to be bundles of energy wrapped in a four-dimensional, space-time continuum. Sometimes these bundles behave like hard little pellets, and sometimes they behave like ocean waves or the vibrations of a guitar string, depending upon how the observer chooses to see them.

Even curiouser, these bundles do not exist with certainty at definite places or times, or in specific ways. Rather, they have the tendency to exist and to occur, and are expressed as mathematical probabilities. The probabilities themselves do not represent things at all, but rather probabilities of interconnections: interconnections between the various processes of observation and measurement, and interconnections with the whole universe.

So in both Einstein's cosmos and Heisenberg's microcosmos, matter dissolves into energy, and energy fades into shifting patterns of interconnections between things unknown. And the connections are not causal because, in the time-space continuum, no time is attached to them: no 'before' and no 'after'.

And though the forward direction of time is dominant, as American author Gevin Giorbran explained in his book *Forever Everything*, the general flow of time since the Big Bang splatters in all directions, moving both forward and backward, and in various directions at right angles to the past and the future.[22]

Hence, the universe turns out to be a complicated web of relations between various parts of a unified whole. As Heisenberg had remarked: 'The world thus appears as a complicated tissue of events in which connections of various kinds alternate or overlap or combine and thereby determine the texture of the whole.'[23]

Einstein, a man who strongly believed in nature's inherent harmony, despaired: 'God does not play dice.'[24] But he was searching for an answer to how the parts impact on the whole. Quantum physicists, however, had discovered that the whole impacts on the parts.

In some ways we are like the hobbits in J.R.R. Tolkien's *Lord of the Rings*. We inhabit Middle Earth, a middle-sized world where everything seems solid and tangible and real. Our minds make it seem so. But as we venture beyond our world, the universe starts to look very different. Those who have travelled beyond the borders of our world—mystics and seers, physicists and cosmologists—have returned with mind-blowing reports. 'The universe begins to look more like a great thought than a great machine,' said British physicist James Jeans.[25] In other words, consciousness, not matter, seems to make the universe what it is. Arthur Eddington, Jeans's compatriot, hit the nail on the head when he said: 'The stuff of the world is mind-stuff.'[26]

And I'll venture to add, this is the stuff of our vital force.

Beyond your doctor's philosophy

Such quantum and cosmic connections, whether causal or acausal, were never dreamt of in your doctor's medical philosophy. But once we accept that both causal and acausal connections co-exist, then we're on the road to gaining a far greater understanding about how things impact on our health. More importantly, we can begin to work with, rather than against, the flow of things, and can learn to change the only thing in the universe we do have some control over: ourselves.

Chapter 9

The Vital Force 2: Spinning Energies

*In every culture and in every medical tradition before ours,
healing was accomplished by moving energy.*
Albert Szent-Györgyi, Nobel Laureate in Physiology or Medicine, 1937
(1893–1986).

A Chinese perspective

The second principle of the vital force is that of energy: that nothing is ever static. Wherever we look, everything is moving, changing, and becoming transformed into something else. Our hearts are beating, our lungs are breathing, the electrons inside the atoms of a rock are spinning, the galaxies are spiralling, photons of light are darting everywhere, and vibrations of air are striking our ears. Even our eyes are flickering at about 100 movements every second as we gaze at the world.[1] In fact, the directional changes in the oscillations of Foucault's pendulum were caused by the spinning energies of the universe.[2]

Yin and yang

In Chinese philosophy, the cycles of change are identified as aspects of yin and yang. Originally, yin referred to the shady side of a mountain and yang to the sunny side. These polar pairs refer to qualities and relationships, tendencies and patterns, not to quantities or absolutes. They are comparative terms that refer to things being more or less, darker or lighter, and so on. And because yin and yang are on a continuum, they cannot be separated.

If you approach the concept of polarities with the sensibilities of a poet, keeping in mind the Eastern advice that the finger that points to the moon is not the moon, you'll have no problems applying this to your health. Table 5 presents some of the qualities of yin-yang continuum. Use your imagination to conjure up others.

We can observe polarities in everything. Wintertime, for example, is the yin season relative to summer's yang. Despite our efforts to cocoon ourselves from the colder, shorter days of winter by heating and lighting our houses and offices, we can still expect—because everything is interconnected—our own energies to follow the same yin patterns. We'll be more lethargic and perhaps sleep longer hours than we would in the summertime yang.

We can also apply the polar pairs to foods, lifestyles, and our own bodily functions in sickness and in health. Even cities and nations reflect differing tendencies of polar energies. The tranquil city of Adelaide, for example, with its low skyline, is more yin than the hustle and bustle of cosmopolitan Sydney with its towering skyscrapers.

Anything that doesn't change, whether it's our bodies, cities, ideologies, political parties, languages, or even people's rigid adherence to fad diets and exercise programmes, holds the seeds of its own destruction. Just ask failed weight-loss dieters.

The polarity of yin and yang, however, is not simply a philosophical concept by which we can passively observe the shifting patterns of things. It is also a tool we can use to change those things we do have some control over, such as the foods we eat, our lifestyles, and how we deal with our illnesses. Even town planners and politicians could use it to help balance the energies of cities if those places are excessively yin or yang. But to use the yin-yang polarity, we need to understand how they relate to each other and function together.

Table 5: Yin-Yang attributes

Yin	Yang
Dark	Light
Cold	Hot
Wet	Dry
Internal	External
Female	Male
Soft	Hard
Gentle	Forceful
Yielding	Firm/controlling
Pliant/flexible	Rigid
Still	Moving
Slow	Fast
Descending	Ascending
Low	High
Passive	Active
Heavy	Light
Substance	Function
Empty	Full
Bust	Boom
Cleanse	Nourish
Deficient	Excess
Weak	Strong
Fat	Thin
Back	Front
Left	Right
Less	More
Hidden	Open
Turned down	Turned up
Wood, water, and earth	Fire and metal
Vessel	Contents
Ground	Figure
Field, or void	Energy
Blood	Qi
Completion	Creation
Receptive	Invasive
Synthetic	Analytic
Subjective	Objective
Earth	Heaven
Moon	Sun
Past	Future
Winter	Summer
Chronic/degenerative disease	Acute disease
Traditional medicine	Modern medicine
Herbs	Acupuncture
Negative	Affirmative

How yin and yang dance together

Divisions all the way down

Firstly, everything can be divided and subdivided into two polarities.

Take, for example, a fever. From your doctor's perspective, if your body's temperature rises above 37 degrees Celsius (98.6 degrees Fahrenheit) you have a fever, nothing more, nothing less. Consequently, you would possibly be prescribed aspirin or paracetamol to reduce your fever, and an antibiotic to knock out any bacterial infection. Of course, if the culprit is a virus, antibiotics are useless.

From a traditional Chinese medical perspective, however, though you may show some signs of heat (a faster pulse rate, for example), you may also have signs of coldness (cold and pale skin, perhaps goose flesh, little thirst and feeling chilled). Treatment would thus be very different to that if your body showed signs of excess heat (hot and flushed skin, sweating perhaps, a strong thirst and feeling hot). In other words, fevers can be divided into hot or cold fevers. The hot and cold fevers can in turn be divided into sweating and non-sweating fevers. (The treatment for each type of fever is presented in Volume 2).

Control and balance

Secondly, yin and yang control and balance each other. Heat controls cold, just as cold controls heat. If you apply the polarity of hot-cold to your diet you may notice that in the heat of summer you tend to eat more cooling foods, such as green-leafy salads and fresh fruits—which just happen to be in season at this time—and drink more fluids. In wintertime, you're likely to eat more heating foods, such as cooked foods in general, and root vegetables and meats in particular, and to prefer hot drinks. And thus a balance is achieved.

However, if yin is too weak then it can't control yang, and vice versa. Similarly, if yin is excessive, then yang may not be able to control it. The converse also applies. If such imbalances continue, eventually yin and yang will separate and the entity that possessed these polarities will cease to exist. If it's a person, then he or she dies.

To understand the dynamics of this more clearly, imagine an open fire. The wood is yin and the flame is yang. Unless both work together, there is no fire. When the fire is first lit, the yin of the kindling wood must be commensurate with the yang of the spark. If you tried to ignite wet wood or a log, which are very yin, the fire simply wouldn't start. A blazing fire is a balance of wood and flame, of yin and yang. As the wood dwindles, so does the flame. And if, perchance, you douse the fire with paraffin, which is excessively yang, then the wood will burn out even more rapidly.

Now apply the analogy of the wood and the flame to yourself. The yin is the force field within which your life blazes. It's also the vessel of your body; it's the substance and the nourishment. It's the infrastructure. The yang is your body's energy and the mental and emotional sparks that arise from chemical processes throughout your body. If you continually throw paraffin onto your fire by rushing through life in the fast lane, then your yin will be rapidly depleted. Some people call this adrenal burnout. Unless you know how to nourish your yin then, hey presto, you end up like an exhausted fire. You're burnt out. If, however, you lounge around and eat excessively, your yin overwhelms your yang energy and activities. Eventually, you end up as a couch potato with a dulled mind and sluggish organs. And should you continue on either path then sooner or later your yin and yang will separate, and you'll leave this mortal coil.

Smooth qi

Thirdly, to achieve health and vitality, the movements of living energy that flux between yin and yang must flow smoothly. This vital energy is known as qi (pronounced chee). In the analogy of the wood and the flame, qi is like the air that ensures the fire burns well. The oxygen in the air is both an element of matter and the energy of the fire itself. Qi thus refers to the interchangeable nature of energy and matter. This idea surfaced in modern times in physics, when Einstein formulated his special theory of relativity, encapsulated in the formula $E=mc^2$, meaning that energy and mass are interconvertible.

If qi is blocked in any part of the body we're likely to experience aches and pains, or an impairment of an organ's functions. Imagine a fire in a fireplace with a blocked chimney, with smoke wafting everywhere, except, that is, up the chimney. The house would be a smouldering mess. Well, that's the effect that blocked qi creates in our bodies. If, however, qi is deficient in any organ—not enough air getting to the fire—then it won't function as well as it should. And if qi is deficient throughout our bodies, we'll experience lethargy and perhaps even a lack of mental clarity.

Using yin-yang polarities to assess and treat illness

Although there are as many polar pairs, as you can see from the chart on yin-yang attributes, Chinese physicians focus initially on four pairs of polarities to make a diagnosis: yin-yang, interior-exterior, cold-hot, and deficiency-excess.

Yin-yang polarity encompasses all the attributes in Table 5, as well as the other three pairs:
- Yin patterns of illness comprise interior, cold and deficient signs and symptoms. Yang patterns consist of exterior, hot, and excess signs and symptoms.

The interior-exterior pair identifies the location and depth of disease:
- Internal syndromes affect the internal organs and bone, and are associated with chronic diseases, poor diet, psychological disturbances, and fatigue.
- Exterior patterns affect the skin, hair and muscles, and are associated with acute illnesses of short duration.

The cold-hot polarity identifies the characteristics of disease:

- Cold patterns are evident when functions of the body slow down—no thirst, feeling chilled, pallor, cold limbs, poor circulation, loose stools, clear profuse urine, slow movements, withdrawn manner, and a preference for warm drinks. These can arise from excess yin (too much wood) or deficient yang (not enough flame).
- Hot patterns are evident when functions of the body speed up—a strong thirst, feeling hot, having a flushed face, hot limbs, high fever, constipation, dark scanty urine, restlessness, and a preference for cold drinks. These can arise from excess yang (too much flame) or deficient yin (not enough wood).

And the deficient-excess pair identifies weak or excessive functions:
- Deficiency patterns are evident when functions of the body are weak or frail—general weakness, tiredness, shortness of breath, little appetite, weak voice, inactivity and passivity, dizziness, listlessness, mental irritability, pain relieved by pressure or massage, incontinence, a weak pulse. Contributing factors include congenital weaknesses, poor diet, lack of physical activities, long-term emotional disturbances, and prolonged illnesses.
- Excess patterns are evident when bodily functions are hyperactive—ponderous movements, pain made worse by pressure or massage, heavy breathing, profuse phlegm, mental confusion or delirium, constipation, difficulty in urinating, forceful pulse. These are associated with acute illnesses and crises.

Why use these polar pairs in the assessment of health and disease? Because recognising the continuous flux of energies in our bodies, provides an insight into how to treat our illnesses.

Take anxiety, for example. It's a feeling of worry, of nervousness, of uneasiness, which can surge to feelings of panic. And it can be very exhausting. The medical profession's point of view is that anxiety is a hyperactive condition of the mind. And since the mind equates to brain, at least in the mindset of medicine, anxiety equates to an overproduction of certain neurochemicals in various parts of the brain. Thus modern medicine views anxiety as a yang-excess condition. Consequently it employs yang-reducing drugs—sedatives or tranquillisers—to quell the fire of anxiety.

However, anxiety, particularly if it's long continued, may well be a yin-deficient condition—irritability and grumpiness over the slightest concern is the clue. In other words, the flame of worries is not being controlled by the nourishment of wood—all the human needs we deal with in Volume 2. Hence, Chinese physicians may prescribe yin-nourishing remedies—such as calming the breathing and eating underground root vegetables, Chinese dates and sesame seeds—rather than employing herbs to quell the fire.

Unfortunately for patients, the medical profession has no concept of yin. Instead, its focus is on yang, on pushing or pulling bodily functions, on opposing the vital force (See Figure 5). Certainly, if you're suffering from an excess condition, such as acute inflammation or fever, it may be necessary to quell functions to preserve your life or prevent irreversible damage to tissues. But because modern medicine has no concept of yin, it also employs such contrary remedies even when you have deficient conditions, such as long-term illnesses, even when you have cold conditions such as osteoarthritis. And if your functions are under-performing—constipation, fluid retention, depression—it uses contraries to drive them into action. But alas, the yin, and all that it encompasses, is ignored.

In Figure 5, you can see the yang continuum, which consists of increasing or decreasing bodily functions. The yin continuum—the one that modern medicine is blind to—consists of cleansing and nourishing the vital force. Unlike the yang continuum, however, nourishing and cleansing cannot be pushed or pulled. In essence, if you satisfy your human needs (see Volume 2) then the yin goes about both cleansing and nourishing your body and mind at a pace determined by your vital force.

Then there's the vital force continuum. We can't stimulate the vital force because it works in its own smooth, impeccable rhythm. And that, in turn, is determined by both the yin and yang continua. But we can certainly sedate it. Why would anyone want to sedate the vital force? To quell the spontaneous energy of life. If you're running a prison camp, or a whole society, fear-mongering, alcohol, and fluoride in tap water will do the trick. And in hospitals, administration of morphine has the same effect. Perhaps the only thing that does boost our vital force is laughter and joy.

Figure 5: Approach to treatment

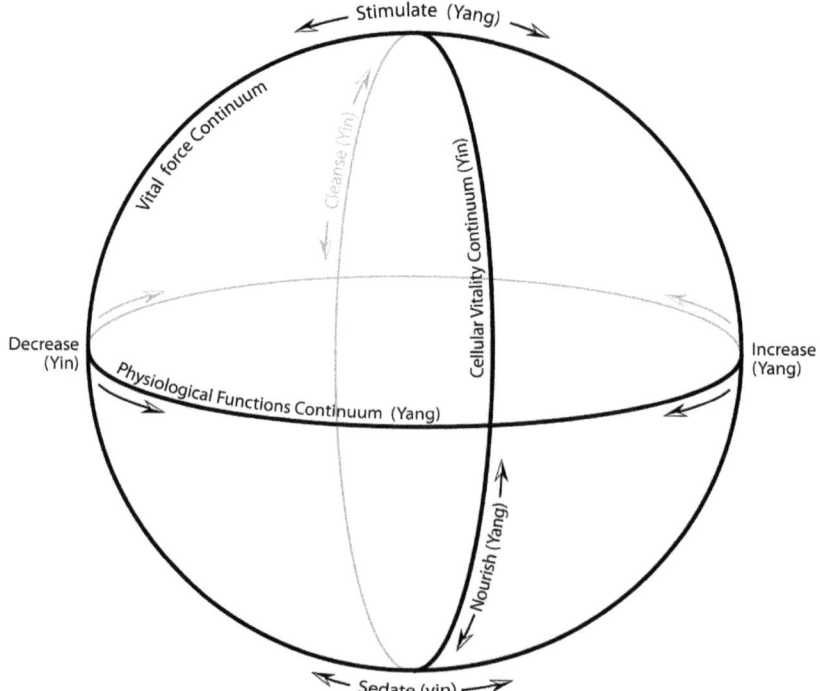

- 150 -

Indian and Ancient Greek perspectives

In Ayurveda, the traditional Indian system of medicine, energy is thought of as the workings of the conscious divinity in the material world. Known as *prana*, it animates all life and generates the movements of all substance. The Chinese equivalent is qi; the Greek is *pneuma*; and all of these terms mean 'breath' or 'air'. Because Ayurveda holds that the divinity animates our lives, it offers a further insight into disease. Every chemical process, and every function that our body's cells and organs perform—even when we're ill, even chronically ill—manifests the universal life force.

This sanguine view of illness—a health crisis—had been adopted by Swiss psychologist Carl Jung, at least in relation to psychological crises. He is reputed to have said to one of his patients who was spiralling into a psychological crisis: 'Let's open a bottle of champagne! You are at the bottom, now we can begin to climb up and out!'[3] Rather than viewing a health crisis as a disaster, Jung was suggesting it was an opportunity for change. Moreover, a Chinese proverb states: 'Crisis is an opportunity riding the dangerous wind';[4] indeed, many people in the West have proferred this as an elegant translation of the two characters in the Chinese language that signify 'crisis': 'danger', and 'occasion'. By claiming that illness is part of the journey to perfection, Chinese physicians had taken the same stand to a physical health crisis.

If illness is an aspect of the vital force, as Ayurvedic and Chinese physicians had claimed, perhaps our bodies aren't necessarily going wrong when we're sick. Perhaps they're doing something right. Perhaps our vital force is trying rectify something. Perhaps it's even trying to tell us that we need to make some changes. But because modern medicine is blind to the polarities of energy in sickness and in health, and because it views a crisis as a disaster, we never learn what to change. Instead, we fight disease.

Interestingly, from the Ayurvedic point of view, the movement of the universal life force generates heat. Thus illnesses with signs and symptoms of heat—inflammation and fever which accompany most acute illnesses—reflect a strong vital force. In ancient Greece this was known as a *sthenic* response; and in Chinese medicine as a yang, condition. Conversely, illnesses with cold symptoms, usually chronic illness, reveal a weakened vital force. Again in Greek medicine this was known as an *asthenic* response; in Chinese medicine, as a yin condition.

And what does modern medicine do to acute illnesses? It tries to prevent them through vaccinations, and to quell their energies if they do arise.

Throwing light on spinning energies

Another manifestation of the movement of the life force is light. Light, in essence, is energy. Paradoxically, light can never be seen. Only the objects it illuminates can be observed. And because light travels at the maximum speed possible (the speed of light, of course) it has, following Einstein's equation ($E=mc^2$), no mass. It is immaterial. Do you recall the *Oxford English Dictionary*'s definition of vital force? 'An immaterial force or principle.' And the explanation for gravity and the movement of Foucault's pendulum? Gravitons, which also travel at the speed of light but have no mass or electrical charge.

It is illuminating to realise that in our universe, where matter and energy are interchangeable, the human species has been primed to be far more sensitive to energy than to matter.[5,6] In fact, one thousand billion billion billion times more sensitive. The peripheries of our retinas, where cells primed for night vision are clustered, are sensitive to less than five quanta (or photons) of radiant energy in the visible spectrum of light. This is about 10^{-10} ergs (an erg is a unit used in physics to calibrate energy). Our skin, however, can only feel the gravitational effect of matter when a weight of at least 0.1 of a gram falls on it. This is about 10^{20} ergs. Compare this with the sensitivity of the tendril of a climbing plant: it responds to a weight of 0.00025 of a gram, 400 times lighter than we can feel. And our muscles are even less sensitive to feeling the weight of an object.

The eyes have it

For the poets, the eyes reveal the soul. For lovers, the eyes reveal passion. For Chinese and Indian physicians, the eyes reveal our consciousness. Clearly, eyes tell us a lot about what's going on inside us. In fact, eyes are the best place to see the vital energies of a person. The sparkle in the eye, known to traditional Chinese physicians as *shen*, is the best indicator of clear and full consciousness and awareness in both body and mind. Dull eyes indicate that the vital force in our bodies is weak. Mad eyes, which dart about or stare menacingly, reveal a disturbance of consciousness and awareness: check out the eyes of your political leaders.[7] And blank eyes, as seen in the eyes of a corpse, indicate the absence of consciousness.

From time to time, all of us experience temporary flights of consciousness, when we stare into space, unaware of our surroundings, recharging our vital energies. During such reveries, and also when we're asleep, our eyes reveal that all lights are on but no one's home.

Clearly, when it comes to energies, conscious energies, the eyes have it.

Chapter 10

The Vital Force 3: Signs of Intelligence

The chance that higher life forms might have emerged in this way is comparable with the chance that a tornado sweeping through a junk-yard might assemble a Boeing 747 from the materials therein.
Sir Fred Hoyle, British astronomer (1915–2001).

Of one mind

The third principle of the vital force is that of intelligence. This principle implies that a mind, or consciousness, is intrinsic to everything. And if a universal mind pervades everything then, *ipso facto*, there should be evidence of this mind's intelligence everywhere. So where is the evidence?

Think of human intelligence. How would an extra-terrestrial know our species has a modicum of intelligence? Or, for that matter, how do we know that any ET is intelligent? This, after all, is the task of astronomers involved in SETI, the Search for Extra-Terrestrial Intelligence.

Let's firstly qualify this quest by accepting that our species' intelligence and range of senses is going to limit our understanding and observations. That said, the first sign of intelligence likely to grab our attention would be some form of communication. Next would be the design and construction of anything that mind had created. We'd be looking for how the things it has created work and interact with other things in their environment: whether its creations can move and react to changes in their environment, or even manipulate other things; whether they can maintain their own order and stability and thus continue to exist; and whether they can re-create themselves.

Babble, or communication?

Now let's apply this to our world by focusing on communication. All animals, birds and insects communicate effectively with other members of their species. To do this they use all manner of squeaks and squawks, and signals that range from brilliant colours, bodily movements and eye contact, to chemical emissions, including powerful pheromone sex signals.

For us, our verbal language can be a great means of communicating intricate details about what we know, think and feel. It *can* be. But it can also be used as much to deceive ourselves and others as to communicate. Far earlier in our evolutionary development is our body language. Hence we have spatial comfort zones, eye movements, pupil dilation or constriction, and other subliminal cues that are far better indicators of what we really think or feel.

The next time you watch politicians prattling on about policies, watch for facial tension and the fixed, unblinking stare. You'll know they're stressed—possibly there's a disparity between what they say and what they know. And when you see, if only momentarily, a kaleidoscope of facial twitches, darting eye movements and rapid blinking, their bodies are telling us they're lying through their teeth.

Communication is not limited to animals, however, for plants also communicate, ostensibly with insects, birds and animals. They repel marauders and attract pollinators by displaying various colours, and by secreting all sorts of chemical compounds that smell or taste disgusting or delicious. Evening primrose, for example, opens its bright-yellow flowers at night, thereby attracting the particular moths that facilitate pollination.

Amazingly, plants also communicate with each other. Acacias are a classic example of talking trees.[1] When an animal browses on acacia foliage, the tree not only increases its tannin content to deter the marauder, it also emits a chemical messenger: ethylene. This volatile chemical travels at least 50 metres downwind, alerting other acacias of the attack. Within 15 minutes, they, too, have increased their foliage's levels of tannins. Any animal foolish or hungry enough to continue eating acacia leaves dies within two weeks because high levels of tannins inactivate liver enzymes. Giraffes defy the talking trees by browsing upwind. But antelopes, and specifically wildebeest, which graze mainly on grass and move downwind, die in huge numbers during droughts when they switch to eating acacia leaves. They simply haven't learned the trick of moving upwind.

Plants also use non-chemical signals to talk with one another. Though the mode of signalling is unknown, lie detectors have recorded electrical responses in individual plants when an experimenter damages or destroys nearby plants. This also happens when an experimenter even intends to do so, as American polygraph expert Cleve Backster discovered.[2-4] And if one of the experimenters is the perpetrator, plants know who the murderer is. Human emotions of love and affection, including a couple's sexual raptures, also set them off. So if you're wondering what goes on behind closed doors, don't bother with wishing you were a fly on the wall; plants seem to provide far better eye-witness reports.

Nor is life's ability to communicate limited to talk between species; nor is it restricted to information about the environment that we pick up through our senses and nervous systems, and that plants gather through their receptors. Communication also happens inside our bodies, between cells and organs. Cells speak to each other through neural transmitters, hormones, and a host of other living chemical messengers. Sometimes they encode their chatter in electrically charged molecules, sometimes in whole organelles (little organs inside cells) that scoot between cells through minuscule tunnels.

Even our DNA talks. Despite the persistence, particularly amongst the genetic engineering buffs, of the old dogma that there is a one-to-one correspondence between a gene and a protein, that our genome is the linear text that controls our physical structures and processes, we now know that genes are dynamic and fluid.[5] The record for a talking gene goes to the fruit fly—one of its genes generates 38,016 variant protein molecules.[6] DNA molecules not only talk to messenger RNA, they talk to proteins and they talk amongst themselves.

But it's not a one-way system of communication. As British geneticist Mae-Wan Ho argues, our genes perform their own genetic dance of life to the rhythms of quantum jazz, ever responsive to our environment: talking amongst themselves, expressing themselves in different ways, even changing their own structures, and all the while keeping in sync with the whole.[7]

Thus there are two environments within which life communicates: the external one that we inhabit, and the internal one where the components of our tissues live. In both environments, communication is integral to life's design and construction. In the former, it is essential for a species' survival. In the latter, cellular chatter ensures our individual health and survival.

Stability in the midst of apparent chaos

At the planetary level, communication, albeit founded on chemical interactions, ensures a relatively stable environment for life on Earth. The levels of atmospheric oxygen, for example, have remained constant, at about 21 per cent for millions of years. How do we know this? Because there is evidence of forest fires in ancient times. If oxygen made up less than 16 per cent of the air, fuel would not burn. If oxygen levels were higher than about 30 per cent, explosions would have erupted.

So how is the constancy of oxygen maintained? From satellite imaging, marine biologists have discovered that phytoplankton, which produce about 70 per cent of atmospheric oxygen, proliferate in the oceans when oxygen levels dip, and then reduce their numbers when the oxygen levels are restored. The explanation? Researchers at the University of Texas at Austin discovered that when oxygen levels in the atmosphere drop, so do levels of free oxygen at the ocean bottom.[8,9] The seabed picks up the message and releases phosphorus, which is a nutrient for plankton. Hence plankton numbers increase. However, when phytoplankton are abundant, the raised levels of oxygen in the atmosphere increase the levels of free oxygen at the ocean bed. And the seabed releases less phosphorus. For phytoplankton, that means less food and so their numbers decrease.

Inside our bodies the same stabilising forces exist. Every moment, billions of messages are being sent on our internal telecommunication networks from cell to cell and organ to organ. But unlike many of our telephone conversations, which can descend into discordant babble, our cellular messages are coordinated and synchronised. Even though every one of the estimated 100 trillion cells in an average-sized adult body lives and moves and functions as an independent citizen of the body-state, it still works in harmony with the other citizens for the body's good. And, just as seven billion humans and the Earth's other teeming life forms communicate to ensure some sort of stability and order on our planet, so do the cellular citizens of our internal, microscopic worlds.

Without the stability of the liquid environment that circulates and bathes our cells, we'd rapidly perish. To survive the impact of our ever-changing environment and the things we do to ourselves, our bodies must maintain the constancy, or homoeostasis, of our internal oceans. To do this, whole cities of cells are beavering away at different tasks. Some, like the cells of our vital organs, are constantly on the go. Others, like our hunter-killer cells, are in cruise mode, ever ready to spring into action to remove cellular debris and foreign invaders. From modern biology's mechanistic point of view, such stabilising functions are called homoeostatic mechanisms. From the vitalistic perspective, however, they reveal life's intelligence.

Like miniature nation-states, our bodies depend for their survival on specialists. Our bodies' specialists control temperature and chemical balance; provide fuel and energy; they clean, and export rubbish; they import fuels and building materials; they transport materials and move our bodies through our environments; they observe the outside world. They also work to defend and communicate, repair and reproduce. And as the supreme commanders and coordinators, our brains filter and ration our consciousness. Otherwise, we'd be swamped with information.

Everywhere, cells are listening and responding to the chatter from other cells. But unlike nation-states, in which fearful or greedy citizens are often embroiled in conflicts, and in which political leaders rant on about 'sending a powerful message' to their enemies, our bodies are geared to their common needs and the common good. Thus intelligence, unsurprisingly, is more readily apparent in our bodies than in our body politic.

To bridge the apparent gap between the world out there and the one inside our bodies, life has provided us with many lines of communication. The gentlest messages come from the quiet duo of gut instincts, or intuition, and feelings. Most of the time they hum along merrily, guiding us ever so gently towards things that are important to our wellbeing, and alert us to dangers.

Why do we tell our children to trust their feelings about strangers? And why, for that matter, did Obi-Wan Kenobi in *Star Wars* advise Luke Skywalker to turn off his computer and fly by the seat of his pants? As he said: 'Turn off your computer, turn off your machine and do it yourself, follow your feelings, trust your feelings.'[10,11] And he pressed the issue: 'Let go, Luke. Feel, don't think.' Why? Because feelings provide far better messages about things that are important to our survival—if not in the confines of a cockpit, then at least in the world of nature—than rational thought or computer systems ever can.

The loudest messages come from instincts and emotions. They are usually so powerful that we simply can't ignore them. But whether we're driven to act depends on the intensity of our instincts and emotions on the one hand, and the power of another set of messages, the social mores and beliefs we've learned, on the other. Thus, if someone annoys us, most of us will either ignore that person or limit our actions to a verbal encounter. But when our lives, or those of our loved ones, are threatened, we'll spontaneously fight, or flee. And if we're completely overwhelmed by fear, we'll freeze on the spot.

Life finds a crafty way

One of the most powerful instincts, though not for self-preservation, is our libido, our sexual urges that bellow through a bullhorn from puberty onwards. Whether accompanied by love or lust, they guarantee the continuation of our species. But life is not satisfied with simply continuing. It makes sure the fittest win. And to do this it often employs crafty means. Thus, people in long-term relationships that are built on trust and love and economic necessities may find themselves sexually attracted to someone else; and despite vows of fidelity, they may even be driven to have extra-marital sex. Why?

Two British biologists, Mark Bellis and Robin Baker, who have extensively researched sexual strategies, believe it's because life has programmed us in this way.[12] Men are programmed to conquer and monopolise, and women are programmed to diversify the genetic input for their offspring. Far below a woman's awareness, her body is alert to potential mates whose characteristics may offer her offspring a better chance of success than those from her long-term partner. And men, ever willing to conquer, are invariably obliging. Hence, 10 per cent of all children aren't fathered by their 'fathers', even though their non-biological fathers may be better providers and mentors than their biological fathers could ever be.

As Bellis and Baker discovered, a woman is indeed more likely to conceive during a casual fling than through sex with her regular partner. There are a number of reasons for this. Firstly, a woman's body 'times' the encounter to coincide with the fertile phase of her cycle, even though she is unaware of exactly when it occurs. Secondly, life bypasses rational thinking; hence she is less likely to use or insist on the man using contraception on such occasions; and he is unlikely to argue the point. Thirdly, in a biological ploy Baker calls 'sperm wars', her vaginal mucus encourages some sperm and blocks others. And fourthly, her lover's sperm count is at least double that of what it would be in routine sex with his long-term partner. In this way, the intelligence of life finds a way for the bodies of lovers to increase the chances of conception.

Made to order

Another set of strident messages makes sure we satisfy our bodies' daily needs. Undoubtedly the most urgent of these is our bodies' incessant demand for air, and specifically oxygen. As we've seen, the atmospheric oxygen levels just happen to have remained constant for millions of years. But the messages also include such bodily sensations as temperature, hunger, thirst, tiredness, and bowel and bladder fullness.

In essence, our bodies are primed for energy—in the form of air, water and food, and warmth from sunlight—to flow through us. Moreover, those energies are stable, not chaotic. Air is stable not only in its oxygen content but also in its content of ionised molecules, which, as we shall see in Volume 2, are essential for life. The molecular structure and shape of water is stable, without which no life could exist. And sunlight, which drives the growth of everything, including our foods, is stable. As physicist Erwin Schrödinger had once written: 'An organism [has an] astonishing gift of concentrating a "stream of order" on itself and thus escaping decay into atomic chaos—of "drinking orderliness" from a suitable environment.'[13]

Accident or design?

Order, not chaos, is the essential feature of all life and of the universe. The current dogma of neo-Darwinian evolution, however, claims that life is accidental; that random mutations and recombinations of genes, together with the natural selection of those characteristics that are useful, is the basis for all life. In other words, Darwinian evolution, as Arthur Koestler mused, 'appears as a game of blind man's buff.'[14]

In the 1950s the eminent British biologist Conrad Hal Waddington, who had never been satisfied that evolution could be explained as the shuffling of mutated genes through natural selection, had been driven to write: 'To suppose that the evolution of the wonderfully adapted biological mechanisms has depended only on a selection out of a haphazard set of variations, each produced by blind chance, is like suggesting that if we went on throwing bricks together into heaps, we should eventually be able to choose ourselves the most desirable house.'[15]

Admittedly, American biologists Harold Urey and Stanley Miller had demonstrated in their laboratory in 1953 that amino acids, the basic building blocks of life, could have been created in the primeval oceans through electrical discharges of lightning or ultraviolet radiation.[16-18] But the chance of life evolving from a random assortment of amino acids into the myriad life forms we see today is ludicrously small. Even the odds against amino acids combining in a particular order to form a single protein are staggeringly small. To get some idea of this, let's consider what these odds actually are.

The odds of the random formation of life

The 22 known amino acids are the 22-letters of the alphabet that forms the meaningful words and sentences from which are composed the entire literature of life's proteins. Our bodies, for example, consist of perhaps 85,000 different proteins, though some estimates are as high as 500,000.[19-22] (At present, nobody knows the exact number because the focus of biologists in recent years has been on unravelling the human genome.) Proteins form not only the structural fabric of our bodies but also much of our internal communication systems—our genes, enzymes and many hormones—and, as haemoglobin barges in our blood stream, the transport system for oxygen. And the number of amino acids composing each of these 85,000 or more proteins? The smallest is just over 20;[23] the largest is over 27,000.[24]

The odds against insulin alone being created by blind chance have been calculated by James Coppedge, the author of *Evolution: Possible or Impossible?* to be 10^{106} to one.[25] That's a 10 billion trillion trillion trillion trillion trillion trillion trillion to one chance.

Adding to the fluke of life is the fact that all except one of the 22 amino acids—glycine—have a side group of molecules attached to the backbone of the building block, like a sidecar that's attached to a motor bike. In the parlance of chemistry these are *isomers*. In experiments like that conducted by Urey and Miller,[16–18] the side group occurs with equal probability either as a left-handed or right-handed configuration. But, fascinatingly, in all living tissues only left-handed configurations exist. So the probability of a particular sequence of only left-handed forms of amino acids joining together through blind chance to form a small sized protein of 410 amino acids is one in 10^{123}.[25]

James Coppedge calculated that the probability of an average-sized protein of 400 amino acids resulting from a chance arrangement of those building blocks is one in 10^{287}. And the probability of a minimum set of proteins (239) for a living organism being formed is one in $10^{119,879}$. The chance of that happening in the entire history of the Earth, in the past 4.5 billion years, is $10^{119,775}$ to one. To put these mind-boggling figures into perspective, since the moment when time, space and matter began, since the time of the Big Bang 15 billion years ago, roughly 10^{18} seconds have elapsed.

And we haven't even taken into account the probability of the chance formation of DNA and its translating system. Our 38,000 genes, comprising three billion nucleotides—the 'words' of genes—is equivalent to a 460-volume encyclopaedia, with each volume comprising 2,000 pages. Without the double-helixed molecule, that minimum set of proteins would not have been able to duplicate itself; and that would have been the end of the line for life. But as cosmologist Paul Davies noted about the probability of the spontaneous assembly of DNA, 'There are so many combinations of molecules possible that the chance of the right one cropping up by blind chance is virtually zero.'[26]

Certainly, genetic mutations do occur. But only those changes that satisfy physical, chemical and functional conditions for each organism are able to survive. Natural selection takes care of that. Thus, in a process that some scientists call micro-evolution, species adapt to their environments. Bacteria, for instance, readily adapt to antibiotics in their environment. And fish that possess genes for smallness survive in today's overfished oceans because they can swim through fishing nets, while human net-and-dinner-plate selection kills off the big fish.[27–29]

Missing from Darwinian theory is the intelligence of every organism. Life itself has internal control mechanisms—correctors and proof-readers, editors and publishers—that eliminate harmful gene mutations and correct, repair and coordinate useful mutations. In other words, there is a whole hierarchy of internal controls that govern the selection of physical, chemical and biological fitness.

Let's crank up this exercise in improbabilities to the cosmological level. The odds against life, the universe and everything appearing by accident have been computed by cosmologist Roger Penrose to be $10^{10^{30}}$ to one.[30] That's a one followed by a million, trillion, trillion zeros. And the time for such an absurdly improbable accident? According to cosmologist Paul Davies, a mere $10^{10^{80}}$ years![26] That's a one followed by one hundred million trillion trillion trillion trillion trillion zeros! This is fine if the universe is infinite in age, but according to cosmologists it came into existence a mere 15 billion years ago.

Let's leave the final comment about blind chance and life to astronomer Sir Fred Hoyle. In true British style, Hoyle clearly understated the issue when he remarked, 'The chance that higher life forms might have emerged in this way is comparable with the chance that a tornado sweeping through a junk-yard might assemble a Boeing 747 from the materials therein.'[31]

Other explanations

Was the universe and life created through divine selection? Could it have been that out of possibly $10^{10^{30}}$ universes, a transcendent God chose to create this one? Many followers of the Judaeo-Christian and Islamic religions, and certainly those Christians who take a literal interpretation of the Book of Genesis, believe so.

Or is it that an infinite number of universes have come into existence throughout infinite time, and that ours, an ordered aberration, is but one? And that in the fullness of infinite time, long after our universe has been crunched, and after possibly $10^{10^{30}}$ Big Bangs and Big Crunches, we'll all return to live in an identical version of our universe, again and again and again? Ludwig Boltzmann, the pioneer of statistical thermodynamics, believed so.[26]

Perhaps there is only one spatial universe, within which there are many, if not an infinite number of parallel universes, each with its own time and space, matter and energies. Some scientists believe this is the case.

Or are deeper forces at work? Is there something in the dynamics of natural physical processes throughout the universe, as well as here on Earth, that creates order? On the issue of the evolution of life, Waddington and other prominent mid-20th-century scientists, including astronomer Sir Fred Hoyle, physicist David Bohm, biologist Sir Peter Medawar, and anthropologist Gregory Bateson, certainly believed this.[31-35]

Do morphogenetic fields, 'memories' of endlessly repeated forms and patterns of organisation from earlier times, as in the Hundredth Monkey Phenomenon, orchestrate patterns of organisation in biology, physics and chemistry, as British biologist Rupert Sheldrake hypothesises?[36] Or is evolution simply learning transposed to a higher gestalt level, as the British anthropologist Gregory Bateson believed?[35] Could it be that, as Bateson argued, 'mind is immanent in certain sorts of organisation of parts,' in ecology, in thought and learning, in evolution and life itself?[37]

Perhaps the universe is founded on algorithms, on sets of mathematical rules that spontaneously generate dynamic order when complex systems with enormous numbers of components are thrown together haphazardly without any design or selection. Perhaps creativity is intrinsic to the natural world. Scientists who map the laws of complexity with number-crunching computers believe so.[38]

Perhaps the answer is to be found in the very nature of the fundamental constants of the universe: the dynamics of gravity and electromagnetism; the strong and weak nuclear forces, the structures of subatomic particles and atoms, and the warp and woof of space and time, as Paul Davies believes.[26]

Perhaps the penultimate answer will be discovered in superstring theory, in 'loops of superstrings and oscillating globules, uniting all of creation into vibrational patterns that are meticulously executed in a universe with numerous hidden dimensions capable of undergoing extreme contortions in which their spatial fabric tears apart and then repairs itself,' as physicist Brian Greene conjectures.[39]

But why such constants exist or were 'chosen' is, of course, the ultimate question.

Perhaps consciousness, or the divinity, or God, or whatever you wish to name it, not only started the whole shebang but also is inherent in the universe. Eastern mystics and pagans, shamans and witch doctors, and the priests of all except the Judaeo-Christian-Islamic religions believed so.[40]

Thankfully there is not an infinite number of theories on the creation of life, the universe and everything from which to choose. But whether the explanation is God, blind chance in an eternity of universes, blind chance in an infinity of parallel universes, the warp and woof of the fabric of space-time-matter and the dynamics of natural processes, or cosmic consciousness, or any other explanation that arises from asking the 'why' of things—as Aristotle had alluded was the wont of men in his time[41]—the fact remains that order, and, with it, intelligence, pervade our universe.

Does intelligence jump ship when we're sick?

Let's return to Earth. Up until this point your doctor may have generally agreed with the ideas presented in this and the previous two chapters, though perhaps putting a different slant on them. After all, the evidence for the principle of unity is compelling; the movements of energy and matter, though perhaps strange from our middle-sized world viewpoint, do offer an insight into how everything functions; and the intelligence of life is undeniable.

With illness, however, medical science and the vitalistic approach part company. As we've seen, medical science views illness, with its various signs and symptoms and biochemical processes, as bad and wrong. But if we accept the argument that intelligence pervades not only the universe but also our bodies, then why would it suddenly depart when parts of our bodies begin screaming in pain or discomfort? Why would intelligence fly out the window when we experience changes in our bodily functions?

Well, from a vitalistic viewpoint it doesn't; life's intelligence doesn't suddenly desert us when we're ill. The symptoms of acute illness announce not only changing functions but also changing needs. Without illness our bodies couldn't ensure their internal stability, and without the symptoms, our bodies couldn't warn us to change or to grow.

Which leads us to another outstanding expression of life's intelligence, one that is central to our understanding of health: its ability to adapt, to grow and to evolve. This ability informs and directs each species' continuum. In Chapter 12 we will examine this in relation to the human continuum. In Chinese medicine, our ability to reach our full human potential is called *jing*, or essence. In modern parlance we could say it refers to our genetic, bodily, psychological, and spiritual potential to grow.

As we've seen, despite the thermodynamic principle of entropy—which states that energies in a closed system become increasingly disordered and, when applied universally, leads to the idea that all matter becomes increasingly disordered—it is obvious that life defies this principle. Paul Davies, and American theoretical biologist, Robert Rosen, both indeed question whether a closed system can exist in nature.[42]

To state the bleeding obvious, our bodies are not falling apart. Nor are they becoming increasingly disordered. From the moment of conception until birth, as our bodies grow in size, the embryonic tissues of our bodies are transformed into increasingly complex organs and systems. And though our bodies continue to grow from birth until adulthood, our minds continue, or at least have the potential, to grow and flourish until we die.

Thus, for any life, human or otherwise, an individual's life force is revealed by its ability to reach its full potential, as a member of that species—known to Buddhists as its 'Buddha nature'—and also as a unique individual. For us, it is evident not only in our ability to survive, but also to grow and flourish in all facets and dimensions of human life. Though it's reflected in our libido and the sparkle in our eyes, it is also expressed in our aptitude for happiness, our moral strength and mental equilibrium, our power to struggle, to create and to love. And for each one of us, to be truly who we are.

On that lofty note, let's leave the vital force to its own wiles and revisit the meaning of health and disease from a vitalistic point of view.

Chapter 11

Health and Disease Revisited

The more I work with the body, keeping my assumptions in a temporary state of reservation, the more I appreciate and sympathize with a given 'disease'. The body no longer appears as a sick or irrational demon, but as a process with its own inner logic and wisdom.
Dr Arnold Mindell, American physicist, psychotherapist and writer.

What is health?

Health is not the same as wellbeing. Though many people use the two words interchangeably, 'health' implies wholeness. And 'wellness', well, it means goodness, for goodness' sake. Sometimes, paradoxical as it may seem, we need to be ill to be healthy. But the more we satisfy our human needs the more likely we are to feel happy and well.

Health is a process, not an entity or a state of being. Perhaps the reason for thinking health is a state lies in fact that 'health' is a noun; that we either have it, or we don't. But our bodies and minds consist of a myriad of continous events and processes that are ever changing.

Moreover, given that the word 'health' derives from the Indo-European root word *kailo*, meaning whole or intact—as do other words in *kailo*'s lineage: 'hail', 'hale', 'hallow', 'holy', 'whole', and 'heal'—it expresses a *quality* of wholeness.[1] And qualities are defined by their relationships. Hence in many ways, 'health' could be construed as being closer to an adjectival verb (which does not exist in Indo-European languages) than a noun.[2]

And most importantly, health is a positive process at that. It encompasses our whole being, body, mind and spirit. Though we can conceptually fragment ourselves into a body, a mind and a spirit, in reality they cannot be separated. They are indeed the essence of what it is to be human. Hence the whole is greater than the sum of our parts. How we view this interconnectedness depends on our own philosophy and religion, though the belief that we are spiritual beings having a human experience is a good place to start.

Health also encompasses our society and environment. If our land and people are ailing, as they were in the mythical story of Parsifal, then it is going to be harder to be healthy.

Health is the process of maintaining stability when all about us is changing. This includes environmental challenges and the abuse we inflict, often unknowingly, on ourselves. Stability does not mean stasis, however. It is our ability to swing from yin to yang while pivoting around an imaginary centre. Sometimes, striving to maintain stability requires our bodies or minds to endure extra-functional activities, which we know as health crises. Thus resistance to change is an indispensable force keeping us in balance. But take heart. A Chinese proverb counsels us that 'a crisis is an opportunity riding the dangerous wind'.[3] In other words, disease is a time for change. If we don't change, then our vital force makes the correction for us.

Health is the process of stretching the bounds between yin and yang. The narrower the confines of these two, the poorer our health; the broader the range, the stronger we become. If life didn't push the boundaries, we wouldn't grow and our lives would be as bland as unflavoured sago. The reason Indians called measles a 'visitation of the goddess', for example, is because this childhood illness kick-starts a child's strength so that it can thrive in our germ-filled world.[4] The same happens with the psychological and social crises we all encounter at various stages of our lives. They either kill us or make us stronger.

This is why stress is important for health. Without stress we as a species would not evolve and adapt. However, if we simply cope or adjust rather than adapt to stress, then we, individually or collectively, have reached the limits of our continuum. So distress—excessive or long-continuing stress—can kill.

What is disease?

From the foregoing chapters, you know you have a choice here. You can either take the pessimistic view that disease is bad, or adopt the positive approach that disease is part of the journey to perfection. The former view leads to war on disease; the latter to the diplomatic path of trying to understand, firstly what's happening in a disease process; secondly why it's happening; and, finally, how you can help your vital force. Fighting life should be the last straw, and invariably ends in tears; the diplomatic path is far more conducive to life.

Diseases have been classified by modern medicine in all manner of ways, from the traditional disease syndromes that are identified by abnormal signs and symptoms to the more recent scientific classifications based on abnormalities in cellular biochemistry or the presence of microbes. But one factor is common to all. They are all based on the idea that there is a norm, and that any deviation from norm is a pathology. Hopefully, we'll cut through the pessimism and norms and identify what disease is all about.

Disease is dis-ease. It's unpleasant. Often we suffer. It's the opposite of wellness. If wellness is the sunny side of health then disease is the dark side. But disease is not the opposite of health; indeed, it is essential for health.

Disease is part of life. There's not a person alive who hasn't been ill at one time or another. Indeed, from 50 to 65 per cent of our population's illnesses disappear without any need for medical intervention.[5–8]

Disease, as with health, is a process, not a state of being. And it's a process of our vital force. The vital force's purpose in disease is to maintain or restore internal stability. When we're well, it is continuously doing this. But during disease it makes an extra effort to restore stability.

The two phases of disease

Disease has two phases: the resistive/eliminative phase—some would call it the destructive phase—and the reconstructive/recuperative phase. The first we readily recognise because it disrupts our daily activities; the second, no less important, slowly builds us back up so we can return to our daily activities.

In the first phase of disease, the vital force makes an extra effort to resist harmful environmental factors and to rid our bodies of anything disturbing internal stability. Things that harm or disrupt our internal stability include metabolic wastes; accumulated toxins from foods, water, the air, and skin contact; and micro-organisms, many of which thrive on the garbage that has accumulated in the 'soil' of our bodies.

During the first phase of disease, our vital force diverts much of its energy from normal bodily functions to focus on resisting and eliminating harmful factors. Hence the physiological functions involved in digesting food—as well as absorbing, metabolising, assimilating and eliminating food substances—are less efficient than when we're well. The strength of our mental and physical functions is also reduced. For us, disease therefore means time-out from our normal daily activities. Pain and discomfort warn us against soldiering on.

The resistive/eliminative phase of disease processes is yang in nature. If we return to the analogy of our bodies consisting of wood and flame, the flame or activity of eliminative processes is flaring. The wood or substance of our bodies is being reduced, and the by-product of this, the ash or metabolic waste, is being cleared out. This means that fever and inflammation are at the heart of the eliminative process.

Fever can be viewed as a generalised inflammatory process, and inflammation, in whichever tissue it occurs, is simply a localised fever. During a fever, for every 0.55 degrees Celsius (one degree Fahrenheit) that our temperature rises above normal—37 degrees Celsius (98.6 degrees Fahrenheit)—our metabolic rate increases by about 7 per cent. Therefore, at 40 degrees Celsius (104 degrees Fahrenheit) our bodies are burning fuel and wastes nearly 40 per cent faster than normal.

From biology's perspective, the first phase of disease is characterised by catabolic processes. Sometimes called the destructive phase of metabolism, catabolic processes break down complex molecules into simpler ones. When we're well, catabolic and anabolic (the constructive phase of metabolism) processes are equally balanced. In disease, however, in the organs and tissues affected, catabolic processes forge ahead of anabolic processes. Not only do catabolic processes break down micro-organisms and other foreign and harmful substances, they also consume our bodies' ailing cells. Thus, at the end of the first phase of disease we can expect our weight to have reduced.

The danger during the first phase of disease is that catabolic processes may destroy extensive amounts of vital tissues, such as those of the brain, kidneys and heart, thereby endangering our lives. Or they can result in irreversible damage to such organs as the eyes or the inner ear. This is why it is important either to assist the vital force to quickly drain away fluid wastes—and not feed the inflammation with fuel (foods)—or rely on drugs to suppress its processes and destroy micro-organisms. But at the end of the day, even if drugs are needed, they don't remove the underlying cause. Incidentally, radiotherapy and chemotherapy are modern medicine's equivalent to the vital force's eliminative phase, though their destructive power is indiscriminate and far greater.

The junk that is rapidly liberated from tissues by feverish and inflammatory processes must still be detoxified, filtered and excreted from the body; otherwise we'd drown in our own wastes. The main organs that do this are the liver and kidneys. The liver detoxifies the bloodstream, and the kidneys filter out the deactivated garbage. Because catabolic wastes are acidic, the lungs (by exhaling carbon dioxide), together with the kidneys, work overtime to ensure the blood's acid/alkaline balance—the blood must remain slightly alkaline—remains stable.

Other organs also enter the fray, depending on the location of inflammation. The skin, and the mucous membranes, which line the hollow organs (lungs, nasal passages and middle ear canals, gastrointestinal tract, urinary passages and bladder, uterus and vagina), provide a huge surface area for ridding the body of wastes. During fevers in general, and with lung afflictions in particular, the skin clears out rancid wastes by sweating. With inflammation of the gut, the bowels jettison their load through diarrhoea, and stomach irritants are ejected through vomiting. Vomiting also reflexly stimulates the lungs to clear catarrh (excessive build-up of mucus).

During the second phase of disease the focus of the vital force is on rebuilding tissues. For us, time-out from normal daily activities continues; or rather, should continue. The recuperative phase is a time of rebuilding the wood, or yin, of our bodies. If we get into the fast lane before this is completed, more than likely we'll recover more slowly, or not return to our former state of wellbeing. This is a time for focusing on supplying our own human needs, not our financial or family needs.

Positive, tolerant, and negative disease processes

A disease process may be positive, tolerant or negative. Which of these courses it follows will depend on the strength of our vital force, the abuse we have done to our bodies, and the degree to which we help or hinder the vital force when we're ill.

A positive disease process reveals the intelligent and integrated functions of a strong vital force. Known to ancient Greek physicians as the *sthenic* response, such an illness is characterised by strong, energetic processes. Fever and inflammation, together with extra-functional activities of eliminative organs, come to the fore. A rapid onset, and signs and symptoms of heat identify this as acute illness. In complementary medicine this is called a healing crisis. The illness typically runs a fast course and is followed by a quick recovery and improved health—that is, if we assist the vital force. If, with each passing illness, we suppress the *sthenic* process or continue to soldier on, or we don't change our lifestyles to meet our needs, then eventually we run headlong into tolerant disease processes.

In a tolerant disease process, the vital force is struggling to resist and eliminate noxious influences. It is characterised by a weaker response, which, you will recall, Greek physicians called the *asthenic* response. In the wood/flame analogy, the flame is not strong enough to adequately clear out the ash. Modern medicine calls this subacute illness. Consequently, signs and symptoms of heat are less pronounced, but are of longer duration. And recovery—renewing the wood—is invariably slower than in a positive disease process. Total recovery may even elude us. Perhaps we feel weaker and less well than we had previously. Certainly the functions of our affected organs and tissues become weaker. Periodically, extra-functional activities will flare up, announcing, through discomfort or pain or disruption to our daily life, that yet another attempt at a healing crisis is in progress. But if we continue to ignore or suppress each recurring illness, and still deny our bodies their needs, then eventually our health tumbles into negative disease processes.

A negative disease process occurs when the vital force is flagging under a heavy load of long-term distress. Typical of this process are the degenerative changes to organs and tissues in chronic and degenerative diseases. Invariably, such diseases are characterised as being cold in nature, even though from a medical perspective inflammatory processes may be present. From the Chinese viewpoint, both yin and yang, wood and flame, are deficient. Because the gap between yin and yang has been narrowed, small challenges to life, whether they arise from breaking a limb, catching a germ, or encountering changes in weather, can lead to a cascade of problems in other organs and systems. They can even kill us. Although doctors sometimes dismiss such problems as being part of the aging process, particularly if the person is elderly, they more truly reflect the way we have thwarted the vital force.

But no matter how weak the vital force is, it continues to keep us alive. Even in the worst disease, it still tries to improve our lot, particularly if we respond positively to its messages. And though the limits to recovery will be bound by the extent of damage, our vital force can still be strengthened.

PART THREE

THE HUMAN CONTINUUM AND BEYOND

Chapter 12

The Human Continuum

Life is a sexually transmitted disease with a hundred per cent mortality.
Ronald David Laing, Scottish psychiatrist and writer (1927–1989).

Time to take stock

We started this book by tackling the popular belief that our health has never been better, and discovered that, despite massive government funding for our national disease-care systems and the plethora of drugs many of us are taking, our collective health has never been worse. We have learned that modern medicine is not only failing to halt, let alone curtail, the onslaught of the diseases of civilisation, but that it is adding to the toll of death and disease. We identified some of the reasons for the harm inflicted by modern medicine, including the fact that the training doctors receive is all about disease, not health. And we found that improvements in nutrition, sanitation and hygiene, not drugs and vaccines, were the main reason for the rapid decline in infectious diseases. It is probably safe to conclude that not only are many of us are sick, so too is modern medicine.

We have been on a journey to discover the underlying reasons for modern medicine's failure to prevent modern illnesses. Our first sojourn was in realm of knowledge. There we encountered the mechanistic and reductionist mindset of modern science, which has been brilliant in creating modern technologies, but has been an abysmal failure in preventing modern diseases because it is blind to the interconnected and multifaceted nature of life. We also identified medical science's belief that illness is bad and wrong, and hence why it wages war on disease. We then went on to explore the territory of the very thing science has rejected, the vital force. We saw how using the concept of the vital force could not only change our beliefs about life, health and disease, it could also help us to work with, rather than against life to improve our health.

Now we come to the very reason for the modern epidemics, something our culture, and medicine in particular, has by and large chosen to ignore. What is it? Not genes or germs or other gremlins. No. It's the human continuum. Or rather, the distance we've travelled beyond the human continuum.

The human continuum is the place we humans came from, evolved in and adapted to. It's the place to which our bodies and minds are primed. In a nutshell, the human continuum is all about human needs.

The setting

Though we are made of star stuff, as American astronomer Carl Sagan used to remind his television audiences in the 1980s *Cosmos* series, our time here on the shores of the cosmic ocean is but a mere fraction of the Earth's history—about three ten-thousandths of a per cent.[1] Certainly our living roots, as with all life, extend back at least 3.5 billion years, to the time when life somehow found a way. And though the Earth experienced at least five mass extinctions, life continued.

Well before our species was even a twinkle in nature's eye, the world was teeming with life. Despite the diversity and varied complexity of these early forms of life, they all had the same cellular structures, the same helical strands of DNA, the same needs for food, water, reproduction and stability. Year in, year out, bacteria and algae, insects and reptiles, amphibians and birds, mammals and plants continued to merrily reproduce, weather storms, soak up the sunshine, find nourishment, and excrete wastes, just as their antecedents had done for eons. Those species that adapted to the ever changing environment continued. Those that failed died out.

So when humankind arrived, perhaps first in the guise of Homo habilis, perhaps two-and-a-half million years ago, and then later as Homo erectus, the world was much the same as it is today—that is, if you exclude the devastation we have inflicted on the environment during the past century. The world had much the same germs, plants and animals; though admittedly many of these are becoming extinct as we propel the planet towards the sixth mass extinction. Back then the world had the same sunshine, air and water, the same infuriatingly changeable weather and the same rivers, lakes and oceans as it does today.

At least 99.6 per cent of human time span has been spent in the world's wilderness as hunters and gatherers. Even if we figure the emergence of Homo sapiens at 125,000 years ago, as many anthropologists suggest, then more than 90 per cent of our modern species' existence has been lived in the wild. This then is the setting for the human continuum.

Primed for the wild

We not only evolved in the natural world, our whole being is primed and geared to surviving and thriving in the wild. Our very design is the result of the experiences our lineage of antecedents encountered, and indeed expected to encounter, in the natural world.

As Jean Liedloff, author of *The Continuum Concept* , has argued, our waterproof skin is designed in expectation of rain; our reflex mechanisms are an expectation of the need for speed in emergencies; our eyes are an expectation of specific wavelengths of light that bounce off things that are important to the survival of our species.[2]

But having a well designed body is not sufficient for survival. Wild animals don't just lounge around waiting for the world to impact on them. They seek out food, they mate, they suckle their young, and they either flee or fight when danger looms. Even our domesticated dogs and cats, however easy their lives may be, must still interact with their environments.

Trial and error, or instincts?

How do animals know what they need in order to survive? What orchestrates their behaviour? How, for instance, do they know what foods to eat, or when to mate, and how? Not from textbooks, obviously. And not by imitating other animals. If survival was based on learning, then solitary animals and our pets, which are taken from the litter early in their lives, wouldn't know how to survive and reproduce. But they do.

As we saw in Chapter 10, animals' primary instructions for living have been hard-wired into their bodies, as instincts. Learning through trial and error certainly refines and hones the survival behaviour in each particular circumstance, but without instincts life would have failed.

Rats and pigeons that are cloistered in a Skinner cage—a contraption designed by psychologists to prove that trial and error learning is not the exclusive domain of humans—quickly learn how to strike a bar to obtain pellets of food. Even octopuses and cuttlefish learn that fishing nets are a great place to find crabs. Undeterred by the apparent barrier, they learn how to squeeze into the net to get to the food. But without their instincts they wouldn't know which foods to eat.

According to current dogma, however, human beings are an exception; all human knowledge, the dogma claims, has been acquired through trial and error, through observation and experience alone, not instincts. Beginning in the first half of the 20th century and still dominating the teaching of psychology today, this dogma arose from the American school of psychology known as Behaviourism. Leading proponents of Behaviourism included the American psychologists, John B. Watson, Edward L. Thorndike and B.F. Skinner. Watson, the founder of Behaviourism, claimed that nothing is instinctual; rather, everything is built into a child through its interaction with the environment.[3] Thus according to this theory, nurture, not nature is the only factor in human knowledge. Tellingly, the ideas of these psychologists arose not from working with wild animals, but from experimenting on animals in human laboratories and, particularly, from running rats in mazes.

Interestingly, the notion that learning is acquired through random trials and errors echoes the theory of Darwinian Evolution, that life evolved through a series of random trials and errors. Strictly speaking, random behaviour never occurs in any living system, whether in an organism, a society, or an eco-system; the reason being that all living systems display varying degrees of order, as we've seen in Chapter 10, and order and stability provide a limitation on choice.

Nevertheless, the philosophical origins of the idea that human beings are born with a *tabula rasa*, (a blank slate) or a blank mind, upon which all subsequent experiences and observations become 'inscribed' knowledge, began with Aristotle in his book *De Anima (On the Soul)*.[4] The idea was also propounded during the 10th and 11th centuries AD by the Persian philosopher Ibn Sina (known in the West as Avicenna), and the Spanish-Islamic philosopher Ibn Tufayl (also known as Ebn Tofail).[5,6] The idea also appears in the writings of Francis Bacon.[7]

But the greatest impetus for the idea that we have no innate learning, that the only knowledge we have is that acquired through observation and experience, came during the 17th century from the British Empiricist philosopher, John Locke. He called the new-born mind a 'blank sheet'.[8] His idea was quickly adopted by other philosophers, including George Berkeley and David Hume.

But there have been many opponents of this idea, beginning with Plato and Socrates, both of whom acknowledged that human beings have innate 'appetites'.[9-13] René Descartes too believed that humans have innate knowledge;[14] indeed he founded his philosophy for science on his innate knowledge of reasoning: that he was thinking, and hence that he existed (*cogito ergo sum*).[15] He in turn influenced several other 17th century Rationalist philosophers including the German philosopher Leibniz, and the Dutch philosopher Spinoza.

Today, many scientists are challenging the 'trial and error' theory of learning; and they're challenging the theory based on their own observations and experiences, as well as experiments. American psychologist Robert Fantz, for example, noted that newborn babies instinctively prefer looking at a stylised drawing of a human face to the scrambled features of a human face drawn willy-nilly on a face-shaped card, or to a solid patch of black on a face-shaped card.[16,17] As Fantz noted: 'Lowly chicks as well as lofty primates perceive and respond to form without experience if given the opportunity at the appropriate age of development. Innate knowledge of the environment is demonstrated by the preference of newly-hatched chicks for forms likely to be edible, and by the interest of young infants in kinds of form that will later aid in object recognition, social responsiveness and spatial orientation.'[16]

Another researcher to challenge the notion that we are born with a blank slate is Howard Gardner, an American developmental psychologist.[18] His revolutionary ideas have had a profound impact on educators, particularly in the United States, though his ideas have by and large been ignored by psychologists. His theory claims that human intelligence, rather than being a single structured entity, as behavioural psychologists contend, consists of innate multiple intelligences: linguistic, logical-mathematical, musical, bodily-kinesthetic, spatial, interpersonal, intrapersonal, and naturalist. Though the human intelligences are autonomous, they are tightly linked together; and each of us differs only in how easily and how swiftly our particular intelligences develop.

But the researcher to pull all of the evidence for innate intelligence together is Steven Mithen, Professor of Archaeology at the University of Reading in Britain.[19]

He begins his treatise by stating: 'We can only ever understand the present by knowing the past. Archaeology may therefore not only be able to contribute, it may hold the key to an understanding of the modern mind.'[20] Using the analogy of a cathedral to describe the architecture and evolution of the human mind, he has proposed that general purpose intelligence (that of the ability to employ trial and error and associative learning) is equivalent to the central nave of a cathedral. It is a form of intelligence that we and other animals are born with, but it is too slow to enable quick decision-making that was necessary for survival in the wild. To respond rapidly to the environment, animals and people need other innate intelligences.

Over the past two million years Homo habilis, then Homo erectus, and finally Homo sapiens evolved with separate intelligences, like separate chapels to the side of the main cathedral, though initially not linked by doorways to it. Borrowing from the ideas of American linguist Noam Chomsky,[21] who suggested that the speed with which children develop language skills, particularly skills in grammar, cannot be accounted for by trial and error, Mithen has proposed that innate linguistic intelligence is clearly evident in Homo sapiens, and was also evident in Homo Neanderthalis.

The evidence compiled by Mithen further suggests that that there are at least five other knowledge domains than seem to be intuitive and fully active in a child by the age of about three; and were undoubtedly present in early members of our species: An intuitive understanding of living things versus inanimate objects; of recognising that a different set of rules applies to living things versus inanimate objects. An intuitive understanding of physics; of understanding the concepts of solidity, gravity and inertia, all of which are 'hard-wired into the child's brain'.[22] An intuitive technical intelligence used in tool making. An intuitive social intelligence, necessary for interacting with others and managing social relationships, thereby keeping the clan or tribe intact. And finally, an intuitive intelligence about natural history; the ability to create mental maps of the characteristics of the environment (experimental psychologist Edward Tolman had recognised such mental maps in maze-running rats[23]); the ability to identify from visual, gustatory and olfactory cues edible, medicinal and poisonous plants, and the food value of, and the dangers posed by, various animals, insects and spiders; and the visual cues, such as footprints or circling buzzards, for locating animal prey.

Incidentally, the Swiss psychologist Carl Jung had considered such instincts, and all instincts in all life forms, to be an aspect of each species' collective unconscious.[24]

Mithen argues that both technical and natural history intelligence advanced dramatically in the early members of the Homo species because of their need to adapt swiftly to the harsh and ever changing environment.[19] Social intelligence advanced rapidly too in order to meet people's needs for food and to defend themselves against predators; after all, large clans or tribes are better at finding food and defending their members than small groups.

The factor that distinguishes Homo sapiens from earlier members of the Homo species, according to Mithen, is the interconnections that were made between these separate intelligences during the past 30,000 to 60,000 years, as if doors had been created and opened between the chapels of separate intelligences and the cathedral proper. This integration of intuitive cognitive domains ushered in human creativity, flexibility, sensitivity and new activities, evident in cave paintings, artifacts for personal decoration, the creation of totems, and, evident from burial rituals, a belief in the supernatural.

Our intuitive mental modules therefore provide a 'kick-start' for the development of our cognitive abilities. And the integration of various, previously separate, intelligences has created our cognitive fluidity. In other words, we are hard-wired to recognise certain things in our environment that will improve our chances of survival. The role of trial and error learning, as Edward Goldsmith, founder and a former editor of the *Ecologist* commented, 'is not to alter innate behavioural tendencies so much as to enable them to be satisfied with ever greater precision.'[25]

Stone Age instincts

As we have seen, it is clear that our ancient ancestors survived because of their human instincts. Hidden within the unconscious mind, instincts held the tried and true recipe for survival and wellbeing. And through the human senses of smell, taste, touch, sight and hearing, that instinctual wisdom informed our forebears of what they needed.

Carl Richter, one-time Associate Professor of Psychobiology at Johns Hopkins University School of Medicine in Baltimore, Maryland, USA, captured the critical importance of instinctual wisdom when he wrote: 'These forces [dietary drives, or dietary instincts] have their origin in the deep biological urge of mammals to maintain a constant internal environment.'[26]

Today we tend to ignore or forget the importance of instinct in ensuring our health and wellbeing. Instead, we give pride of place to learning, intellect and ingenuity. Certainly, the human intellect is a distinctive feature of our species. We call it 'rational' for it is brilliant at reasoning. It is also adept at scheming up new ways of doing things, and slicing to the heart of many a problem we encounter, thereby helping us to manipulate and control our environment. We see its splendid work in every facet of our civilised world.

The intellect can also be crafty, for it often finds ways to thwart our instincts—like making yourself drink six glasses of water a day, not because you're thirsty, far from it, but because someone said it would be good for your health. The intellect can even rationalise instinctual behaviour that our culture deems taboo—like rationalising human slaughter by calling it 'war' or, even worse, 'collateral damage', or 'a technical failure'. As you can see from these examples, the intellect is readily seduced by ideologies of whatever ilk.

But like the typical doctor we visited in Chapter 3, the human intellect hasn't got a clue how to ensure our health. It has no reference point, no secret recipe. And unlike our ever-active unconscious mind that can perform any number of observations, calculations, syntheses and executions simultaneously, our conscious thinking mind can only focus on one thing at a time. And only when we're awake.

British medical herbalist and one-time public relations officer of the National Institute of Medical Herbalists (UK), Ann Warren-Davis has noted in reference to traditional medical systems in general, and to ancient Egyptian medicine in particular: 'The Egyptians had little respect for cerebral knowledge so highly prized in our Western civilisation, for this type of knowledge dies with the head. They stressed what they called "knowledge of the heart", knowledge which has to be experienced by careful observation. Cerebral, parrot-like knowledge without the intervention of *instinctive* observation easily becomes meaningless dogma.'[27]

And yet, despite the attempts of our civilised intellect to smother our instincts, they are still alive today. Beneath the many health-threatening habits we have learned, it still tries to guide us.

In selecting foods, for instance, the colours, smells and tastes still determine what we eat. If a food is black, blackish-green or violet we may feel uncomfortable about eating it. And with good reason, too, because these colours occur in the flowers, berries and leaves of many poisonous plants—poisonous to humans, not necessarily to other species—including hemlock (*Conium maculatum*), monkshood (*Aconitum napellus*), ivy (*Hedera helix*), dogwood (*Cornus spp.*), herb Paris (*Paris quadrifolia*), pivet (*Ligustrum spp.*), hellebore (*Helleborus spp.*), deadly nightshade (*Atropa belladonna*) and other species of the nightshade family (*Solanaceae*).

For our ancestors, that instinct was essential for survival. In the modern world that instinct is harnessed by fast-food restaurants—they dish out food on white or yellow plates. To use black would spell disaster for their businesses.

Try adding black colouring to your mashed potato and see how you react. More than likely you'll cringe. Now check out the colours and tastes of the foods you eat. You'll soon discover that most of them are white, orange, yellow, green and pink. And the taste is mainly sweet, sour and salty, and to a much lesser extent spicy, acrid, bitter and astringent.

Even though we do eat green leafy vegetables, the excessive bitterness and astringency of the wild varieties have been selectively bred out of them. Unlike the instincts of herbivores and gorillas, ours deter us from eating large amounts of very bitter-tasting or astringent foods. (Though, as you'll discover in Volume 2, small amounts of bitter-tasting foods are essential for health). Besides, cooking leeches out much of the bitterness and astringency.

And red, the colour of hot coals, is still a warning sign, as you'll notice next time you stop at traffic lights; but it also indicates that the red berries of many plants are poisonous: woody nightshade (*Solanum dulcamara*), cotoneaster (*Cotoneaster spp.*), yew (*Taxus baccata*), cuckoo pint/lords and ladies (*Arum maculatum*), lily of the valley (*Convallaria majalis*), black bryony (*Tamus communis*), holly (*Ilex aquifolium*), jack-in-the-pulpit (*Arisaema triphyllum*), red baneberry (*Actaea rubra*), spindle tree (*Euonymus europaeus*), butcher's broom (*Ruscus aculeatus*), daphne (*Daphne odora*), and honeysuckle (*Lonicera japonica*).

During the Middle Ages this age-old method of identifying the possible therapeutic effects of plants from their colours, smells, tastes, and even their distinguishing shapes and features, and locale, was called the 'Doctrine of Signatures'.[28–30] It meant that God or nature had given humankind a sign that pointed to the therapeutic, or poisonous, effects of each plant. Trial and error, together with observation and experience, simply confirmed the wisdom of their instinctual suspicions and hunches, and eventually led to traditional herbal lore that was passed down through the generations.

Babies, stone-agers, and wild animals

Babies' bodies are the least affected by civilisation. Babies are also the only members of our species who are totally unencumbered by learned habits. Nevertheless, their raw instincts of suckling and imitating, and crying when they are hungry or feeling abandoned, ensure their survival. The squawking baby is powerful enough to trigger the mother's instinct to pick it up and cuddle it.

For a few years young children retain that connection to the human continuum. Eventually it becomes a crusty relic of our personal and collective past. But if we strip away our modern garb, our technological marvels and the social institutions that dominate our lives, as well as the 'shoulds' and 'shouldn'ts' that have been rammed into us by our culture, we find that we are still Stone Age people.

Many of our instincts may be rusty, but we inhabit the same bodies, we look out through the same eyes, and our anger produces the same physiological effects. The difference is that we're surrounded and dominated by the trappings of our man-made world. And many of those things are harming us.

Therefore, the secret to what we need—rather than what we *think* we need—for health and wellbeing resides in those hard-wired instructions we call instincts. And the best place to identify those instincts is in Stone Age people, babies and young children. And, for some instincts, in wild animals.

The problem is, babies are dependent on their enculturated parents for satisfying their needs. So at the very least, babies' dietary instincts, and their postural instincts for sleeping tummy-side down—incidentally, most animals sleep either on their sides or front, never on their backs[31] (known in yoga as 'the pose of the corpse')—are repressed by their parents who have been taught that laying the baby flat on its back will prevent sudden infant cot death. Still, we can observe some of their instincts, such as the way they continue to nose-breathe even when they have snuffly head colds—nose-breathing, as you'll discover in Volume 2, is essential for satisfying our cellular need for oxygen from the air.

As for Stone-agers (Stone Age people) they're almost extinct thanks to our culture's 'guns, germs and steel'—as Jared Diamond so aptly entitled his book on the short history of everyone for the last 13,000 years.[32] So unless you're an anthropologist, you'll have no chance of observing them in the wild. But we can glean ideas about their lifestyles, about the way they satisfied their needs, and about the success of those lifestyles, by reading the journals of early explorers. And we know for certain that Stone-agers had none of our technologies, our chemically and electromagnetically polluted environments, our synthetic drugs, our lifestyles. (See Table 6: 'Lessons from the human continuum')

We can also glean ideas about instincts that engender health by observing wild animals in their natural environments. Remember the story in Chapter 2, of zoologist Mike Huffman observing a sick chimpanzee eating the inner pith of the stems of a wild plant? It recovered; and later Huffman discovered that the local Tongwe people also used parts of the plant for intestinal problems.[33] Well, that's an example of how humans can borrow ideas from the instincts of wild animals. Admittedly not all animal instincts and needs are the same as ours, but many are.

The health of hunters and gatherers

Because fragments of bones don't talk, there is little direct evidence about the health of our Stone Age ancestors. Snippets, however, do emerge from time to time. Palaeopathologists now believe that iron-deficiency anaemia, for example, was non-existent, and that osteoarthritis was rare, until the advent of the agrarian revolution about 10,000 years ago.[34–37]

But because bones are unaffected by most diseases, we still don't know the types of diseases Stone-agers had. They were certainly aware of medicinal plants. A grave site that was unearthed in the 1980s in southern Iraq revealed that our Neanderthal cousins were using at least eight genera of medicinal herbs, seven of which are still used by modern-day herbalists.[38,39] As for their longevity, there is some evidence, as we've seen in Chapter 4, that many hunter-gatherer people did reach grandparenthood.[40–45]

However, we do know about the health and longevity of people who continued to live as hunters and gatherers in the wilds for tens of thousands of years, until recent times, when their ways of life were shattered by the onslaught of civilisation.

Aboriginal health

Australia's Aboriginal people had thrived in the continent's harsh and often hostile environment for at least 60,000 years before the European invasion just over 200 years ago. At that time, it is estimated there were up to 750,000 indigenous inhabitants, and around 250 distinct languages, each with several dialects.[46,47]

On their first encounters with the indigenous people, European naturalists had noted the stark contrast between the health of their own kin and that of Aboriginal people: the frail health of the former; the robust health, athleticism and strength, vigour and joyful nature of the latter.[48,49]

Few, if any, of the Aboriginal people had such chronic diseases as arthritis, diabetes or cancer.[50] And though the estimated life span was only about 40, death by injury being the main cause of death, many Aboriginal people did live healthy lives to a ripe old age.[51,52]

A sad indictment of modern ways is the fact that since the arrival of Western civilisation's guns, germs and steel, Australia's indigenous population has plummeted by nearly 80 per cent, from 750,000 to 170,000; 65 per cent of its former 250 languages have become extinct, and a further 25 per cent are under threat; many of its communities are fragmented; and its health ranks lowest in the developed world.[47]

Tellingly, a study on 10 middle-aged, diabetic Aboriginal men from the urban Mowanjum community in the far north of Western Australia, found that after they reverted to living as hunters and gatherers for only seven weeks, all of them had a profound improvement in all of the metabolic abnormalities of diabetes and all the risk markers for heart disease.[53]

Professor Kerin O'Dea, one of the researchers who conducted this study, recently remarked: 'But in addition, I was struck by changes which I could not measure at the time: wonderful changes in people's demeanour. When the people in this study went back to their own land—even for a few weeks—they changed greatly. They were confident, competent and articulate practitioners of their traditional lifestyle. They seemed to physically grow in stature! What I was witnessing was the dramatically positive impact of mastery and control.'[54] In other words, the men's seven-week stint as hunters and gatherers had dramatically improved not only their physical health but also their psychosocial health.[55] Why? Because they had returned to the tried and tested healthy lifestyle of the human continuum.

Yekuana health

One of the last remnants of the Stone Age continuum is the Yekuana tribe who live deep in the jungles of Venezuela. In the 1970s, American author Jean Liedloff spent two-and-a-half years living with these people, investigating their child-rearing practices.[2] She too noted the stark contrast between civilised and Stone Age people, though her attention was drawn to social and psychological factors rather than physical health issues. Unlike most of her fellow New Yorkers, the Yekuana were, and still are, a closely knit tribe who live in harmony not only with their surroundings but also with themselves.

Leidloff recounts the lessons she learned from these people, attributing their joyous and fearless natures to their child-rearing practices. Regardless of a Yekuana mother's daily tasks, children, she noted, were continuously held and cuddled. And as they grew and began to crawl and, later, to play, they, unlike their civilised counterparts, were allowed unfettered space and unlimited time in which to do so.

Though such reports on the psychological and physical health of native people, not only in Australia but wherever they were first encountered by literate Europeans, are sparse, they do provide proof that hunters and gatherers enjoyed robust health.

We can therefore assume that our ancient Stone Age forebears were equally as resilient, as healthy, and as successful in meeting their basic needs as Aboriginal and

Yekuana people were. Our forebears resisted germs and wild beasts, gave birth to babies and suckled them, and recovered from diseases. They even survived a spate of ice ages. If they hadn't been successful we wouldn't be here today. It's as simple as that.

Moving beyond the continuum

As you can see from Table 6: 'Lessons from the human continuum', our modern lifestyles clearly have little in common with those of our forebears. And if the limits to what we, as a species, can tolerate are defined by the circumstances to which our antecedents had adapted, then modern man is rapidly moving beyond the human continuum. In other words, we're in new territory. And there's overwhelming evidence that it's wrecking our health.

Table 6: Lessons from the human continuum

Stone-agers	Us
Evolved and lived in the wilds of nature	Evolved in the wilds of nature, but cocoon ourselves in man-made structures, in towns and overcrowded cities
Lived in clans and tribes	Live in nuclear families, or on our own, in fragmented communities
Behaviour was dominated by instinct and tribal customs	Behaviour is dominated by intellect, market forces, and political and religious ideologies
Lived by the rhythms of the sun, moon, and seasons	Live by the clock
Were physically active	Typically, sit for much of the day
Slept when night came	Turn on lights and sleep according to tomorrow's dictates
Were exposed to the weather and the seasons	Protect ourselves with housing, air conditioning and central heating
Breathed fresh, ion-filled air	Breathe ion-depleted air with a top up of aromatic hydrocarbons, phthalates, brominated flame retardants, and untold other man-made chemicals
Drank pure water	Drink chlorinated, fluoridated water, more than likely with a top up of herbicides, pesticides and xenoestrogens
Ate fresh, wild, whole foods	Eat limited range of 'scientifically-improved', commercially bred, chemically-fertilised, herbicide- and pesticide-sprayed foods that are often processed, with the addition of some chemical colours, flavours, enhancers and preservatives. Recently, genetically engineered concoctions have been added to the menu
Treated their sick people with herbs, or fasted	Give sick people poisonous drugs and hospital food
Protected babies from penetrating wounds	Inject ours with vaccines

Chapter 13

Beyond the Continuum

I do wonder whether there will come a time when we can no longer afford our wastefulness—chemical wastes in the rivers, metal wastes everywhere, and atomic wastes buried deep in the earth or sunk in the sea. When an Indian village became too deep in its own filth, the inhabitants moved. And we have no place to which to move.
John Steinbeck, American, Pulitzer Prize-winning novelist (1902–1968).

An idea whose time had come

Perhaps it was because our cerebral cortexes swelled and we started scheming. Or perhaps it was because someone somewhere was fed up with the untamed life of hunting game and collecting wild plants, and came up with the idea; and then told other clan members about the idea; and the idea then jumped to other clans and tribes until, like the hundredth monkey phenomenon, the idea took hold everywhere. Or maybe it was simply an idea whose time had come.

For whatever reason, about 10,000 years ago, just as the snows of the last ice age were melting, the idea of cultivating crops and farming animals took hold. Across the world, in Asia, the Middle East, Europe, Africa, and Central and South America, people started to abandon their nomadic lifestyles in favour of farming and village communities.[1–6]

We, as a species, were embarking on a new adventure. It was one that would lead to the creation of city states and, later, of empires that would rise and then crumble like children's sandcastles. Ours, with its skyscrapers, nuclear bombs and symphonies, is but a sequence in that saga.

But at what cost to our health? The evidence suggests that the further we strayed from the human continuum, the worse our health got.

The benefits
Human enclaves certainly afforded more protection against an often hostile environment than the old ways. The basic needs of food, water and shelter were more assured. With such security the population would grow more rapidly, and human enterprise would flourish.

Thus, by the beginning of the Christian Era 8,000 years later, the world's human population had increased from an estimated 5–10 million to 300 million; and by the beginning of the Industrial Revolution 1,750 years after that, there had been a further increase of 500 million.[7]

Grains, which were rarely consumed by most hunters and gatherers, except as starvation foods and by those living in arid and marginal environments,[8] became the primary staple foods: rye, oats and barley in the colder regions of Asia and Europe; millet and sorghum in the warmer regions of Africa and India; maize, quinoa and amaranth in central America; rice and millet in China and South East Asia; and wheat became almost universal. In Indonesia and Peru, however, root vegetables became the staple.

For the first time, milk from domesticated sheep, goats and cows became a component of the human diet—at least for the people of the Middle East, Europe, and the pastoralist groups of North and East Africa, and southern Asia.[9-13] There were also psychological benefits from the new diet. Wheat, oats, rye and barley, and milk, contain exorphins, chemicals that, when eaten, elevate mood.[14]

The agricultural revolution also generated new roles for people: farmers and miners and woodcutters collected the raw materials for artisans to craft, and for merchants to trade and sell. They still exist in today's world, though in a more sophisticated form.

The costs

But there were disadvantages too. One that has largely been ignored by medical pundits, perhaps because of its insidious nature, was the impact of the new diet.

Previously, hunters and collectors had eaten a wide variety of wild plants and animals. If the diet of bonobo chimpanzees, who are closest to us genetically, is anything to go by—they eat about 10 different species of food a day, 40 a month—then we could expect that Stone Age people were eating over 200 species of plants, insects and animals throughout the year.[15,16] Certainly wild chimpanzees, which are genetically the second closest animal to humans, eat up to 184 different species of plants and animals throughout a year, according to British primatologist Jane Goodall.[17]

This wide-ranging diet was replaced by a far more limited range of foods, primarily grains and tubers. Aside from the health implications, which we will examine in the Volume 2, being dependent on a limited range of foods was risky. Any crop failure could be disastrous, as the Irish discovered when the potato blight struck during the 1840s. Even today, humankind is dependent upon about 15 species of plants as its primary source of food, and a crop failure in any one would be catastrophic.[18]

Another trade-off for the settled life was the relative loss of freedom that the hunter-gatherers had enjoyed. Primitive farmers had to do more work, and regular arduous work at that, for the same amount of food.[14] Through time, particularly after the rise of the city states about 6,000 years ago, many human societies became more like ant hives. The former custodians of the land, the clans and tribal communities who worshipped the Mother Goddess,[19-31] were swept aside or forgotten. Land ownership, possessions, the patriarchal God, and political, legal and administrative controls, all crowded onto centre stage.

But civilisation was a cruel taskmaster, for it rode on the backs of slaves, soldiers, poor workers and women. And in the wings, psychological and social stresses began piling up. The misery of poverty, squalor, wars and exploitation, both human and environmental, have continued unabated right up until today.

A far more dramatic impact on health was that of infectious diseases. Germs often run amok in densely populated communities, especially if there's plenty of dead and decaying material around. And for many of them sewage is the ideal breeding ground. So if drinking water became contaminated by sewage, epidemics of infectious diseases could easily whip through communities. Added to that was the likelihood that pests and micro-organisms would attack and infect stores of foods, particularly granaries.

The advent of city states magnified these hazards. But there is plenty of archaeological evidence to suggest that people in ancient times were aware of these hazards, because sanitary systems of sewage disposal, and technology to supply unpolluted drinking water, had been created in the first civilisations: the Mesopotamian empires of Assyria and Babylonia, 4,500 years ago, and their antecedent Sumerian and Akkadian states;[32,33] the Aegean civilization on the Island of Crete, 5400 years ago;[32,33] the Norte Chico civilization in Peru, 5,000 years ago;[34] the Indus Valley civilization in the western part of the Indian subcontinent, 5,000 years ago;[35] and the Egyptian civilization, 2,000 years ago.[33] Evidently, even the people living at Skara Brae on the west coast of the Mainland of the Orkney Islands, north of the Scottish mainland, understood the importance of the sanitary disposal of human wastes via latrines and drained outlets; and that was 5,200 years ago.[36]

The importance of sanitation and hygiene was also understood by the ancient Greeks and Romans, who had built aqueducts and other water piping systems, elaborate public bathhouses, as well as efficient sewerage systems.[32,33] And until the decline and fall of Rome in the fourth and fifth centuries AD, the same intelligent approach to sanitation and hygiene prevailed throughout the Roman empire.

But all that changed when the Church of Rome took the helm. Under its rule, the extensive aqueducts and plumbing systems throughout Western Europe fell into disrepair and then vanished; toilets and indoor plumbing disappeared.[37] As California sanitary and hydrology engineer Harold Farnsworth Gray had written of the whole sorry saga: 'Medieval and even modern Europeans, so far as sanitation was concerned, were certainly not above the savage level, and even fell below it.'[38] During Medieval times, human excreta in chamber-pots was hurled from open windows into streets and lanes, making them foul with filth; and in the houses of the wealthy, human excrement from indoor latrines fell through chutes into under-floor cesspools. In England, wealthy lords had installed latrines that jettisoned the excreta of the castle's inhabitants and visitors into the castle's encircling moat. Indeed, a common practice of the time was to urinate and defecate in public places.

Adding to Mediaeval sanitary woes was the fact that because orthodox Christians taught that all aspects of the flesh should be reviled, bathing was discouraged. Even though Roman spas and bathhouses continued, clerics of the

Church made every effort to close them, claiming they were dens of iniquity and disease; stamping out immorality, licentiousness, and depravity had always been high on the Church's agenda. During the 16th century, Church officials even banned public bathing in an unsuccessful attempt to halt epidemics of syphilis from sweeping through Europe.[39]

Consequently, disease became commonplace, and for hundreds of years, towns and villages were decimated by epidemics. But the greatest toll on human life occurred during the fourteenth century when the Black Death (bubonic plague) swept through Europe. It had done so before, during the dying years of the Western Roman Empire, from 541 AD to 590 AD (the Justinian Plague), wiping out up to half of Europe's population. The bacterium, *Yersinia pestis*, was carried by fleas, which thrived on black rats, which in turn thrived on the squalor and filth of Medieval Europe. Peaking between 1347 and 1351, the Black Death claimed 45 to 50 per cent of Europe's population; in Italy, the South of France, and Spain an estimated 75 to 80 per cent of the population perished.[40]

The plague, and the epidemics of cholera, typhoid and smallpox that swept through the overcrowded cities of Europe during the 18th and 19th centuries, were simply the result of poor public sanitation.

Adding to the death toll in Mediaeval times was the ergot fungus, *Claviceps purpurea*, which can contaminate rye. Rye was absent from the diet of the ancient Greeks and Romans, and not until the Christian Era was it introduced into Western Europe. Therefore it was not until the Middle Ages that written reports of a syndrome known as St Anthony's fire are found, the first report being in Germany in 857 AD.[41] The syndrome was characterised initially by burning sensations in the extremities due to the constriction of peripheral blood vessels, later leading to gangrene, and by convulsions, manic episodes and hallucinations due to the neurotoxic effects of the LSD-like chemicals in the fungus. Ergot poisoning was therefore another scourge of Mediaeval Europe, killing untold numbers of people, particularly pregnant women and their unborn babies.

Not until the 19th century, nearly six thousand years after the rise of the first cities, did European civilisation finally get the message that the mix of food and drinking water with excreta, decomposing bodies, and rodents, and poorly-ventilated granaries, is a recipe for disaster.

Adaptations

Nevertheless, the inherent intelligence of the human body did enable it to adapt to local environments. Our skin, for example, changed its pigmentation according to the local sunlight.[42] Those who have the fairest skin, like the Irish, come from regions that have the least number of sunshine hours each year. This adaptation enables their bodies to receive a modicum of ultraviolet radiation for the production of vitamin D which is essential for healthy bones.

Dark skin, which is ideal for the sunny climes closer to the equator, reduces the skin's absorption of the sun's rays. Thus in cold and cloudy regions, dark-skinned children are more likely to suffer from rickets, and adults from osteomalacia (softening of the bones), than their fair-skinned counterparts. However, white-skinned people who lived for much of the year indoors, or away from direct sunlight down in the dark narrow lanes of European cities, were not spared from these diseases either.

Adaptations also occurred in our digestive systems. Normally, only baby mammals produce lactase, an enzyme that facilitates the digestion of their mother's milk. However, when cow's milk became a major component of the diets of people who lived in the cold regions of the northern hemisphere, and of the diets of pastoralists in North and East Africa, and southern Asia, this enzyme continued to function.[13] This was the result of a genetic mutation about 7,500 years ago.[11–13] Today, nearly 80 per cent of the European population carries this gene, and is therefore lactose tolerant.[43] But those whose ancestry can be traced to the indigenous people of the equatorial regions of the world are more likely to have digestive intolerance to cow's milk.[44] Hence, about 70 per cent of the world's population today is lactose intolerant.[45]

Our bodies adapted even to local parasites and germs. Because the viruses that cause measles, mumps, and chickenpox have co-habited with many of world's populations for millennia, these illnesses became minor childhood illnesses, except, of course, for those children who were already unwell or poorly nourished.

In India, measles was even called 'a visitation of the goddess', because the inhabitants realised that it kick-started a child's immunity, thus enabling the child to live a healthier life thereafter.[46] For the indigenous peoples of America, Australia, and the Pacific Islands, however, who had never encountered European germs until the European invasions, these diseases were deadly, killing up to 80 per cent of their populations.[47]

Again, many sub-Saharan Africans, who had lived with the perennial problem of malaria for tens of thousands of years, adapted to this mosquito-borne disease. Genetic changes in their blood cells, which can cause sickle-cell anaemia if a person inherits two of the alleles (mutated genes), had enabled many of those who inherited only one allele to become resistant to the clumping of blood cells that produces malarial paroxysms in other people.[48] Today, from 30 to 40 per cent of the indigenous population of sub-Saharan Africa carry a single gene (sickle-cell trait) that confers resistance to malaria.[49] Having the gene confers on a person about a two-fold reduction in the risk of malaria-fever, and a 10-fold reduction in the risk of severe malaria.[50,51] Nevertheless, according to the World Health Organisation, malaria kills about one million people each year, mostly children in sub-Saharan Africa.[52]

Such adaptations prove that every facet of our bodies, including our genes, are integral components of our ability as a species to adapt. But this only happens within certain limits.

Moving towards the cusp

As civilisation advanced, the aptly named diseases of civilisation began to enter the equation. First there was osteoarthritis—thought to have been rare in Stone Age people—which became prevalent in those who lifted heavy loads, such as farmers and builders, and in those with repetitive tasks.[53-56]

As time went on, new materials and new technologies brought new diseases: lead poisoning in plumbers, potters and painters; cancer, in chimney sweeps; gangrene of the jaw from phosphorus, in match makers; manganese madness, in metal workers; and mad hatter's disease, from mercury.

Nevertheless, the mechanical power for machines came, as it had done for thousands of years, from human and animal effort, from the wind, and from flowing water.

Then the coal-fired Industrial Revolution arrived. For the following century the human race lingered on the cusp, where a 10,000 year experiment with a primarily agrarian lifestyle was coming to an end, and a scientific and technological rampage was about to begin.

Up until this point, the human race had lived within the limits of the human continuum. Now it was closing the door on microbial pollution and the misery of infectious diseases that had flowed from that. And although the promise of an era filled with material goods lay ahead, the new experiment would soon bring far more deadly forms of pollution that would tax our species' ability to adapt.

The chemical deluge

The first populations to be hit by the deluge of new chemicals that rained from the skies and spewed into the waterways, were those living in the industrial towns and cities of Europe and North America. Foreshadowing the epidemics of the 20th century, new diseases began to appear.

Often each disease was named after the physician who first identified it: Parkinson's disease, first identified in 1817; Bright's disease, 1827; Addison's disease, 1855; Still's disease, 1897. Hayfever was first identified in 1819 by London physician John Bostock, in himself as it happened. Systemic lupus erythematosus, 1851; locomotor ataxia, 1858; and multiple sclerosis, 1868. And though rheumatoid arthritis undoubtedly existed in previous centuries, the syndrome was first described by a French medical student, Augustin Landré-Beauvais, in 1800. By the end of the 19th century, however, rheumatoid arthritis, as well as various cancers, were becoming commonplace.

Medical apologists will of course argue that there really wasn't a spate of new diseases; that they had always been around; that it was just that doctors hadn't previously recognised them. That argument, if it is an argument at all, is predicated on the premise that the powers of observation of physicians in earlier centuries were somehow poorer than those of their 19th century counterparts—after all, X-rays, blood tests and microscopy, which added a new dimension to diagnosis, were not available to doctors until the 20th century. Or it's simply the cynical ploy of shooting the messenger when the message is unpalatable, and casting doubt about 'an inconvenient truth', be it the cause of disease or the cause of global warming.[57] Besides, as we saw in the Introduction, the incidence of such diseases has continued to rise unabated, even during the past 25 years. Remember the flimsy argument medical pundits proffer for this inconvenient truth? The ageing of the population.

Up until the end of the 19th century, coal continued to power steam engines that drove industry, though it was also beginning to be used in power stations to generate electricity, which in turn would soon become the power behind all industries. Texas crude, discovered mid-century, continued to provide lighting. And the chemical wastes from the revolution in manufactured goods gushed into the environment.

Within 20 years of the dawning of the 20th century, oil had found a gigantic outlet in the burgeoning motor vehicle industry, the horse was permanently put out to graze, and hydrocarbon emissions were skyrocketing.

An ingenious idea

Perhaps spurred by the discoveries of industry boffins who had created paraffin, kerosene, creosote, aniline dyes, plastics, rayon, DDT, even aspirin, from coal-tar derivatives, some astute European and American businessmen alighted on an ingenious idea: rather than simply supplying the fuel to power industry and transport, and making things from the by-products of coal and oil, why not use the by-products to tamper with life itself.

Scientists had already realised the deadly nature of chlorine and such chlorinated compounds as mustard gas and phosgene. These gases had been hideously effective against human foes in the trenches on the Western Front during the First World War. They had also been deadly, by way of collateral damage, to comrades-in-arms. So, under the Geneva Convention, the wartime use of such weapons of mass destruction would henceforth be banned. Though the chemical ruin on the Western Front would foreshadow the collateral damage from man-made chemicals on wildlife and human populations later in the 20th century, the idea of killing life with chemicals, whether it was germs, unwanted insects or even pesky weeds, took hold.

Did this idea arise from the swelling of someone's cerebral cortex? Undoubtedly not. A vision of a swelling bank account was all that was necessary. And so, with the spirit of conquest in their sails, the capitalist vision of massive profits ahead, and war against foes as the common mission, the agro-chemical, pharmaceutical and weapons industries began to crank into action.

By mid-century man-made chemicals were being deliberately dumped on crops, prescribed to sick people, injected, as vaccines, into well people, and made into even more hideous weapons.

Never before, not in its 3.8 to possibly 4.4 billion-year history,[58] had life encountered pesticides or the chemical concoctions churned out by the burgeoning drug industry. Nor had life ever experienced the vast quantities of chemical fertilisers that were being dumped on fields, or the gases from vehicle exhausts that permeated city air, or the levels of radioactive emissions that resulted from meddling in nuclear affairs.

Unsurprisingly, new diseases arrived in tandem: hyperactivity, 1902; Alzheimer's disease, 1906; food intolerance, 1907; Crohn's disease, 1932; amyotrophic lateral sclerosis (Lou Gerig's disease), 1942; and autism, 1943.

But as we know, the chemical deluge was not about to stop. Government and industry made sure of that. They would seduce populations, as they still do, into believing that science and technology would cure, even prevent, all ills, and create a world full of goods undreamt of by our forebears. The good times were about to roll.

The war on pests

Nowhere can the dangers and extent of the chemical deluge be seen more starkly than in the war on pests. The Second World War had provided Nazi researchers with the perfect opportunity to develop and test, ostensibly on insects, chlorinated hydrocarbons and organic phosphates. Even though less than one in every 1,000 of the estimated 750,000 species of insects are harmful to humans, animals or crops,[59] these elixirs of death had been employed in the post-war years against all manner of insects, in fields and households, schools and swamps. Indeed during the 1960s and '70s, they became the Green Revolution's Grim Reaper for all manner of life-forms (see Chapter 15).

By the early 1960s, however, the hideous error of using organochlorine pesticides—DDT, chlordane, dieldrin, aldrin, endrin, lindane and heptachlor—was coming to light. Besides the damage to wildlife that US biologist Rachel Carson had highlighted in her book *Silent Spring*, they were being implicated in childhood brain tumours, leukaemia, and other cancers, and were known to interfere with our reproductive, nervous and immune systems, as well as our liver and kidneys.[60]

DDT was the worst offender. Its widespread use in combatting such pests as mosquitoes and termites, together with its nature of accumulating in fatty tissue, meant that it readily passed down the food chain. By 1986, not a single living species on the planet was free from traces of it.[61] Though Germany, Hungary and Norway had banned its use in the 1960s, and most other European nations and the US had done so in the 1970s, Australia did not impose a ban until 1987—and not because of health reasons, but because it had been identified in beef sold to the US and therefore threatened Australia's beef trade.[62]

Even today, Australia and many third-world countries continue to allow the use of the deadliest organochlorines—heptachlor, chlordane, aldrin and dieldrin—for crop application and, in the building industry, for the prevention of white-ant infestation. Understandably, Canadian environmentalist David Suzuki would describe Australia as 'an ecological disaster characterised by a squalid history of greed, short-sightedness and ignorance.'[63]

As if insects didn't have enough nightmares to contend with, the organophosphates were added to the human arsenal to make their lives hell. Unlike the organochlorine pesticides, which persist in the environment for well over 20 years, the organophosphates—dichlorvos, chlorpyrifos, diazinon, maldison, malathion, parathion and fenitrothion—are more transient, their half-lives being measured in weeks, not decades. However, they are amongst the most deadly of all chemicals, enacting their lethal effects by disrupting the brains and nervous systems of insects, and of any other being that possesses a nervous system. Seven drops of parathion applied to the skin, for instance, will kill a human adult.[62] Even a single exposure to certain nerve agents, such as chlorpyriflos, can cause permanent damage to our brains.[64]

And yet, these nerve poisons are present in household pesticide sprays, powders, animal collars and shampoos to kill all manner of pests, including fleas and flies, ants and spiders, cockroaches, bees and wasps, headlice and tics, slugs and snails, aphids and caterpillars. In fact, anything alive that's considered an enemy.

In sprays, up to 20 per cent of the residues of these hellish delights, as well as the accompanying solvents, spreaders and preservatives, drift on the air, waft indoors, and are traipsed inside on shoes and clothes.[65] They collect on carpets, furniture and house dust, and persist in these environments for up to a year. Out in the fields, farmers spray their crops, dip their sheep and douse their cattle with them. And so, such chemicals turn up in our foods.

In New Zealand, for instance, 23 of the 26 species of fruits and vegetables sampled in a government-funded survey in 2003–2004, harboured residues of at least one pesticide.[66] Grapes fared worst, with a cocktail of 13 different pesticides. Cucumbers were next with 11, and apples and celery came in third with residues of nine different pesticides. Of the 54 chemicals tested, 18, according to the New Zealand Green Party, are linked to cancer.[67]

As for wheat, up to 64 per cent of pesticides applied to it may end up unaltered in bread; that's hardly the staff of life, is it?[65]

Back in 1973, the World Health Organisation estimated that every year three million people suffered acute poisoning from pesticides, and that as many as 220,000 died as a result of pesticide use.[68] By 1990, the environmental organisation Greenpeace put the annual figure for acute pesticide poisoning at about 25 million, the worst culprit being parathion.[69] Today, the San Francisco-based environmental group Pesticide Action Network North America (PANNA) estimates that as many as 39 million people are poisoned by pesticides every year.[70] But the toll from acute pesticide poisoning, as with the evidence from bio-monitoring studies—that human tissues harbour residues of hundreds of man-made chemicals—merely highlights the tip of the toxic iceberg.

And the quantity of pesticides used throughout the world? Today, it equates to about a two glasses of pesticide per person each year.[71]

Synthetic pyrethroids, the most recent weapon to be added to the pesticide arsenal, have been touted as being as harmless to mammals, as are natural pyrethrins from chrysanthemums. However, of the synthetic pyrethroids, some cause human chromosomal abnormalities, others disrupt male hormones, and yet others cause permanent brain damage in young mammals.[72–76] It's not surprising really, considering that the mode of action of synthetic pyrethroids is similar to that of organochlorine pesticides.

The war on weeds

Just as the battlefields of the First World War had been the testing ground for chemical weapons against human foes, and just as the Nazi concentration camps had been the domain for testing weapons against insects, the jungles and rice paddies of Vietnam became the testing ground for weapons against plants. The weapon? Hormone weed-killers that had been developed by the US military during the 1940s.

During the Vietnam War, US military forces drenched the nation with about 45 million litres (12 million gallons) of a dirty concoction known as Agent Orange, which included the hormone-disrupting and carcinogenic herbicides 2, 4-D and 2,4,5-T,[77] enough to cover a football field to a depth of 3.8 meters (more than 12 feet) of liquid death. Though the purported military intention was to defoliate the forests, the Vietnamese people and many Vietnam veterans were later to discover that these defoliants, which have high levels of the most deadly of all poisons, dioxin, caused cancer and birth defects.

Since then, a vast arsenal of herbicides have been developed but, like the pesticides, are proving to be dangerous, long after government authorities have approved their release. Glyphosate, for example, which is one of the most widely used herbicides (its global use each year equates to about three teaspoons for every person on the planet),[78] has been implicated in non-Hodgkin's lymphoma.[79] It has also been discovered that glyphosate damages DNA in mice, reduces sperm motility in rabbits and humans, and disturbs immune function in fish.[80–83]

The triazine herbicides, such as atrazine, cause breast cancer in animals and have been implicated in human breast cancer.[84,85] The acetanilide herbicides, such as atachlor, are probable carcinogens and are thought to disrupt the human hormone system.[86–88]

Life fights back

Despite the war on pests and weeds and, for that matter, germs, the enemy fought back. Indeed, as in all protracted wars of foreign aggression, the resistance mounted as the war continued. In 1938 only seven species of pest were immune to pesticides; by 1978 the tally of resistant bugs was 305;[89] by 1985, it was 447; and nowadays it's over 500.[90] Weeds, too, mounted their own defences. Today, 186 species of weeds have become resistant to herbicides.[91]

As for the war on germs, within four years of the mass production of penicillin in 1943, some strains of the golden staph bacteria (Staphylococcus aureus) were becoming resistant to the antibiotic.[92] So, too, by the 1960s were the Shigella bacteria, which cause dysentery.[93]

Drug companies in turn mounted another offensive by deploying penicillin's chemical cousins, methicillin, neomycin and tetracycline, among others. But the golden staph soon began to resist these too.[94–96] By 1967, strains of Streptococcus pneumoniae, or pneumococcus (which can cause infections in the lungs, heart, brain, ears and bones) and Neisseria gonorrhoeae (those bacteria that cause gonorrhoea) hit back. They were becoming resistant to these antibiotics too.[97,98]

Enterococcus faecium (which can infect the bowels, heart, brain and urinary tract) joined their ranks in 1983, not only in humans but also in farm animals.[99,100] The reason? From the 1970s onwards, antibiotics had been fed to intensively-farmed, food-producing animals to increase their growth. This practice has been particularly common in the pig, poultry and feedlot cattle industries, and also in the aquaculture business. In Australia, for example, of the 700 tonnes of antibiotics imported into the country each year during the 1990s, 36.4 per cent was used in human medicine, and 7.8 per cent in veterinary medicine.[101] But a massive 55.8 per cent was mixed into stockfeed to fatten up animals. So if meat was on the human menu then the antibiotic-resistant bacteria could jump into the human gut, or their genes could be transferred to the bacteria inside the human gut in a process called horizontal gene transfer (see Chapter 15, 'Chilling Warnings'). And in farmyards and feedlots, the genes can be transferred to farmers through breathing the air.[102] This would suggest, therefore, that inhaling air in a hospital ward where antibiotic-resistant bacteria are wafting, would be less than ideal for modern antibiotic therapy.

And today, the golden staph and enterococci superbugs have managed to defeat the medical weapon of last resort, vancomycin.[103] Indeed antibiotic-resistant superbugs present a clinical super-challenge to a system that has been founded on fighting disease and destroying pests.[104–108]

Has the war been worth it? In terms of efficiencies or savings or human health, clearly not. Despite a 10-fold increase in the use of insecticides in the US from 1945 to 1989, crop losses to insects nearly doubled from seven to 13 per cent.[109] Indeed, US Professor of Entomology David Pimentel has calculated that despite the war on pesky insects and weeds, 13 per cent of crops are lost to insects, eight per cent to weeds, and 12 per cent to pathogens or plant diseases.[110] In total, 33 per cent of crops are lost to one pest or another. And even if all pesticides and herbicides were banned, Pimentel estimates that crop loss would increase by only nine per cent.

In terms of energy efficiency, modern farming practices expend about 10 calories of energy for every single calorie of food produced, whereas traditional farming practices produced 10 calories of food for every calorie expended.[111] And in economic terms, many environmentalists contend that for every dollar spent on the killer chemicals, five to 10 dollars worth of human and environmental damage ensues.[112]

Drowning in man-made chemicals

Today, 70 years after the chemical revolution first cranked into action, over 80,000 man-made chemicals have been created, turned into consumer products, or unleashed into the environment, either deliberately or as by-products of our technologies.[113] Every year, the global production of man-made chemicals has escalated, from about 10 grams (just over a third of an ounce) for every person alive in 1935 to about 40 kilograms (88 lbs) for each person today.

The US alone, which according to the World Watch Institute in Washington, DC, produced 150 million kilograms of chemicals in 1935, and accounted for 34 per cent of global production,[114] now produces 1.5 billion kilograms of chemicals, 19 per cent of global output.[115] That 1,000-fold increase is enough to supply every man, woman and child in America today with half a ton of chemicals every year.

Every week, another 40 synthetic chemicals, on average, enter the marketplace.[116] They're in our shampoos and cosmetics, our clothes and furniture, our household products and appliances and cars. They're in our children's toys. They're sprayed on crops, added to processed foods, and packaged in everything from cheese and cooking oils to takeaway foods.

As an illustration of this, the CAS Registry, a US database of chemical substances, lists over 49 million organic and inorganic substances, of which 35 million are commercially available. Twelve thousand new substances are added to the registry every day.[117]

The tip of the toxic iceberg

For years environmental scientists have been warning us that many man-made chemicals have polluted the environment and entered the food chain, often with devastating effects to wildlife.

Now, thanks to modern analytical methods, scientists are discovering that many chemicals, unsurprisingly, have found their way into us; that we're as polluted as the environment; that our bodies, unlike those of our great-grandparents, are contaminated with a cocktail of hundreds, if not thousands, of toxic man-made chemicals.

In the largest bio-monitoring study ever undertaken, conducted by the US Centers for Disease Control and Prevention (CDC) in 2001–2002 on the blood and urine of 2,400 US residents aged 6 and upwards, researchers discovered that all people's bodies harboured residues of pesticides, plastics and industrial by-products.[118]

Regardless of where they lived or worked, people were contaminated by residues of industrial metals, including cadmium, mercury and lead; a number of phthalates (chemicals that make plastic flexible), some at four times the US Environmental Protection Agency's 'safe levels'; and a range of dioxin-like chlorinated chemicals which are by-products of industrial bleaching and incineration.

Chemicals that had been banned 20 years earlier, but still persisted in the food chain, also turned up in most people: the pesticides DDT and chlordane, and other chlorinated chemicals such as the polychlorinated biphenyls (PCBs) that had once been used in the manufacture of electrical insulators and lubricants.

Admittedly, the residue levels of some chemicals—notably DDT, which had been banned because of environmental concerns, and lead, which had been removed from petrol because of human health concerns—had declined from levels found in a previous CDC study. But residues of the new generation of pesticides, the synthetic pyrethroids, were identified in over 75 per cent of people.

According to scientists at the US-based Pesticide Action Network North America (PANNA), who analysed the pesticide data, more than 90 per cent of those tested were contaminated by a mixture of organochlorine pesticides, organophosphate pesticides—including chlorpyrifos, parathion and permethrin, all of which are also used in Australia—and synthetic pyrethroids.[119]

So what risk do these chemicals pose to human health? Even though many are linked to cancer, or are known to disrupt sex hormones, or cause developmental problems in children, the CDC report simply states: 'The presence of a chemical does not imply disease.'[120]

Other scientists, however, believe this study, along with other bio-monitoring studies, highlights the tip of the toxic iceberg. Mount Sinai School of Medicine, New York, for example, recently found a total of 167 chemicals—the same chemical groups measured in the CDC study—in the blood and urine of nine volunteers.[121] Each person on average was contaminated by 91 toxic industrial compounds and pollutants.

The Washington-based research organisation Environmental Working Group (EWG), which collaborated in the study, warned that 76 of the contaminants are known to cause cancer, 79 cause birth defects or abnormal development in children, and 96 are toxic to the brain and nervous system.[121]

In the UK, every one of the 155 people tested in 2003, in a study commissioned by the World Wildlife Fund (WWF), were contaminated with residues of the long-banned organochlorine pesticides and PCBs—again, known to be carcinogens and hormone disruptors.[122] They were also contaminated with brominated flame retardants. These are present in many modern textiles, electrical appliances and sofas.

A follow-up study on three generations of seven families found that every child was polluted with the same range of chemicals as parents and grandparents.[123] More worrisome, the residue levels in children of flame retardants, and perfluorinated chemicals—present in non-stick pans, coatings on takeaway food packaging, and treatments for carpets, furniture, clothing and footwear—were as high as, if not higher than, levels in their elders. Both these chemical groups accumulate in the food chain, disrupt sex hormones, disturb child development and are linked to cancer.

Recent studies in Australia have also identified residues of organochlorine pesticides, flame retardants and dioxins in all samples of breast milk collected from women across the nation.[124] The studies, funded by the Environment Protection and Heritage Council, found that although the residue levels of pesticides were low compared to findings from international studies, the levels of dioxins were well above the 'tolerable monthly intake' for babies. In fact, they were 17 times higher, according to the Australian-based environmental group National Toxics Network.[125] Again, dioxins are known to cause cancer and disrupt hormones.

Even more ominous are the findings from a recent bio-monitoring study, spearheaded by the EWG.[126] The blood from the umbilical cords of 10 babies born in US hospitals in 2004, collected by the Red Cross, and tested by two major laboratories, contained a total of 287 chemical contaminants. This is an average for each child of 200 chemicals.

Their blood harboured nearly 30 by-products from the burning of fossil fuels and garbage, dozens of consumer product chemicals—including phthalates from plastics, flame retardants, and perfluorinated non-stick chemicals—over 20 pesticides, and 200 chemicals that had been banned or severely restricted in the US.

Of the 287 chemicals detected, 180 cause cancer in humans and animals, 217 are toxic to the brain and nervous system, and 208 cause birth defects or abnormal development in animals.[126]

Exactly how each specific chemical infiltrates our bodies is as yet not known. That is one of the criticisms of bio-monitoring studies. Nevertheless, it's patently clear that the total onslaught is coming from traces of chemicals in foods, water, air, and from skin contact with modern products. And as shocking as the findings from these bio-monitoring studies are, scientists estimate that our bodies harbour over 700 man-made contaminants.[127,128]

Scientific uncertainty

Government and industry have long argued that government regulations, which are based on international standards and policed by regulatory watchdogs, ensure that the foods we eat, the water we drink, the air we breathe, even the things that come into contact with our skin, are all safe.

The public, lulled by government assurances, and largely oblivious to the modern chemical deluge, continues to reap the material rewards, if not the disease burden, of the chemical revolution.

Certainly, government authorities regularly check for chemical residues in foods and water. But traces of them, well below levels of analytic detection, are likely. According to biochemist Alfred Poulos, former Chief Medical Scientist at the Women's and Children's Hospital in Adelaide, it is almost inconceivable that traces of herbicides and pesticides aren't in foods.[129,130] The same applies to chemicals from food and drink packaging, particularly plastics, which US regulatory authorities classify as 'indirect food additives'.

Drinking water undoubtedly also harbours traces of hundreds, if not thousands of man-made chemicals, though regulatory authorities are loathe to announce this. Adelaide's tap water, for example, is likely to contain chemicals from farms, factories, vehicles and treated septic waste water—because from 40 to 90 per cent of its water, depending upon rainfall, is pumped from the Murray River. The Murray Darling Basin does, after all, drain one seventh of Australia's landmass; and though the local water authority treats and filters Murray River water by conventional means, it does not yet use membrane filters (reverse osmosis treatment is known to remove almost all chemicals).

Government authorities are tight-lipped about the health implications of the findings from bio-monitoring studies—perhaps because they don't know. The reason? Very few chemicals have been tested for adverse health effects. According to Philip Landrigan, Professor of Pediatrics at Mount Sinai School of Medicine, New York, where many bio-monitoring studies have been conducted, only 43 per cent of the 3,800 high production chemicals have ever been tested for their toxicity to humans.[131,132] And only 8 to 10 per cent have been tested for their effects on babies and children.

In fact, a report in 1984 by the US National Academy of Sciences (NAS), following a four-year study into the need for toxicity studies for chemicals in US commerce, concluded that 78 per cent of the high production chemicals used in the US at that time lacked even the minimal information about toxicity.[133] By 1997, when researchers at the Environmental Defense Fund (EDF) updated the NAS study, there had been little change.[134] According to the EDF researchers, 71 per cent of the high volume chemicals didn't even meet the minimum testing requirements outlined by the Organisation for Economic Co-operation and Development (OECD).

Adding to the scientific uncertainty is the scarcity of studies on chemical synergism—the multiplicative effect of chemicals interacting with one another, thereby magnifying, many-fold, the effects of chemical cocktails. Hence, regulatory authorities are clueless to the synergistic effects of the thousands of agricultural and veterinary chemicals farmers use. Or to the synergy of the 350 commonly-used chemicals and thousands of flavourings that food manufacturers deliberately add to processed foods.

The trade-off between health and profits

At the heart of scientific uncertainties about health risks lies the long-held policy that man-made chemicals should be assumed to be innocent of human toxicity until the weight of scientific evidence proves otherwise. If risks are identified, initially through animal tests, then industry, together with regulatory authorities, establish protocols and 'safety margins' to minimise them. In other words, it's a trade-off between risks and benefits.

Canadian scientist John Bonine, Professor of Environmental Law at the University of Oregon, captured the essence of the issue when he remarked about pesticides: 'If the costs of using the pesticide are considered to be 90 cents worth of cancer and the benefits are estimated at a dollar's worth of profits, the pesticide is registered.'[135]

Because profits take preference over health, scientific testing and data collection are often skimped. In 1984, a report from the US National Research Council estimated that only 10 per cent of pesticides and 5 per cent of food additives had had complete health and exposure assessments.[136] And a US government enquiry submission estimated that only 20 per cent of registered pesticides had ever been tested for carcinogenicity, 35 per cent for birth defects, and 9 per cent for genetic damage and mutations.[135,137]

Yes, there are international standards, whether for 'minimum residue levels' of registered agricultural chemicals and veterinary drugs in farm produce, or for the 'allowable daily intake' of chemicals in foods, or for 'water quality'. But they are all based on animal studies. The standards are set— in the main, arbitrarily, according to Alfred Poulos—by a 'safety margin' of between a 10th and a 1000th of the dose at which experimental animals no longer show signs of acute adverse effects.[138] Tests on chronic low-dose toxicity, however, are rare. Hence 'guesstimates' form the basis for food and water quality regulations.

In essence, these standards—where indeed they do exist for a chemical—permit traces of that chemical, measured in parts per million, to be present in food and water. Recent evidence, however, suggests that hormone-disrupting chemicals may exert their effects at parts per trillion (one part per trillion is a million times lower than one part per million).[139–142] This figure equates to a few drops of a chemical dissolved in a 20-meter column of liquid covering a cricket oval or a baseball stadium.

According to US biologist Professor Frederick von Saal of the University of Missouri, who has been investigating the effects of synthetic chemicals on wildlife and humans since 1976, synthetic chemicals can trick the human body into responding the same way it does to sex hormones.[143] That can lead to changes, particularly in embryos. 'Whether you're a rat or a human, it takes one-tenth of a trillionth of a gram (of a sex hormone) to stimulate cells,' von Saal told a reporter from the *St Louis Post-Dispatch*. 'That is a level of sensitivity that is really mind-boggling.'[143]

As Peter Dingle, Associate Professor of Health and the Environment at Murdoch University in Western Australia, has warned, 'We have standards to justify the presence of a toxic chemical in our food with very little understanding of the toxic properties of the chemicals and our real exposure to these chemicals and the multiple interactions.'[144]

Even though many studies have identified health risks from many chemicals, governments persist with the mantra that all is well. Not until the weight of scientific evidence proves conclusively that specific chemicals are dangerous, they argue, will they ban them.

And yet there is overwhelming evidence that some of the chemicals used in water treatment are linked to disease: aluminium to nerve damage;[145–147] the by-products of chlorine to birth defects and cancer;[148] sodium fluoride to nerve damage and bone abnormalities.[149]

As to food additives, many nutritionists contend that of the 600 commonly used chemicals, only about one third are safe.[150,151] The safety of 200 others are questionable, and about 200 others, particularly many of the artificial colours and preservatives, are downright dangerous. At least 50 have been linked to cancer, 64 to hyperactivity in children, and 91 to asthma.

Sir Richard Doll, one-time Regius Professor of Medicine at Oxford University, estimated that various components in our diet account for about 35 per cent of all deaths from cancer, and that food additives on their own are responsible for one per cent of all cancer deaths.[152]

However great the risk of this toxic burden is to adults, children are far more vulnerable. For their weight, children drink more fluids, eat more food and breathe more air than do adults. And with their rapid rates of growth, underdeveloped barriers to toxins, and immature body systems, children are wide open to attack from the chemical onslaught. Peter Dingle warns: 'Over the past 40 to 50 years we have increased the number of synthetic chemicals we use with virtually no extra thought as to how vulnerable children are to these chemicals, or how little we know about their subtle and accumulative toxic effects.'[153]

Dingle believes that one of the reasons for the reckless disregard for children's vulnerability is the erroneous assumption that children are just smaller versions of adults. But, as he points out, the US Environmental Protection Agency holds that 2- to 16-year-olds may be three times more vulnerable to gene-damaging chemicals than adults, and the under-twos 10 times more vulnerable.

Despite assurances by government and industry that man-made chemicals pose little or no danger to public health, there are warning signs. There have been for years. Since the 1940s, throughout the developed world, the incidence of various cancers, autoimmune diseases, infertility, autism, childhood developmental and behavioural problems, and asthma, to name just a few, has skyrocketed. Today, thanks to industrialisation and market forces the same disease trends are emerging in the populations of all nations.

Chapter 14

Drowning in a Sea of Electropollution

During times of universal deceit, telling the truth becomes a revolutionary act.
George Orwell, English novelist, essayist and journalist (1903–1950).

Basking in electromagnetic fields

Our adventures beyond the human continuum have not been limited to playing with chemicals. In tandem, we began tampering with one of the four known forces of nature: electromagnetism. Except for the visible spectrum, we're blind to this force, and deaf—and some would say dumb. If it were otherwise we'd probably be blinded by the blitz, and deafened by the roar from modern day electropollution. Certainly we'd be shocked at how pervasive it is.

For millions of years all life forms had been humming along merrily, basking in the electromagnetic fields from the earth, and space, and the air in between. Except for a few geomagnetic micropulsations at extremely low frequencies (the Schumann resonances) these were DC (direct current, or electrostatic) fields.

Until recent times we were exposed only to a very weak magnetic force, far weaker than a refrigerator magnet, emanating from the molten core of our planet. And to bursts of static electricity, at frequencies centred at 10,000-hertz (cycles per second), that bounced around the world from hundreds of thunderstorms raging at any one time. And to small amounts of X-rays and gamma rays, and a few weak radio waves, from the sun and outer space. And perhaps, depending upon where we lived, to ionising radiation emitted by radioactive minerals in rocks. But the most abundant form of electromagnetic energy we were exposed to was ultraviolet and infra-red radiation and light.

Awash in a sea of electropollution

About a hundred years ago we figured out how to generate and harness electricity. The first city to light up, thanks to Thomas Edison's DC electric system, was New York. Then in 1893, Nikola Tesla successfully employed an AC (alternating current) generator to light up the Chicago World Fair. In so doing, he set us on the road to electrifying cities, nations, and eventually the whole world, with a form of energy that had never before been encountered by life. For unlike DC currents, which are surrounded by steady magnetic fields, AC currents reverse their direction in push-pull fashion many times a second, thereby whipping their magnetic fields into a jitterbug frenzy.

In 1901, another of Tesla's inventions, used without acknowledgement by Guglielmo Marconi, sent a radio message across the Atlantic. By the 1920s, man-made electromagnetic waves from the first commercial radio stations, and magnetic fields from overhead transmission lines, substations, and household electric wiring were silently buffeting human tissues. Of course no one could see these energies so their impacts on health were ignored. Not that anyone, at least in the West, bothered to investigate the issue.

Then in the 1930s we began bouncing ever shorter radio waves off the planet's atmospheric ceiling, the ionosphere. The age of long distance communication had arrived.

Soon afterwards, long distance human communication broke down, and the world was again at war. But as we've seen, war fosters human ingenuity. Not only did the chemical revolution get a military boost from the Second World War, so did the electromagnetic revolution. Microwave radar was developed and deployed. This gave the Allies a military advantage over their enemies. It also added pulsed microwave frequencies to the atmospheric fray. But this was only the beginning of the microwave blitz.

Immediately after the war we began deploying the first microwave phone relay towers, and radar installations for the burgeoning commercial aviation industry. Then in 1947, the first television signals, also transmitted by pulsed microwaves, hit the air waves. By the '60s, signals from television masts that dotted city skylines, transmogrified by television sets into entertaining images and sounds, had revolutionised family life. So, too, did a raft of household electrical appliances and gadgets. But unbeknownst to most of us, they were also revolutionising our environment by breaking the pristine silence of large parts of the Earth's energy spectrum.

By the 1980s our lives were again being revolutionised, this time by personal computers and information technology. The habit of staring at a screen for hours on end, a habit that had started when television sets became part of the furniture, became widespread, especially amongst office workers. And with it came a further drenching from the invisible waves.

Not to be outdone by previous decades, the '90s brought us the mobile and cordless phone, and the towers. Like spawns of the Tower of Sauron in Peter Jackson's cinematic rendition of Tolkien's *The Lord of the Rings*, they began to litter the skyscape, peering over buildings and trees, their 'eyes' searching for the faintest signal, their 'ears' straining for the faintest whisper. And because the spawning still continues apace thanks to the roll-out of wireless broadband technology, the levels of electromagnetism in the microwave and extra-low frequency (ELFs) spectra continue to rise unabated (See Tables 7 and 8).

Table 7: Characteristics of Electromagnetic Radiation

Name	Wave Frequency (cycles per second)	Wave Length (meters)	Comparative Size of Wavelength	Natural DC (Electro-static) Fields	Man-made AC(Pulsing) Fields
Cosmic rays	$10^{22}-10^{19}$	$10^{-17}-10^{-14}$	Electron	Galaxies; solar flares,	Nuclear affairs
Gamma rays	$10^{19}-10^{16}$	$10^{-14}-10^{-11}$	Hydrogen nucleus	Radioactive isotopes	Food irradiation
X rays	$10^{16}-10^{14}$	$10^{-11}-10^{-9}$	Water molecule		X-rays, CT scans
Ultraviolet radiation	$10^{14}-10^{12.25}$	$10^{-9}-10^{-7}$	Protein molecule	Sunlight	UV lamps, fluorescent lights
Visible light	$10^{12.25}-10^{11.5}$	$10^{-7}-10^{-6}$	Bacteria	Sunlight	Lighting
Infrared radiation	$10^{11.5}-10^{9}$	$10^{-6}-10^{-3}$	Cell	Sunlight	Halogen lamps, lasers, electric lights
RADIO WAVE SPECTRUM	300GHz–30MHz				
MICROWAVES					
EHF (extremely high frequency)	300GHz–30GHz	1mm–1cm	Fly speck		Microwave transmitters
SHF (superhigh frequency)	30GHz–3GHz	1cm–10cm	Tennis ball		Radar, cordless phone
UHF (ultrahigh frequency)	3,000MHz–300MHz	10cm–1m	Dog basket		Radar, cordless and mobile phones, microwave ovens
VHF (very high frequency)	300MHz–30MHz	1m–10m	House		FM radio, TV, analogue phones
HF (high frequency)	30MHz–3MHz	10m–100m	Football field		Shortwave radio; US HAARP Project
MF (medium frequency)	3,000kHz–300kHz	100m–1km	Airport runway		AM radio
LF (low frequency)	300kHz–30kHz	1km–10km	Small city		
VLF (very low frequency)	30kHz–3kHz	10km–100km	Large city	Lightning	
EXTREMELY LOW FREQUENCY SPECTRUM	3,000kHz–0.1Hz	10m–3×10^{6}km			
ELFs					
ULF (ultralow frequency)	3kHz–300Hz	100km–1,000km	Intercity trip		Underground communication
SLF (superlow frequency)	300Hz–30Hz	1,000km–10,000km	International trip	The Earth and Sun	Electrical appliances, phone tower pulsations
ELF (extremely low frequency)	30Hz–0.1Hz	10,000km–3×10^{6}km	Lunar flight	Schumann resonances	Electrical appliances, digital radio and TV, emergency services' telecommunications

Table 8: Comparison of intensity of EMFs from various sources

Magnetic Field	microTesla	milliGauss
Planet Earth (not pulsed)	50	500
Threshold of sensitivity for bees	0.0026	0.026
Background in average house	0.01–0.4	0.1–4
Background for office workers	0.1–10	10–1,000
Homes near high voltage power lines	0.5–1	5–10
Computers: 30 cm in front	0.2	2
Computers: 1 metre in front	0.1	1
Homes near substations	0.5	5
Powerlines: within 100 metres	6–40	60–400
Electricity substations	270	2,700
Mobile phone tower within 100 metres	10	100
Household appliances:	150	1,500
In front of microwave oven	24	240
1 metre from microwave oven	2	20
Hair dryer	1,000	10,000
Electric blanket	4.8	48
Clothes iron at 30 cm	0.8	8
Cordless phone	5	50
Mobile phone with poor reception from tower	10,000	100,000

Nowadays nearly every human activity involves an electrical device or appliance. The global economy is, after all, based on the use of unlimited power. According to Dr. Robert Becker, a pioneer in the study of both the beneficial and harmful effects of electromagnetism, and a man twice nominated for the Nobel Prize in Medicine, our use of electricity since the days of Edison has doubled every two years.[1]

Becker estimates that the density of radio waves surrounding us today is 100–200 million times the natural level reaching us from the sun,[2] and that the ambient energy from ELFs alone is several thousand times above the Earth's natural background strength. As he wrote in *The Body Electric*, his brilliant treatise on the subject: 'Today we are awash in a sea of energies never before experienced by life.'[3]

A cautionary tale

So what danger do any of the man-made electromagnetic fields pose to our health? According to government watchdogs, and the power and telecommunications industries, none. Standards, they say, ensure that the magnetic flux surrounding high voltage power lines, electricity substations, household wiring and domestic appliances pose no threat to human health. Nor is public health threatened by the emissions from radar systems, radio and television transmitters, or mobile phone towers. And despite, or perhaps more likely because of, public concern, they continue to swear blind that mobile phones pose no danger whatsoever to users.

But, as we've seen many times before, there's another side to the story. Unfortunately, Western governments and industry have been loathe to fund research into the biological effects of man-made electromagnetic fields, let alone to monitor the health of people living near electromagnetic emitters. Only recently have governments been forced to investigate the effects of mobile phone use because of public concerns (and even then, when research does identify risks, have downplayed them). Therefore, the following is at best a cautionary tale.

As Becker had noted, all matter, whether living or non-living, is ultimately an electromagnetic phenomenon.[4] The cellular functions of all living organisms, from slime moulds to humans, are controlled by their own steady DC fields in the ELF range, in particular between 0.1- and 70-hertz. From the moment of conception, all our biochemical functions, in sickness and in health, when sleeping or awake, when growing and healing, are orchestrated by our own whispering currents. They even regulate our levels of consciousness.

Our whispering cells are directly influenced by natural ELFs (the Schumann resonances: 7.83-Hz, 14-Hz, 26-Hz, 33-Hz, 39-Hz, 45-Hz and 60-Hz), as well as a few higher hertz electromagnetic fields generated by sunspots, solar flares and thunder storms. In essence, ELFs are signals; signals from the macroscopic world out there to the microscopic world inside our cells; signals that our cellular aerials, or receptors, pick up and amplify 100,000 to one million times; signals that are then decoded inside our cells by ion oscillators, and then encoded into biochemical messages. In a nutshell, ELFs are signals that communicate by means of electrical oscillations to our exquisitely sensitive cells, which function like tuned circuits in a radio.[5–7]

Our most electrically sensitive cells are those in our brains and hearts, in our immune systems, and, as you'll soon realise, in the organ that some people call the 'third eye', the organ that acts as the navigational system for migratory birds: the pineal gland.

The circadian rhythms of all creatures, for instance, are governed not only by lunar, solar and seasonal cycles, but also by micropulsations in the natural 0.1- to 50-hertz range, known as Schumann Resonances.[8,9] Even the rate of bacterial growth is influenced by minute variations in magnetic fields emanating from different sectors of our 27.7-day rotating sun.[10,11]

Becker hypothesises that because the first organisms were formed when the Earth was experiencing a 10-hertz discharge, all their descendants, including us, resonate at these extremely low frequencies.

So where are man-made pulsed ELFs to be found? In the forests of human habitation, certainly. Cities are abuzz with ELFs. But they are not the only places. Extra-low frequencies are, in fact, buzzing around everywhere. Because of their long wavelengths, ELFs bounce around the world and penetrate the ground and oceans with ease. And so their magnetic fields envelope almost everyone and everything on Earth.

At the 50- or 60-hertz frequencies (the US employs 60-Hz frequencies, most other countries use 50-Hz) they pour out of high-voltage power lines, substations, street power lines, household and office electric wiring, and electrical appliances. In the three- to 216-hertz range, they surge out of mobile phone towers and phones and wireless computers (as pulsed modulations), surfing the crests and troughs of the raging microwaves. ELFs are also pulsating from the new digital radio and television signals. And because today's environment is a wild sea of crisscrossing waves of signals, the synergistic effects of which are unknown, undoubtedly they are also being formed by the electromagnetic maelstrom itself.

No doubt by now you're thinking: Surely man-made ELFs, let alone every other form of pulsing electromagnetic field, must be safe? Otherwise government watchdogs would have banned them long ago; besides, there are standards.

Well, sadly, as with the chemical revolution so with the electromagnetic revolution: mighty profits, together with our collective craving to have more of the good things in life, win over health every time. And this is despite overwhelming evidence, both scientific and anecdotal, that all electromagnetic frequencies, even at very weak levels, do have biological effects (See Tables 9 and 10).

Table 9: Biological effects of radiofrequency/microwave electric fields

Study	Electric Field microwatts per cm²	Effect
Natural background levels	0.0000000001	All life is adapted to this level
Schumann resonance[8]	0.00000012	Governs melatonin levels
Schwarzenburg study[39,42]	0.001–0.0004	Drop in melatonin levels, sleep disturbances
Phone towers and sparrows[220,222]	0.005–0.17	Sparrows desert the area
Frogs' hearts[146]	0.08	Calcium ions leak out of cells
Sydney TV towers[124,125]	0.25	Incidence of childhood leukaemia 60% higher than normal; childhood death rate from lymphatic leukaemia nearly 300% higher; and 10 year survival rate is halved. For all people, 25% increased risk of leukaemia
Spanish phone tower study[24]	0.015–0.45	Depression, fatigue, loss of appetite, disturbances to memory and concentration, circulatory problems
Israeli phone tower study[227]	0.3–0.53	Four-fold increase in cancers in general, 10-fold increase in breast cancer
Background levels from mobile phone base stations[22–24]	0.018–18	Considered safe by the WHO and ICNIRP (50–50,000 times below ICNIRP exposure guidelines)
Phone towers and storks[221]	0.074	Aggressive behaviour, drastic reduction in number of hatched fledglings
Blood brain barrier[159,160]	24	After two hours exposure, blood proteins, including albumen, leak through blood brain barrier
Mice genome[167]	1,000	DNA damage
Rat, mice and human DNA[161–169]	1,000–5,000	After two hours, messages in human cells become garbled. After 4 hours, single- and double-strand breaks in rats' DNA, and mice DNA after a daily half-hour exposure for 18 weeks. And after 24 hours, genes begin to mutate
Rats' brain cell DNA[166]	2,000	Single- and double-strand DNA breaks
Transgenic mice[170]	260–1,300	After 30 minutes twice daily for 18 months, mice developed lymphomas
Mobile phone emissions[13–19,28,29,172–176,177,179–186,226]	10,000–20,000	Headaches, dizziness, irritability, poor memory, inability to concentrate, burning sensations of facial skin, warmth on or behind ear, nausea, weakness, chronic fatigue, insomnia, disturbances to REM sleep, disturbances to alpha brain waves, decreased libido, chest pains, disturbances to heart rate and slight rise in blood pressure
Mobile phone emissions[2,12,30–41,146,159–169]	10,000–20,000	Calcium leaks from cells, DNA breakage and message disruption after 2 hours of exposure. Proteins leak across blood-brain barrier, genetic mutations after 24 hours exposure. Thyroid depression and adrenal exhaustion, disruption to melatonin levels after 25 minutes on phone each day
Cordless phone and mobile phone emissions[170,187–195,204–208]	10,000–20,000	For cordless phone users, the risk of acoustic neuromas increases by 50% after 10 years of use; for mobile phone users, the risk of acoustic neuro-mas increases by 80–300% after 10 years; and for analogue mobile phone users, the risk of acoustic neuromas increases to 700% after 15 years of use. For cordless phone users the risk of gliomas (brain cancer) increases by 50–200% after 10 years of use; for mobile phone users, the risk of gliomas increases by 120–400% after 10 years of use; risk of lymphomas in rats doubles after 30 minutes twice a day: sperm quality deteriorates

Table 10: Biological effects of ELF magnetic fields

Study	Magnetic Field		Effect
	microTesla	milliGauss	
Bees[211]	0.0026	0.026	Threshold of sensitivity
Chick embryos[155]	0.1	1	Major developmental defects
Denver powerline study[109]	0.2	2	Double the risk of childhood leukaemia and triple the risk of soft tissue sarcomas
Electric blankets[123]	0.2	2	Five-fold increased risk of childhood leukaemia
Swedish powerline study[111]	0.2	2	Over double the risk of childhood leukaemia
Residential ELF exposure[94]	0.25	2.5	50% increased risk of breast cancer, 300% increase in oestrogen receptor-positive breast cancer
Residential ELF exposure[114]	0.3	3	75% increased risk of childhood acute lymphoblastic leukaemia
Rat brain cells[158]	10	100	Single- and double-strand breaks in DNA.
Male rats testes[152]	25	250	Decline in sperm count and testosterone levels
Rat brain cells[157]	250	250	Double-strand breaks in DNA after two hours exposure

Early research, conducted by Soviet scientists from the 1930s onwards, had identified that low-strength oscillating electromagnetic fields do affect brain function in animals and people.[2,12] Common symptoms included: depression, learning impairment, reduction in exploratory behaviour and reaction times, disruption to short term memory, and an increased incidence of suicide.

Foreshadowing the recent discovery of 'microwave sickness' in many mobile phone users,[13–19] and among some people who live near mobile phone antennas,[20–27] Soviet sleuths had also identified 'radiofrequency syndrome', a syndrome that included headaches, fatigue, irritability, sleep disturbances, weakness, decreased libido, chest pains and disturbances to heart rate.[28,29]

Such disruption to biochemical signals had also been identified in the hormonal system: depression of thyroid function; initial stimulation of the adrenal glands (a physiological response to stress) followed by adrenal exhaustion; raised blood sugar levels; and disruption to the pineal gland's secretion of melatonin.[2,12]

The discovery about melatonin alone was portentous. Western researchers, decades later, confirmed that exposure to electromagnetic fields, from high frequency fields to ELFs—including those emitted by computers, shortwave radio transmitters and mobile phones (even those fields arising from disturbances in the Earth's natural geomagnetic fields)—did indeed lower melatonin levels.[30–41] This is not all: researchers would also begin to link low levels of melatonin to sleep disturbances,[42,43] depression,[44–46] suicide,[47,48] miscarriages,[49] cot deaths,[50] cancer in general,[51,52] and leukaemia and breast cancer in particular.[53–59]

Soviet researchers had discovered that blood, too, came in for a battering.[12,18] At magnetic densities one-twentieth of the levels stipulated in current US government safety standards, all radio waves produced a decline in red and white blood cell counts and haemoglobin content. And when animals were exposed to pulsed ELFs, the blood-brain barrier—a defence mechanism that prevents toxins from entering the brain—leaked.

Perhaps the most disturbing discovery was that pulsed electromagnetic fields can increase sperm defects and stillbirths, disrupt immune functions, and increase the growth of cancers six-fold.

Western scientists by and large ignored or dismissed the Soviet findings with typical aplomb: the design of the experiments was flawed, insufficient data were presented, the subjective reports from human subjects were too subjective. But lurking behind their dismissal was a refusal to accept that anything other than heat or shock could affect living tissues.

The reason? Safety standards in the West had been based on the belief that the spate of health problems among radar operators during the 1940s and '50s had resulted from the thermal effects of close exposure to electromagnetic fields. In other words, heat, and nothing but heat, was the culprit—and only in frequencies above 27-MHz (VHF); and only when a person was in close proximity to the emitter of these frequencies. And, damn it, the Soviet findings looked very much like an inconvenient truth.

In an interview in 2000, Dr Becker would say of the engineers and physicists who established Western safety standards: 'Their view in general of what living systems consist of is that the cells are little plastic bags filled with minestrone soup. And you can then, with that sort of concept, calculate the field strength and the frequencies you would need to produce an effect on the minestrone soup.'[1]

And so, while the Soviet Union and Eastern Block countries were implementing strict standards, the West was cooking up guidelines for ELFs, and standards for radio- and microwave frequencies (RF/MW), from the 'minestrone soup' model of harm. Physicists and engineers would identify the levels at which cellular heating begins, then reduce the levels by 10 times—or a 100 times, or any other arbitrarily chosen figure—to establish a safety margin, and, bingo, everyone could be reassured that all was well. Indeed, this approach remains the basis of government standards today.

Alas, our standards had been, and still are, based on a shaky premise.

Harm by any other name

One scientist who had doubted the Western scientific assertion that heat was the culprit for the spate of cataracts among radar operators was Dr John Heller at the New England Institute for Medical Research in Ridgefield, Connecticut. So he and his colleagues, in 1959, tested the theory by exposing a variety of living organisms and objects—including bacteria, amoeba, penicillin spores, red blood cells and garlic-root tips, as well as particles of carbon and silver, starch and polystyrene—to a wide range of pulsed radio waves, from 3- to 29-MHz, below the heating threshold.[60]

Lo and behold, the orientation of objects, both living and non-living, immediately changed. Depending on the frequency, some oriented themselves at right angles to the magnetic field, others in line with the field. This was proof that radio waves did affect cellular behaviour.[61]

More worrisome was the finding that 24 hours after living garlic-root tips had been exposed for a mere five minutes to pulsed radio waves (27-MHz, pulsed at 80 to 180-Hz), they had developed gross chromosomal abnormalities.[62]

The implication was clear: if a range of laboratory-generated radio waves could not only change the behaviour of cells but also damage chromosomes, then the same could be happening to the cells of human populations exposed continuously to the whole gamut of electromagnetic frequencies in our global laboratory.

Did the research findings suggest that long term exposure to electromagnetic frequencies could impact on the incidence of cancer? Or birth defects? Or psychological disturbances? Or any other health problems?

The answers would soon be forthcoming.

Harm at work

From the 1970s onwards, Western scientists began to verify, from both laboratory and epidemiological studies, the earlier Soviet findings. They verified that exposure to levels of pulsed electromagnetic fields far below those that produced a heating effect on tissues, and to frequencies below the VHF band, which are known to have no thermal effects, did have biological effects; and, in many cases, harmful effects. In fact, at intensities thousands of times lower than those in the so-called safety standards (See Tables 9 and 10).

Men who worked in high-voltage electric switchyards in Sweden, for instance, were found to have significantly increased levels of abnormal lymphocytes (immune system cells)—in fact four times higher than in office workers—and a significantly greater number of malformed children than expected.[63,64] Power workers in Quebec and France had three times the expected incidence of leukaemia.[65] Among Ontario hydroelectric workers, it was 11 times greater. And the incidence of brain cancer in these men was 12 times higher than that found in the general population.

In New Zealand, too, the incidence of brain tumours among electrical engineers was found to be eight times higher than the national norm, and among electricians four times higher.[66] Similarly, in the US, the risk of dying from a brain tumour was nearly four times higher for workers exposed to electromagnetic fields in the transport, telecommunications and power industries.[67] And the children of such men also had nearly four times the risk of dying from brain tumours; if their fathers were electronics workers, the risk was nearly 12 times higher.[68]

Indeed, studies were beginning to suggest that anyone who worked in environments churning with electromagnetic fields—electricians, electrical and electronics engineers and technicians, telegraph and telephone operators, lines workers, repairers in the radio and television industries, welders, even computer users—had a significantly increased risk of developing and dying from brain tumours,[69–73] particularly glioblastomas (the most common and most aggressive form of brain cancer), as well as leukaemia,[71,74,75] and non-Hodgkin's lymphoma.[74,76,77] The longer a person worked in such occupations and the higher the exposure levels, the greater the risk.

Moreover, depending upon the study cited, such workers had from twice to seven times the risk of developing amyotrophic lateral sclerosis (ALS), a degenerative disease of the nervous system;[78–83] up to four times the risk of developing Alzheimer's disease;[83–85] even a slight risk of developing Parkinson's disease.[78,81,86] And according to three studies, electric power workers also had an increased risk of committing suicide.[48,87,88]

Occupational exposure to ELFs was also being implicated in breast cancer in both men and women. Again, depending upon the study cited, women whose jobs had exposed them to high levels of ELFs—electrical engineers, telephone installers, repairers and lines workers, telegraph, telephone and radio operators—had from 50 to 400 per cent increased risk of getting breast cancer.[89–97] And for men in such occupations, the increased risk of male breast cancer was, on average, 400 per cent.[98]

The same trend could also be seen in people whose occupations exposed them to radiofrequency and microwave emissions (RF/MW).[52,99] Two US studies found that the incidence of brain cancer in radar operators, and in US Airforce officers, was also significantly higher than expected.[100,101] A Polish study of 70,000 military personnel between 1971 and 1985 found that those who had been exposed to RF/MW radiation had double the national rate for cancers; and five times that rate if they had been exposed to higher levels of radiation, though still deemed 'safe' by national standards.[102]

Nor were the unborn children of workers spared. One US study found that the incidence of Down's syndrome in the children of fathers who worked as radar operators was significantly higher than expected.[103] Another study found that the risk of miscarriages among pregnant physiotherapists who used microwave diathermy in their practices was at least three times higher than expected.[104]

Adding to the microwave woes was a Danish study which had found that the incidence of dead or malformed babies among female physiotherapists was also significantly higher than among non-exposed women.[105] A Swedish study discovered that of the children born to physiotherapists who had been exposed to high levels of RF/MW radiation before or during their pregnancies, only 24 per cent were boys;[106] and that a significant number of the boys were underweight at birth—the inference being that MW/RF radiation was playing havoc with genes and possibly with hormones.

Harm at home

If long-term exposure to electromagnetic fields could damage workers' health, then how would people who live near street power lines fare? Or those living near high voltage power lines?

Not too well, according to a number of epidemiological studies. Children seemed to fare particularly badly.

In 1979, in the first study to examine the impact of magnetic fields on the general population, epidemiologist Nancy Wertheimer and physicist Ed Leeper discovered that children in Denver, Colorado, who lived near street power lines had statistically increased levels of cancer.[107] Their follow-up study found the same applied to adults.[108]

Eight years later, US epidemiologist David Savitz, contracted by the New York State Power Lines Project to investigate the safety of powerline radiation, and no doubt also to see whether Wertheimer's findings were flawed, also found an abnormally high rate of cancers in children living near power lines in Denver.[109] Moreover, he found that the intensity of the magnetic field that doubled the risk of childhood leukaemia and lymphomas, and tripled the risk of soft tissue sarcomas was 0.2 microTesla (2 milliGauss)—this is 500 times lower than the maximum public exposure levels presented as 'safety' guidelines by the International Committee on Non-Ionizing Radiation Protection (ICNIRP), endorsed by the

WHO, and currently used as the basis for ELF 'safety' guidelines in many Western countries.

Further studies then began to identify an association between the incidence of childhood cancer and the proximity of their homes to power lines. In Taiwan, for example, researchers discovered that children who lived within 100 meters of high voltage power lines had nearly three times the risk of developing leukaemia.[110] In Sweden the risk for children living within 300 meters of high-voltage powerlines was three to four times higher than expected.[111] In a survey of 29,000 British children with cancer, UK scientists found that in comparison with children who lived more than 600 meters from high voltage power lines, those living within 200 to 600 meter radius had nearly a 30 per cent increased cancer risk. And those living within 200 meters of the lines had nearly a 70 per cent increased risk.[112] Similar findings were also emerging from US studies.[113–115]

Adding to the evidence for harm has been a recent Australian study, which found that, between the years 1972 and 1980, adults in Tasmania who had lived within 300 meters of high-voltage power lines in their first five years of life had a five-fold increased risk of developing blood cancers. And a three-fold increased risk of cancer if they had lived near the towers at any time in their first 15 years of life.[116]

Whether in Finland or New Zealand, Poland or England or the USA, residential exposures to pulsed ELFs from high-voltage powerlines were also being associated with a significantly increased risk of breast cancer,[117] melanomas,[118] suicide, anxiety and depression.[44–47,119,120] And for people who lived within 100 meters of powerlines, the risk of depression increased four- to seven-fold.[44]

Did the ELF emissions in all these powerline studies fall within international guidelines? Yes indeed they did. About 500 times lower, according to New Zealand environmental scientist, Dr Neil Cherry.[121] Before his untimely death from motor neurone disease in 2003, he had collated the damning evidence from hundreds of studies, presented it to international committees, and warned parliamentary committees in Australia and New Zealand about their governments' reckless disregard for human health.

Moreover, exposure even to the pulsing magnetic fields generated by electric blankets was being implicated in an increased risk of breast cancer and childhood leukaemia.[122,123] And what was the intensity of magnetic fields from electric blankets that increased the risk of leukaemia five-fold? 0.2 microTesla—this is 500 times lower than the ICNIRP's maximum public exposure 'safety' guidelines.

Harm in the shadow of broadcasting towers

People who lived in suburbs close to broadcasting masts seemed to fare little better. In Australia, for example, epidemiologist Bruce Hocking and his colleagues discovered that, from 1972 to 1990, the incidence of leukaemia across all age groups of people living in the municipalities surrounding the three television masts on Sydney's North Shore was about 25 per cent higher than that among the population four to 12 kilometres from the towers;[124] that the incidence of childhood leukaemia was nearly 60 per cent higher; that the childhood death rate from acute lymphatic leukaemia was nearly 300 per cent higher; and that the 10-year survival rate for children with lymphatic leukaemia was halved.[125]

Similarly, in Hawaii, researchers from the State Department of Health discovered significantly higher rates of cancer among people living in eight out of the nine census areas with broadcasting transmitters when compared with people in areas devoid of transmitters.[126] In Rome too, residents living within a six-kilometre radius of Radio Vatican were discovered to have significantly higher than normal rates of leukaemia—in children, six times the normal incidence.[127] And in California, an eight-year study had identified increased rates of adult brain cancer and childhood leukaemia, as well as ALS, in residents living close to broadcasting towers.[128]

In fact, no matter which population epidemiologists investigated—whether it was that living in the vicinity of the VHF-TV towers in Oregon,[129] or near the cluster of radio and television transmitters in Sutton Coldfield near Birmingham in Britain,[130] or near AM-radio broadcasting towers in Korea[131]—they discovered the same trend: an increased risk for all types of cancers, particularly leukaemia, lymphomas and brain tumours, among populations living within a three-to-six kilometre radius of broadcasting towers. The risk was also apparent, according to Neil Cherry, even in studies where researchers had concluded—errroneously, he argued—that there was no increased risk, such as in people living to the west of the Sutro Tower in San Francisco, and among those living near 20 other broadcasting towers around Britain.[132–135]

Epidemiologists had also identified a link between exposure to emissions from FM radio transmitters and the incidence of melanomas (a virulent form of skin cancer). Though Australian doctors have blamed their nation's soaring incidence of melanomas on excessive exposure to solar radiation, Swedish researchers discovered that the 20-fold increased incidence of melanomas in Nordic countries during the past 50 years was linked not to sunlight exposure, nor to travel to sun-drenched countries, nor to atmospheric ozone depletion, but to FM radio emissions.[136–138] In Nordic countries, those emissions began in the late 1950s, in the US in the late 1960s, and correlated directly with the rising tide of melanomas in those countries.

To add insult to injury, emissions were also being linked to psychological and physical disturbances. In Latvia, for example, researchers found that a significant number of school children who lived near the Skrunda radio mast, when compared with children who lived further afield, suffered from attention deficit disorder, reduced memory, slower reaction times and less endurance.[139]

And did the emissions from broadcasting towers fall within international guidelines? Indeed they did. Up to 8,000 times lower, according to Neil Cherry. Proof, yet again, that thermal-based standards were, and are, flawed.

And when scientists studied the health of people and two herds of cows living near a short wave radio transmitter at Schwarzenburg, near Berne in Switzerland, they found that many of the human residents suffered from sleep disturbances and chronic fatigue, and that the bovine residents had lower than normal levels of the sleep hormone, melatonin.[39,42] They also discovered that when—unbeknownst to the residents and, probably, the cows—the power to the tower was turned off for three days, melatonin levels rose and sleep disturbances fell; and that when, in 1998, the tower was permanently turned off, normal levels of melatonin and undisturbed sleep returned to the Schwarzenburg denizens.[43,140]

And did the emissions from the Schwarzenburg transmitter fall within the international 'safety' guidelines? But of course. Five million times lower.

Harm in the lab

The extensive epidemiological findings outlined above should have come as little surprise to government watchdogs. Laboratory studies had, after all, identified that pulsed electromagnetic fields at various frequencies caused calcium ions to either leak out of, or flood into, cells,[141–145] even at intensities 25,000 times below those in the ICNIRP public 'safety' guidelines.[146] Such disruption to cellular functions, together with the known disturbances to melatonin levels, would account for the harm identified also in laboratory studies—harm to animal and human brain functions, harm to reproductive and immune functions, harm to cellular growth and development, and harm to DNA synthesis.

For example, when cancer cells, both animal and human, are exposed to 60-hertz fields for 24 hours, their growth rate increases 6- to 16-fold.[147] Sixty-hertz fields also suppress animals' night-time melatonin levels,[148,149] as Soviet scientists had discovered long ago. Long term exposure suppresses norepinephrine (noradrenaline) and brain dopamine levels,[150] male rat testosterone levels and sperm counts,[151,152] and serotonin levels[150] (in humans, low levels of this neurotransmitter are linked to depression).[153] In fact, after a three-week exposure to 60-hertz fields, animals' serotonin and day-time activity levels are suppressed for months.[154]

When chick embryos are exposed to ELF magnetic fields as low as 0.1 microTesla (1 milliGauss)—hundreds of times lower in intensity than that required to electrically stimulate nerve cells, and 1,000 times lower than that stipulated in 'safety' guidelines—they suffer major developmental defects.[155] So it should have come as little surprise to government watchdogs that researchers would also find that the second and subsequent generations of animals that were continuously exposed to 60-hertz fields suffered high rates of foetal abnormalities and birth defects.[156]

And wouldn't you know it, pulsating ELFs can also damage life's most vital molecule, the double-stranded helix: DNA. US researchers Henry Lai and Narendra Singh, hours after having exposed living rats to a 60-hertz magnetic field for two hours—and at levels that the ICNIRP considers safe for workers to be exposed to for eight hours a day—found that the DNA in the rats' brain cells had a significant increase in both single- and double-strand breaks.[157]

Seven years after that ominous finding, Lai and Singh discovered that when rats are exposed for 24 hours to 60-hertz magnetic fields as low as 10 microTeslas (10 milliGauss)—10 times lower than the limits of exposure deemed 'safe' by the ICNIRP for members of the public—they too develop a significant increase in single- and double-strand breaks in the DNA of their brain cells.[158]

The suspected reason for the damage to DNA? A lack of melatonin. The researchers had discovered that this hormone, which is one of the body's most potent free radical scavengers, which removes toxic substances and damaged tissue, and which fights cancer, also protects DNA from damage accruing from non-thermal levels of electromagnetic radiation.[33] And the magnetic fields from ELFs had sent the rats' melatonin levels into a dive.

Experiments on sacrificial, laboratory animals were also providing an insight into how RF/MW radiation could disturb cellular processes. Indeed many of the studies foreshadowed the recent findings about human exposure to mobile phone technology.

For example, exposure to non-thermal, low levels of both continuous or pulsed microwaves—levels that people who use mobile phones certainly receive and those who live within a 100 meters of some mobile phone towers may receive (24 microwatts/cm^2)—cause proteins, including albumen, to leak across the blood-brain barrier.[159,160] And that's after only two hours exposure. For a molecule the size of albumen to breach the blood-brain barrier means that other toxins would also readily leak into the brain. Which, at the very least, is hardly conducive to a clear-thinking, headache-free day.

And yes, as with their ELF mates, non-thermal levels of microwaves also damage DNA. When mice or rats or human immune-system cells are exposed to emissions that mobile phone users would certainly receive (1,000–5,000 microwatts/cm^2), a significant number of their DNA strands snap.[161–164] That occurs in rat brain cells after a single four-hour exposure,[165,166] and in mice cells after a daily two-hour, 18-week session.[167] In fact, in human cells the messages from the DNA command system start to become garbled after as little as a two-hour exposure.[168] And after 24 hours of continuous bombardment, genes begin to mutate.[169]

Admittedly, DNA is continuously repairing itself because of damage incurred from bodily and environmental toxins. Environmental toxins are ubiquitous in today's world; but when the protective role of melatonin is diminished because of the electromagnetic overload,[34] DNA damage can lead to cancer.

In 1997, in a Telstra-funded study, Michael Repacholi and his Adelaidean colleagues made an inconvenient discovery: when cancer-prone rats are exposed to low intensity (250–1300 microwatts/cm^2) 900-MHz fields for 30 minutes twice a day over a period of 18 months—and many mobile phone users have subjected their brains to such levels for years—their lymphoma rates more than double.[170] Even more inconvenient for 'minestrone soup' boffins and telecommunications corporations, was the fact that, five years earlier, US researchers had found that when rats were continuously exposed, for over two years, to much the same intensities of microwaves, the rats had almost a 4-fold increase in primary malignancies. These included auditory tumours, squamous cell carcinomas, lymphomas, and sarcomas.[171]

The smoking phone

So do mobile phones damage their users? Are they akin to the cigarette of yesteryear, an indispensable accessory for success in the modern world, a product whose dangers are hidden, or ignored, or masked by corporate campaigns of smoke and mirrors? Certainly the evidence for harm is compelling.

Many years ago, long before mobile phones were even a twinkle in technologists' eyes, Soviet and Western researchers had, as mentioned above, identified a syndrome in many radio and radar workers they called radiofrequency or microwave sickness.[28,29,172–175] To recapitulate, the syndrome includes such symptoms as headaches, dizziness, irritability, weakness, chronic fatigue, inability to concentrate, memory loss, difficulties with problem solving tasks, burning sensations on the skin, insomnia, decreased libido, nausea, chest pains, and disturbances to heart rate and blood pressure.[17,176]

Now, according to the British expert scientific group, which in 2000 published the *Stewart Report: Mobile Phones and Health*, the intensity of radiowaves emitted by a mobile phone near a user's ear can range as high as 10,000 microwatts per square centimeter for a 900-MHz phone, and as high as 20,000 microwatts/cm^2 for an 1800-MHz phone.[177] Which means that emissions can be 200 to 400 times higher than levels known to disrupt the blood-brain barrier;[159,160] 60,000 to 120,000 times higher than levels that cause calcium to leak from cells;[146] and 7–14 million times higher than the emissions that disrupted melatonin levels in inhabitants living near the Schwarzenburg tower in Switzerland.[39,42] So it would stand to reason that something untoward is bound to be happening behind the ears of mobile phone users.

Depending on the study cited, from 13 to 70 per cent of mobile phone users certainly do report experiencing one or more symptoms of microwave sickness. Common symptoms reported by users include feelings of warmth on or behind the ear, headaches, dizziness, burning sensations in facial skin, lassitude, and an inability to concentrate.[13–16,18,19] Invariably, symptoms occur within minutes of using the phone, and can last for up to two hours or longer. And the longer the duration of a call, and the greater the number of calls made each day, the greater the prevalence of symptoms.

In the largest study, for example, one which had gathered reports from 17,000 Norwegians and Swedes who used mobile phones in their jobs, nearly 50 per cent of those who were on the phone for more than an hour a day reported getting headaches; and nearly six per cent got headaches merely from being on the phone for a minute or two.[13,15]

Are the reported headaches real? And are they due to mobile phones? According to molecular biologist Dr Allan Frey, who had examined the effects of low-intensity microwaves on military personnel during the 1970s, there is reason to believe the answer to both questions is 'yes'.[178] Why? Because 30 years ago he and other researchers had identified the same cluster of symptoms—microwave sickness—in people exposed to low-intensity microwaves. For the US military, that had been an inconvenient finding because they had withdrawn further funding for such research.

So what is happening inside the brains of mobile phone users? You could suspect that melatonin levels would drop. And that indeed is what one team of researchers found: spending 25 minutes a day on the phone did reduce night time levels of melatonin.[40] But that's only one effect. A slight rise in blood pressure is another.[179] Researchers also discovered a significant reduction in the time people spent in rapid-eye-movement (REM) sleep and the percentage of their REM episodes during the night.[180]

How is a lack of REM sleep likely to impact on phone users daily lives? Well, from sleep deprivation studies during the 1960s, psychologists had discovered that total deprivation of REM or dream sleep will, after four days, induce temporary psychosis. In other words, consciousness becomes scrambled. So, partial deprivation of REM sleep will, at the very least, disrupt the brain's sifting and sorting of information about the previous day's experiences. And that will impact on learning and memory. More than likely it will also make a person feel addle-brained the following day. And what symptoms do many mobile phone users report? Poor memory, poor concentration, irritability, fatigue and being fuzzy-headed.

Several teams of scientists have also discovered that the pulsed modulated signals from mobile phones affect brain waves (as measured by an electroencephalograph), particularly alpha waves, not only during sleep,[181] but also during waking hours.[182-186] The implications for brain function, however, are as yet unclear.

But by far the most worrisome finding has come from a team of Swedish researchers headed by cancer specialist Professor Lennart Hardell. From over a dozen studies conducted during the past 10 years they have found a direct link between the use of all wireless phones—analogue and digital mobile phones, as well as cordless phones—and both benign and malignant brain tumours; specifically, acoustic neuroma (a benign tumour behind the ear) and glioma (a virulent form of brain cancer).[187-195]

No matter which way the researchers examined wireless phone use, whether by cumulative hours or years of use, or by cumulative years of using a wireless phone on the same side of the head as the tumour, and regardless of whether a person used an analogue or digital mobile phone or a cordless phone, or a combination thereof, the message was clear: the longer a person had spent on a wireless phone each day, and the greater the number of years he had done so, particularly if he had used the phone on one ear only, the greater the odds of that person getting a brain tumour.

After 10 years of one-sided use of a cordless phone, for example, a person had up to a 50 per cent greater chance of getting an acoustic neuroma than a non-user.[193] For a mobile phone user, the risk soared from 200 and 300 per cent higher.[195] And after 15 years of using an analogue phone, a person had up to a 700 per cent greater risk of getting an acoustic neuroma than someone who had never used a wireless phone.[190]

The chance of developing brain cancer (glioma), however, was even greater. For a cordless phone user who had used the device for at least 10 years, the chances of getting brain cancer, as compared to the chances for a non-user, ranged from 50 to nearly 200 per cent greater.[187,191,194] For a mobile phone user, the risk is up to 400 per cent higher than for non-users.[195]

Even worse, wireless phone users were at greatest risk of getting high-grade gliomas, the most virulent form of brain cancer.[190,194] The people at greatest risk were the people who undoubtedly have the greatest addiction to wireless phones, those who had started using the devices in their teens: the current 20- to 29-year-olds.[188]

Curiously enough, other teams of researchers—those whose studies have been substantially funded by mobile phone manufacturers and telecommunications operators in what is called the Interphone International Study—failed to find a link between mobile phone use and brain tumours, at least in the short term.

But as with all studies that have been partially or wholly funded by industry, whether they were tobacco industry-funded studies on passive smoking, or pharmaceutical industry-funded drug trials, researchers are far more likely to arrive at pro-industry conclusions than reseachers who are independent of such funding.[196–202] Remember the studies on vaccines we examined in Chapter 5? So it should come as little surprise that a recent review of research conducted during the past decade on the health effects of mobile phones would find that industry-funded research was nine times more likely to come to conclusions that support the telecommunication industry's agenda than do independent studies.[203]

Nevertheless, three of the Interphone studies published to date have found evidence for harm. After 10 years of using a mobile phone on one ear, people have an 80 per cent increased risk of developing acoustic neuromas, according to one study,[204] and another study found a near 300 per cent increased risk.[205] A third study found that people who use mobile phones for more than 10 years have a 120 per cent increased risk of getting brain cancer (glioma).[206]

The most alarming point about these findings is the short time frame of exposure for tumours to develop. Asbestos-related mesothelioma, and smoking-related lung cancer can take 30 or more years of exposure, but for mobile phones brain tumours begin to develop in as little as seven to 10 years.

And finally, to add to the woes of mobile phone addicts, two recent studies have found that sperm quality in males deteriorates in direct relationship to the amount of time a man spends on the phone.[207,208]

The birds and the bees

Today, one third of humanity uses a mobile phone. At any one moment, tens of millions of conversations and messages, not to mention billions of bytes of data from wireless-broadband Internet connections, are being sent and received via the 1.5 million base stations that cover the planet with a fine mesh of microwaves. And the numbers are rapidly increasing thanks to the roll out of the third generation (3G) technology. Hence the background levels of microwaves today are from 150 million to 150 billion times higher than those 100 years ago, when the only sources were the sun and the Milky Way. And everyone is in the crossfire.

In bygone days, before the advent of scientific instruments, miners would rely on their feathered friend, the canary, to alert them to deadly air: when the canary toppled from its perch, it was time to skedaddle. Today, the warning signs that telecommunication emissions may be causing harm come from those creatures that are particularly sensitive to electromagnetic radiation, the birds and the bees.

Bees, for instance, possess minuscule particles of magnetite (iron oxide) in their abdomens that readily absorb microwaves.[209,210] They are also incredibly sensitive to ELF magnetic fields.[211,212] Hence bees are constantly picking up our telecommunications signals. Pulsed ELFs can even send them into a rage in which they sting one another to death.[213, 214] Even more disconcerting is the fact that ELFs around 250-hertz—which just happen to correspond to the pulsed modulations from base stations—are known to disrupt bees' navigation systems, causing their flight paths back to the hive to deviate by up to 10 degrees.[215] Which means, they get lost.

Adding to the evidence that bees can get lost in the microwave blitz are two recent German studies. The researchers found that bees in hives subjected to emissions from a cordless phone on standby mode are significantly less likely to return to their hives than bees from hives spared such interference.[216,217]

So how are bees faring with the microwave onslaught and their accompanying low-frequency blasts?

Well, coincidentally or not, ever since mobile phone towers became part of the landscape, billions of bees have vanished. Britain today, for instance, has lost 57 per cent of its pollinating insects when compared with the number and variety of such insects hovering around in 1980.[218] And the highest loss has been among the busiest of pollinators, the ones who do 80 per cent of the work, wild bees. Ominously, the flowers they pollinate have also declined in number. The news from the Netherlands is even worse. Since 1980 the diversity of its specialist wild bees has declined by 67 per cent.

Meanwhile, over in the United States, many bee keepers began noticing in 2006 that honey bees were deserting their hives. Called Colony Collapse Disorder, the syndrome of vanishing bees has now destroyed 60 per cent of hives on the West Coast, and 70 per cent on the East Coast. The same phenomenon is also happening in Britain, Germany, Spain, Italy, and Greece. The reason? No one knows though the official story is that the Varroa mite is to blame. But there are suspicions that the collapse of bees' immune systems is the result of one factor: the microwave blitz.

Some researchers have noted that the disappearance of bees in North America in 2006 coincided with the four-fold increase in emissions from the HAARP project installation (High-Frequency Active Auroral Research Project) operated by the US Airforce and Navy, in Alaska. Now using 3.6 million watts of energy, and emitting in the 2.5- to 10-MHz frequencies, it is the most powerful transmitter on Earth.[212]

Ominously, honey bees are essential for the pollination of 90 crop species, about 30 per cent of our foods.

As for birds, they too are disappearing, or at least millions of them have winged their way to habitats far removed from the towers. In Belgium, for instance, researchers identified far fewer breeding sparrows within 400 meters of mobile phone towers that in areas further afield.[219] And in the Spanish city of Valladolid, environmental biologist Alfonso Balmori has documented the rapid decline in the numbers of the city's sparrows, white wagtails, kestrels, rock doves, collared doves, bats, starlings, and white storks.[220] The retreat began, despite a reduction in the city's air pollution, with the arrival of the microwave blitz in the late 1990s. Balmori has noted that white storks, which are loath to abandon their nesting places, produce far fewer hatchlings, and are far more aggressive to one another, if they nest within 300 meters of the towers.[221]

But by far the starkest sign of bird dissatisfaction is to be seen in Britain. Since time immemorial, the house sparrow has been the feathered friend of city dwellers. But not any more. About two thirds of them have decided to abandon the places where the microwave blitz is at its most intense, the large cities, and migrate to small towns and other regions with less blitz. London, for instance, in just six years, between 1994 and 2000, lost 60 per cent of its house sparrows.[222]

The news is not all bad, however. By 2001 Scotland had begun to buck the nationwide trend with a 20 per cent increase in its numbers of sparrows.[223] Tellingly, over a third of the Scottish local planning authorities had decided in November 1999 to adopt the precautionary principle and keep mobile phone towers away from schools and residential areas. For house sparrows, that would have come as a welcome relief.

Not that any of this should have come as a surprise, at least to ornithologists. They knew 40 years ago that birds detest non-thermal levels of microwaves, and that they demonstrate their displeasure by escaping.[224,225]

In the shadow of the phone towers

Given that our buzzing and feathered friends are winging their way to other lands, if not other worlds, how are human denizens faring with the microwave blitz? For many of those living within 300 to 400 meters of base stations, not well. At least that's the evidence to date. Again, microwave sickness emerges as the accursed visitor.

No matter which group of towerside-dwellers researchers have questioned—whether it has been those in the French city of Villeurbanne,[20,21] those in Vienna or out in the rural landscape of the south Austrian district of Carinthia,[22] those nestled on the hillside beneath the two towers in the Spanish village of La Nora,[23,24] those cloistered in the Polish city of Łódź,[25] or those in the buildings beneath or opposite the first tower to be erected in the north Egyptian city of Shebin El-Kom[26]—they have found that many of the people experience symptoms of microwave sickness. The closer people live to a tower, the greater the prevalence and severity of symptoms.

According to the French study, for instance, people who lived 300 meters away from towers were 40 per cent more likely to feel tired than people living further afield.[20,21] At 200 meters, the trend was for the added curse of increased headaches and sleep disturbances. As for people who were unfortunate enough to reside within 100 meters of the blasting antennas, they were far more likely to experience not only the above symptoms but also to feel irritable or depressed, to have difficulty concentrating and remembering, and to find that their libidos were wilting. And the people most affected by the rays were women and the elderly.

From the Austrian study, the major finding was that 15 per cent of people who lived near phone towers, and who received microwave intensities on average nearly 1,600 times lower than those deemed safe by the ICNIRP, suffered from cardiovascular symptoms.[22]

Similarly, the Spanish study found that even though people who lived within 150 meters of a tower received in their bedrooms microwave intensities 2,000 to 50,000 times lower than those deemed safe by the ICNIRP, they nevertheless were over 60 times more likely to suffer from depression, and 40 times more likely to suffer from fatigue, than people who lived more than 250 meters from a tower.[23,24] Even when microwave intensities were as much as 1.5 million times lower than those considered safe by the ICNIRP (0.0006 to 0.00128 microwatts per square centimeter), people still suffered from fatigue, depression, sleep disturbances, concentration difficulties and cardiovascular problems.

In fact, concerns about the health implications identified in the Spanish study prompted the government of Salzburg in 2002 to tighten its standards. The permissible emission levels from base stations in Salzburg today are 9,000 times below those recommended by the ICNIRP.

Adding to the weight of evidence for harm are the findings of two experimental studies. The first, a Dutch study, found that a significant number of people feel unwell when exposed to emissions from 3G base stations, though not from GSM stations.[27] In the second study, conducted in the Rudolf Steiner School in Salzburg, 80 meters in the direct line of fire from a mobile phone antenna, researchers were able to directly link disturbances in wellbeing in electrosensitive people to changes in their alpha and beta brain-waves.[226] And that occurred at levels 3,000 times below the ICNIRP's guidelines for public exposure (0.3 microwatts per square centimeter).

Unfortunately, to date only two studies have investigated the incidence of cancer among people living near towers. But both should set alarm bells ringing, if not among health authorities then certainly among towerside-dwellers.

In the Israeli city of Netanya, two doctors discovered that the incidence of new cases of cancer among the people who lived 350 meters from a base station—a base station that had been commissioned only a year before the study began—was double the rate for people living further afield, and four times the national rate.[227] The residents at greatest risk were women who, in comparison with the population at large, had over 10 times the rate of recently-diagnosed cancers.

Meanwhile, a study commissioned by the German Federal Government found that the rate of cancers, including malignant brain tumours, among people who lived within 400 meters of a tower in the Bavarian town of Naila, Oberfranken—a tower than been operating for only five years—had tripled, and occurred at a younger age.[228]

Standards for safety or for profits?

Given all this evidence, it's not surprising that in recent years some nations—notably Switzerland, Italy, Belgium and Greece, as well as the city of Salzburg in Austria—would adopt the precautionary principle and set standards with exposure levels hundreds, if not thousands of times lower than those of other Western European nations. The public health policy adopted by these nations recognises that the dose of electromagnetic fields, even non-thermal doses, to which the public are exposed should be as low as is technically possible. Sixty years ago, China, Russia and other Eastern European nations had, on the basis of their scientific studies, done the same.

Nor should it come as a surprise that at least some government watchdogs would alert their political masters to the dangers of the electromagnetic blitz; that the US Environmental Protection Agency (EPA), having spent two years reviewing the evidence for harm, would conclude in a draft report in 1990— which was leaked to Louis Slesin, editor of the influential newsletter *Microwave News*—that radio-frequency and microwave radiation should be classified as 'a possible human carcinogen', and that power-frequency ELFs should be classified as 'a probable human carcinogen', alongside formaldehyde, dioxins, DDT and PCBs.[229]

It's also unsurprising that the US National Institute of Environmental Health Sciences (NIEH) would, in 1998, evaluate exposure to power-frequency ELFs as 'a possible human carcinogen';[230] that the California Department of Health Services, having acknowledged that EMFs can increase the risk of childhood leukaemia, amyotrophic lateral sclerosis (Lou Gehrig's disease) and miscarriage, would, in 2002, evaluate exposure to ELFs as 'a possible carcinogen';[128] and that the

International Agency for Research on Cancer (IARC), having previously refused to acknowledge any link between magnetic fields and cancer, would, in 2002, finally classify ELFs as a 'possible carcinogen'.[231]

But given the track record of Western governments, of putting profits before health, it should come as little surprise that the administration of President George H. Bush, through the White House Office of Policy Development, would exert pressure on the nation's environmental watchdog, the EPA, to delete from its final report any mention of harm.[232]

It should also come as no surprise that the government of President Bill Clinton would ignore the recommendation of the nation's radiation advisers, the National Council on Radiation Protection and Measurements (NCRP), which had spent nearly a decade reviewing the evidence for harm—and whose report was also leaked to *Microwave News*—to set safety limits for ELF magnetic fields to 0.2 microTesla (2 milliGauss).[233,234] Should the US government have adopted this standard—setting emissions 5,000 times below levels in current US guidelines, and 500 times lower than current international guidelines—it would have greatly inconvenienced power line companies and some manufacturers of electrical goods.

No less surprising is the claim made by New Zealand scientist Neil Cherry, that the WHO and the ICNIRP also systematically rejected or ignored the mounting evidence for harm from non-thermal emissions right across the man-made electromagnetic spectrum.[121]

At least one thing is certain. We are all part of a giant experiment, an experiment that has dragged us even further away from the human continuum.

Chapter 15

The Rape of Life

You can fool all of the people some of the time.
You can fool some of the people all of the time;
but you can't fool all of the people all of the time.
Abraham Lincoln, 16th President of the USA, (1809–1865).

Vanishing varieties

Our missionary zeal for tampering with nature and revolutionising the world would also embrace foods. But unlike the contemporary revolutions in chemistry and electromagnetism, which continue to be announced with great fanfare as a succession of state-of-the-art products roll off assembly lines and flood the marketplace; and unlike the nuclear revolution, which came with a bang, the scientific agricultural revolution (the Green Revolution) arrived by stealth.

The general public, by and large, has remained oblivious to the impact of the Green Revolution on crop diversity, or to the consequent impoverishment of our diets. People are generally ignorant about how, during the past 20 years, Big Business's increasing control of the entire food chain, from seed to supermarket, together with globalisation of food trade, is further severing our links to the human continuum; and they close their eyes to how the current Gene Revolution is pushing life's boundaries by manipulating genes.

For tens of thousands of years our prehistoric ancestors worldwide had lived on wild foods and medicinal plants, perhaps as many as from 10,000 to 30,000 species from the vegetable and animal kingdoms.[1,2] Then, beginning about 10,000 years ago, our agrarian ancestors had selectively bred plants and animals that were adapted to local conditions, that could cope with crises, with floods and droughts, mini-ice ages and infestations. By the beginning of the 20th century, nigh on 500 generations of farmers and pastoralists worldwide had collectively managed to breed millions of varieties of crops from about 7,000 species of wild plants, and thousands of breeds of animals from about 40 species of wild animals.

In the US, for instance, farmers during the 19th century were growing over 7,000 varieties of apples, 5,000 varieties of tomatoes and 2,600 varieties of pears.[3]

But today, only 14 per cent of the American apple varieties still exist.[3,4] Amongst the fallen are those named after bygone presidents: the 'Washington', the 'Jefferson', and the 'Lincoln'. Only 20 per cent of tomato varieties and 12 per cent of pear varieties still exist. Even worse, only 9 per cent of America's traditional varieties of maize, 6 per cent of pea varieties, and 5 per cent of cabbage varieties still exist. In fact, of the 8 major crops grown in the US today, fewer than 9 varieties of each still exist. Overall, 96 per cent of the vast range of vegetable varieties that adorned American dinner plates at the turn of the 20th century have disappeared forever.[5]

The same story of the decimation of crop varieties is repeated in country after country. Mexico, for instance, has lost 80 per cent of the country's tens of thousands of traditional varieties of maize.[3] China has lost 90 per cent of the 10,000 traditional wheat varieties that farmers had been growing up until 1950.[6] And in South East Asia, where farmers once grew 30,000 varieties of rice, only a handful of rice varieties remain.[7,8] In fact, two-thirds of the region's rice paddies have submitted to one variety alone.[4]

Similarly, hundreds of varieties of eggplants that Sudanese farmers once grew have succumbed to the dominance of the US-bred 'Black Beauty'.[4] The vast array of beets that Turkish farmers once grew have been vanquished by the 'Detroit Globe' variety. And thousands of varieties of apples and pears that Belgium farmers once grew have been uprooted in favour of 5 varieties of apples and 3 varieties of pears. The predominant apple? The one that fits neatly into moulded papier mâché cartons and tastes like wet cardboard: the 'Golden Delicious'.

Even home gardens are suffering. In Korea, for instance, only 26 per cent of the traditional varieties of vegetables that were cultivated by home gardeners there in 1985 were still present in 1993.[6]

The rise of the food barons

What caused such a staggering loss of crop diversity? Not climate change nor the degradation of arable land, though admittedly both are beginning to impact on crop diversity today. Nor was the wipe-out caused simply by supply and demand, though on the surface the economic answer is seductive. On the demand side of the equation, so the argument runs, has been the world's ever-growing and increasingly urbanised population. China and India today are perfect examples of that. On the supply side are the technological improvements in plant breeding practices that created higher-yielding crop varieties to feed a hungry world; improvements in food manufacturing practices that could process and package container-loads of industrial foods; improvements in transport systems that would enable the 'improved foods' to be carted rapidly to the global marketplace.

The improvements on the supply side of the equation, however, are merely symptoms of an underlying malady. For it could have been otherwise; humanity could have retained its rich culinary heritage despite, or even because of, its exploding population and its technological prowess. But it didn't. The reason? Profits and power. And on the demand side, a populace ever willing to believe that science and technology could dish out the good things in life and improve on nature.

Mesmerised by the power of the chemical revolution to control pests, and lured by the potential for mighty profits, Big Business and Government, together with their artful bedfellows, science and technology, had, from the 1950s, set out on a mission to revolutionise agriculture worldwide. The promise, as ever, was to create new things bright and beautiful.

In the first foray into the food chain, in what came to be called somewhat ironically the Green Revolution, technocrats from the Ford Foundation, the Rockefeller Foundation, and the US Agency for International Development (USAID) had conned farmers worldwide into replacing thousands of traditional varieties of grains that were adapted to local conditions with one or two 'scientifically-improved' new breeds of higher-yielding and more marketable crops.[9] The new varieties of grains, particularly wheat, rice and maize, had been bred to produce higher levels of carbohydrates and proteins, and would thus feed the world. Or so the argument went. But the programme was as much ploy to counter the spread of socialism with Big Business as it was a humanitarian gesture.[10]

The grocery grab

Then, with the Green Revolution in full swing, the food manufacturing and supermarket giants entered the fray and began dictating to farmers the varieties of foods they would purchase: the new 'improved varieties' of fruits and vegetables, with their uniform sizes and shapes and colours, and resistance to bruising; foods that could be transported and stored and sold more readily than the traditional varieties. Taste and texture, and nutrient content, were cast to the wind. The old varieties of apples, the 'Washington', the 'Foxwhelp' and 'Saint Augustine's Orange' therefore succumbed to the bland-tasting 'Golden Delicious', 'Pink Lady' and 'Fuji'.

Thus by the twentieth century's end, at least 75 per cent of the world's traditional crop varieties had gone the way of the dinosaur.[11] So too had half of Europe's livestock breeds; and of the remainder, 43 per cent are endangered. In fact, globally, nearly a quarter of the 6,300 traditional animal breeds that existed at the beginning of the 20th century are critically endangered, and every week another two become extinct.[12] In effect, the Green Revolution and the corporate appropriation of the entire food chain has shattered our 10,000-year legacy of selective plant and animal breeding.

Not one of the new varieties of crops, however, had been bred for its nutritional value, for its content of vitamins and minerals, for such micronutrients as iron and zinc, copper and selenium, folate and iodine. As it turned out, many of the new varieties, particularly of the grains, are indeed low in essential nutrients, especially iron, zinc and vitamin A.[13]

Adding to nutritional woes has been the advent of mass milling and polishing of grains which strip bran and germ and micronutrients from the already micronutrient-depleted cereals.[14] And, to complete the tragedy of errors, farmers in much of the Third World began to grow fewer pulses, fruits and vegetables, despite a rapidly increasing population, in favour of the new 'scientifically improved' cereals.

How did that impact on people's health? Well, today, more than a third of the world's population face debilitating diseases because their diets are dangerously low in precious micronutrients.[14] Forty per cent of all women and 50 per cent of pregnant women suffer from iron deficiency anaemia, which causes up to 40 per cent of the half-a-million deaths in childbirth each year. And 220 million children worldwide die from infectious diseases each year because their respiratory tracts and immune systems have been weakened from diets deficient in vitamin A. Indeed severe vitamin A deficiency blinds up to half-a-million children each year, half of whom die within six months of being afflicted.

We in the affluent West have also succumbed to the dietary revolution. Four of the leading causes of death—heart disease, cancer, strokes and diabetes—as well as such risk factors as obesity and high blood pressure, are associated with diets high in carbohydrates, fats and sodium, but low in dietary fibre and micronutrients. Even in affluent America, 20 per cent of premenopausal women suffer from iron deficiency anaemia.[14]

To add insult to injury, the higher-yielding crops leach nutrients from soils. Farmers had therefore abandoned their traditional practices of crop rotation and manuring to become dependent on chemical fertilisers. Unfortunately, the highly soluble inorganic fertilisers interfere with each plant's uptake of various micronutrients. Nitrates, for example, interfere with a plant's uptake of boron and potassium; and superphosphates do the same to copper, zinc and potassium. Hence the micronutrient content of the new foods, foods that were already deficient in many of these vital molecules, was further diminished.

Because genetic variation in the new monoculture crops was virtually nil, pests and weeds proliferated in the genetic vacuum. Hence pesticides and herbicides, the dangers of which we examined in Chapter 13, had to be added to farmers' shopping lists.

Once the American-style, mechanised, chemical-intensive, large-scale, broad-acre farming had been foisted onto farmers in the Third World, millions of them could no longer afford their traditional mixed-crop farming. Left to fend for themselves, many of them drifted into poverty and became the core of the world's 800-million starving. Political incompetence and wars simply added to their woes. Still others became poorly paid labourers on the large farms that did survive, those that churned out food commodities for Western markets. And everywhere, farming communities crumbled. Not surprisingly, many farmers throughout the developing world still curse the Western agricultural missionaries.

In the West, farmers fared little better. Some became dependent on government subsidies—the US dishes out crop subsidies, the EU nations pay farm subsidies. Other farmers, squeezed between soaring production costs on one side, and pricing dictates of the food manufacturing and retailing giants on the other, sold out to large farming corporations and drifted into city jobs. And everywhere, farming communities, like the land they once farmed, became eroded.

As the corporate juggernaut gained momentum, small-scale food manufacturers were swallowed up by the industrial giants, and the local corner store lost out to the supermarket chains. In the UK, for instance, three quarters of the nation's 30,000 farm-produce retailers plying their trade there in 1975 had disappeared by 1995.[15]

In effect, the food chain's rich diversity of characters who once formed the hub of food production and trade had been crippled by the new feudal barons. Today 10 transnational corporations control half of the world's seed supplies.*[16] Monsanto alone controls 25 per cent of the global seed market and, with its genetically engineered (GE) seeds, has conquered 88 per cent of the world's GE crop acreage. Three corporations alone control more than 75 per cent of the trade in cereals.†[17] And 10 control 84 per cent of the world's pesticide market‡[16]—4 of them (Monsanto, Syngenta, Dupont, and Bayer) are from the group of 10 transnational corporations that control half the world's seed supplies.

Moreover, 10 corporations control a quarter of the global market in food and drink manufacturing.§[16] And 10 control a quarter of the world's retail sales in packaged foods.¶[16] Indeed in most Western nations fewer than 5 corporations, the supermarket giants, control from 60 to 80 per cent of national food sales.[15] And that includes fresh produce. Australia has the dubious honour of having a duopoly, where Woolworths and Coles control nigh on 80 per cent of the nation's food market.[18,19] Welcome to the lords of our food.

Footnotes

* Monsanto/ Seminis, Dupont/Pioneer Hi-bred International, Syngenta, Groupe Limagrain, KWS AG, Land O'Lakes, Sakata, Bayer CropScience, Takii & Co Ltd, and DLF-Trifolium

† Cargill, Bunge, and Drefus

‡ Bayer, Syngenta, BASF, Dow Chemical Company, Monsanto, Dupont, Koor Trade International, Sumitomo, Nufarm, and Arysta LifeScience Corp

§ Nestlé, Archer Daniels Midland, Kraft Foods Inc, PepsiCo, Unilever, Tyson Foods, Cargill, Coca-Cola, Mars Inc, and Groupe Danone

¶ Wal-Mart, Carrefour, Metro AG, Ahold, Tesco, Kroger, Costco, ITM Enterprises, Albertsons, and Edeka Zentrale AG & Co

As in Mediaeval times, the modern barons are serviced by courtesans, or at least by their latter-day equivalents, the experts and specialists: specialists in plant breeding; specialists in modern farming practices; experts in food processing and packaging, safety and transport; experts in marketing and retailing and international trade.

Given the distance food has to be carted, from the farm gate to the processing plant and then to the supermarket, before it arrives on our dinner plates—in the US, typically between 1,500 and 2,500 miles[20]—it's not surprising we need specialists in food safety. 'Fresh', after all, is the operative word when it comes to food safety. In bygone times food safety had been assured by eating locally grown produce, a lesson Napoleon learned the hard way when, with his armies stretched across Europe, he lost more of his troops to food poisoning than to gunshot and sabre wounds.

But despite the abundance of safe foods found on supermarket shelves—at least 15,000 food lines in large supermarkets—our choice is limited to only about 30 species of plants. Despite the scores of products in the breakfast cereal aisles, for instance, all are limited to one of four cereals: rice, wheat, maize and oats. Indeed those four grains constitute three quarters of human cereal consumption today.[4] In fact, 30 crops provide 95 per cent of the world's food.[1] Three (rice, wheat and maize) provide 50 per cent of our food, and six others (sorghum, millet, potatoes, sweet potatoes, soy and sugar cane/sugar beet) provide a further 25 per cent. And all varieties of these foods have been bred for their commercial, not nutritional, value.

Clearly, food diversity, at least in the West, is an illusion. Unlike people in underdeveloped nations whose dietary needs are supplied by about 3,000 plant species—Javanese farmers, for instance, may grow over 600 species of crops in a single home garden[21]—we survive on sameness, not difference. Perhaps this is understandable given that corporate and government bureaucracy thrives on sameness, uniformity and standardisation.

Strength in diversity

Unfortunately, we forgot that there is strength in diversity. Nowhere can this be seen more clearly than in living systems, whether in the vast range of organisms within any ecosystem, or in the enormous genetic variability between individual members of a species. Greater possibilities and choices, within the ever-changing world, are available and the chances of survival are increased. Conversely, loss of diversity runs counter to life.

The Tasmanian devil, for instance, is in danger of becoming extinct because of an epidemic of facial cancer. The underlying reason? Europeans hunted these aggressive marsupials to the edge of extinction and the remnants lack genetic diversity in their immune systems.[22]

We human beings, however, are a classic example of strength in diversity. Excluding identical twins, each one of us is genetically unique. Even the diversity of our cultures and languages, both of which are inextricably bound to the growing and harvesting and preparing and eating of local foods, has contributed to our strength. But the fact that half of the world's remaining 6,500 languages are threatened with extinction, that during the past 100 years we have lost a language a month thanks to the dominance of Western, and particularly US culture, that the food revolution has been a major player in this decimation, is warning enough of how far we've veered from the human continuum.[23,24]

As for a lack of crop diversity, the Irish well knew the consequences of growing only two varieties of a crop. Over one-and-half million people died of starvation during the 1840s because of the potato blight. But Peruvians, who for centuries have grown up to 3,000 varieties of potatoes, never had to contend with such infestations. American maize farmers and Russian wheat farmers were reminded of such monoculture madness during the 1970s when plagues of pests swept through their genetically-uniform crops.

Thus variety is not just the spice of life, it is the very essence of life.

Frankenfoods

The genie of life

The germ of an idea about how humankind could exert ultimate control over life was born over half a century ago when James Watson and Francis Crick discovered, deep inside the core of cells, the supposed genie of life, DNA.

By the 1970s, as geneticists began to prise open the double-helix and fathom the specific workings of life's blueprints, technologists were leaning over their shoulders, dreaming of new creations. By tampering with genes, so they thought, they could put new life into foods. What nature had failed to do in 5,000 million years, biotechnologists would do in a year. And so the idea of Frankenstein foods was born.

Curiously, for a nation that purports to be Christian—no president has ever dared reveal he doesn't follow the faith—the US was embarking on a programme that would violate God's creations.

To cash in on their new creations, biotechnologists needed to patent their living creations. Previously, legal boffins had steered clear of patents on life forms because of ethical issues. But in 1978 the US Supreme Court granted Ananda Chakravarty, the developer of an oil-eating microbe, the first patent on life.[25] Now that morality had been thrown to the winds, Big Business would soon enter the fray.

That legal decision opened the door to patenting any gene, manipulated or not. Any gene, any protein, in fact any life form that some 'inventor' had tweaked, was now open to corporate grab. For the global stampede to patent anything living, all that was needed was to con the rest of the world into adopting US patent laws. Through the economic clout of the World Trade Organisation, and the Agreement on Trade-Related Aspects of Intellectual Property Rights (TRIPS), that Washington consensus was achieved.

Endearing themselves to no one except their shareholders, giant corporations fell over themselves, buying up seed companies and patenting genes and plants by the tens of thousands. Examples of the plundering include US patents on the wound-healing properties of turmeric, the anti-fungal properties of India's neem tree, the saccharin-like properties of Gabon's brazzein berries, 36 of South America's traditional varieties of quinoa, and a cross-breed of basmati rice.

Even though 90 per cent of the world's biological resources are to be found in developing nations, 97 per cent of the biological patents worldwide are held by developing nations and transnational corporations.[26–28] Thus by the turn of the century, 50,000 patents on genes or gene sequences had been granted or were pending.[29] In the US alone, 20,000 gene patents had been granted, and another 20,000 were pending—more than double the figure for 1990.[30]

By 2005, 20 per cent of human DNA had been patented, thanks to the US Patent and Trademark Office.[31] And who were the patent owners? Sixty-three per cent were corporations; 28 per cent were universities.

Today, the number of patents on human and non-human genes, gene sequences, and gene fragments is estimated to exceed four million;[32] patent applications on stem cells alone are estimated to exceed 2,000.[33]

And remember, anyone who uses a patented commodity, must pay the owner a fee. Think feudal system.

The procedure: raping the genie

Before biotechnologists begin the procedure of manipulating an organism, they sit down and dream of characteristics they hope to confer on the targeted life form: a plant that is herbicide-resistant, or pest-resistant, or bruise-resistant; or perhaps one that is frost-resistant or vitamin-enriched; or has anti-cancer, anti-aging, memory-enhancing, or weight-loss properties; a supersized salmon; a cow that produces pharmaceutical drugs in its milk; a self-lighting Christmas tree with genes from fireflies; a self-peeling apple. Even a master race of humans. The possibilities are only limited by the biotechnologists' imaginations.

Next, they hunt down the organism that has those characteristics. Then the procedure of genetic engineering begins. Like surgeons performing miniature organ transplants, biotechnologists first slice sections of DNA from the donor organism's cell. Then, in anticipation of switching on this genetic slice once it has penetrated the recipient's own genes, they latch on another gene, a promoter gene. Invariably this is the highly reactive, cauliflower mosaic virus. Then a third gene, one from a bacterium that is resistant to antibiotics, is hooked up to the other two. Later, this 'marker gene' will help the human manipulators identify which plants received the whole gene train—those plants that are doused with antibiotics and die did not conceive; those that survive have been successfully impregnated.

Now the rape begins. One technique is to stick the gene mix to gold or tungsten bullets and fire them with a miniature shot gun into the victim's nucleus. The other method is to hitch the gene mix to a parasite (either a virus or a bacterium). The parasite then hacks its way through cellular membranes, dragging the genetic invasion force behind. Where the whole concoction lands among the recipient's chromosomes, however, is anyone's guess.

Nonetheless, the position of the gene mix is of critical importance to how an organism manifests the new gene sequence.[34] If, for instance, a gene-laden bullet or a gene-dragging parasite strikes chromosome 13 of a potato's 48 chromosomes (two more than in humans), the characteristics of the potato will be very different to if the gene mix became hitched up to chromosome 45, or 21, or any other chromosome. Even its specific location within chromosome 13's double-stranded DNA, will impact on the potato's characteristics. Hence, the 'gene expression' of the engineered and newly inserted gene mix depends upon its specific location within a species' genes.

Once the antibiotic dousing has killed off the losers, the successfully violated cells divide, and divide again and again. Eventually a new, seemingly ordinary, plant appears. But it's not. The genetic concoction resides in every part of a genetically engineered (GE) plant—roots, leaves, pollen, the lot.

Unfortunately, genes do not work in isolation; they chatter amongst themselves. So, with the invasion of a foreign, genetically-engineered, whizz-bang concoction there is every likelihood that there will be unknown, unpredictable and unexpected changes in the host's cellular functions.

Moreover, the cauliflower mosaic virus promoter (CaMV 35S) has a weak spot that is prone to break and recombine with other genetic material. In other words, it can wreak havoc on genetic codes. Unfortunately for all life, that virus can happily work in the genes of all living organisms and act as the promoter for many other viruses as well as bacteria.[35] The consequences of unleashing virulent bacteria and viruses on the world would of course be catastrophic.

Lying dormant inside the cells of all organisms is so-called 'junk DNA'. Some of this is dormant genetic material for producing internally-made viruses (virogenes) or cancers (oncogenes)—not the sort of genes you would want switched on by some virus you ate in your GE meal.

The lie

The US Food and Drug Administration (FDA) animal and human health scientists, who in 1991–92 were assessing the then unregulated, unapproved GE foods, had warned FDA policy makers of the recognised potential for bioengineering to produce unexpected and unpredictable toxins, allergens and carcinogens.[36,37]

Notwithstanding the scientific expertise underpinning the reports, the official policy of the FDA, released on 29 May 1992, stated: 'The agency is not aware of any information showing that foods derived from these new methods differ from other foods in any meaningful or uniform way.'[37]

That was a lie. But so long as the public—who rely on government regulatory authorities to tell them the truth, who are used to thinking that if an object looks like a tomato, feels like a tomato, smells like an tomato, and tastes like a tomato, then it probably is a tomato; so long as they remained ignorant of the cutting and pasting procedure, they would be none the wiser.

The truth is that GE plants are radically different to ordinary plants. The difference hinges on their respective modes of reproduction. Since time immemorial, and regardless of human agricultural and animal husbandry practices, plants and animals have reproduced sexually within their species; occasionally, for some plants, with closely related species of the same genus. Such reproduction involves vertical gene transfer. In essence, it's all about sex.

Genetic engineering, however, enables scientists to breed across genuses, orders, phyla, even across kingdoms. Such horizontal gene transfers, by genetically breaking down species' barriers, have never happened before. Since the violation of life with laboratory concoctions does not equate to the age-old practice of sex, GE foods are not biologically the same as other plants.

So why would the FDA's policy contradict the warnings of the Agency's scientists? Because Presidents Reagan and Bush (Senior) had given orders to government regulators in the departments of environment, agriculture and food to streamline the development and approval of GE foods.[38] Come hell or high water, domination of the world's food market was, after all, in the nation's interest. To facilitate the order, Bush had appointed Michael Taylor to the new position of Deputy Commissioner for Policy at the FDA. His task was to develop policies on GE foods.[37]

Tellingly, Taylor was a lawyer who had previously represented biotechnology companies, including Monsanto, on regulatory issues.[37] Records subpoenaed from the US FDA—in a lawsuit undertaken in 1998 by the Alliance for Bio-Integrity against the FDA for not regulating GE foods—revealed that during 1991–92 warnings from FDA scientists were persistently overridden and policy statements contradicted their findings. And on completion of his policy work with the FDA, Michael Taylor whipped back through the revolving door and became Monsanto's Vice President for Public Policy.

And so it came to pass that GE foods were classified in the US as 'substantially equivalent' to conventional foods; indeed, that lie is still the basis for US government policy today. To ram home the message that GE foods are safe, biotech companies would conduct their own short-term animal tests—which is akin to letting the fox guard the hen house. And as we've seen in Chapter 3, ('Clinical Tests'), basing the safety of any food or medicine on animal tests is a scientific absurdity.

Hence there has been minimal independent peer-reviewed research on the safety of GE foods. When the Alliance for Bio-Integrity took legal action against the FDA for not regulating GE foods, three of the plaintiffs, who are eminent scientists, declared under oath that to the best of their knowledge, at that time (28 May, 1999), there was no report in the peer-reviewed scientific literature of any study establishing the safety of even a single GE food.[37]

As a sign of things to come, the first food to be approved under the policy of 'substantial equivalence' was the slow-rotting 'Flavr Savr' tomato, engineered by Calgene, its corporate creator, for longer shelf life. But though it looked and felt and smelt and tasted like a tomato, it wasn't a normal tomato. In tests conducted by Calgene, rats that were fed these 'tomatoes' showed a repeated pattern of stomach lesions. But despite requests from FDA scientists that more tests be conducted, none were.[36,37]

GE glee

In North America, farmers took to the GE herbicide-resistant, and pesticide-producing crops with glee. The former could be doused with herbicides with impunity; the latter spared farmers the expense of spraying pesticides. Biotech companies were gleeful too, for farmers were not only purchasing their patented seeds, but also their herbicides.

However, the patented seeds required farmers to pay licence fees and royalties, and hence removed their traditional practice of collecting seeds for the following year's sowing. Even farmers whose crops had been contaminated by pollen and seeds from neighbouring farms had to pay royalties to the corporate owner.

This disturbing legal precedent on patent rights occurred in 1998 when the biotech giant, Monsanto, sued a Saskatchewan farmer, 69-year-old Percy Schmeiser, for 'stealing' its GE canola seeds (rapeseed) and infringing its patent.[39] Previously, Monsanto had sent private investigators onto Schmeiser's property to take snippets of his canola. Investigations of the DNA revealed that in some fields adjacent to a road along which trucks carried the canola harvest, Monsanto's 'Roundup Ready Canola' was growing—in western Canada about 40 per cent of canola farmers grow Monsanto's 'Roundup Ready Canola', for which they sign an agreement preventing them from saving, selling or re-planting the company's patented seeds. Despite Schmeiser's claim that the seeds he collected from each year's harvest had been contaminated by Monsanto's GE canola seeds, despite the judge's finding that Schmeiser had not intentionally grown GE crops, despite the fact that he gained no commercial advantage from the contaminated crop, and despite the ruination of the canola variety that three generations of Schmeisers had bred; despite all this, on 29 March, 2001, a Canadian judge found that Schmeiser had violated Monsanto's monopoly patent.[39] And the punishment? He was ordered to pay Monsanto $15,000 for licence fees and to negotiate with Monsanto to pay up to $75,000 from the profits of his 1998 harvest.

GE gloom

Clearly, biotechnology companies were riding a winner. If they could seduce governments into supporting them, entice farmers into growing their patented crops, and ruin those farmers whose fields they contaminated, all that remained was to con consumers into accepting their Frankenstein monsters.

In the US and Canada that was easy. With no requirements for segregation of

GE crops, and no food labelling laws, government, together with Big Business, would guarantee that the public remained clueless about the foods they were eating. Today between 70 and 75 per cent of processed foods on grocery shelves in the United States and Canada contain GE ingredients or are derived from animals that have been fed GE foods.[40,41] Mostly, these occur as the oils and meal components of GE soy, corn, and canola. In fact, the US is the only nation to approve the use of Monsanto's genetically-engineered bovine growth hormone on dairy cows.

Elsewhere, populations didn't buy the lie. The greatest condemnation came from populations in Europe, India and Japan. The British in particular had cause for concern. After all, they had had to contend with bovine spongiform encephalopathy (BSE), better known as mad-cow disease. It is a disease that destroys the nervous systems not only of cows but also of many people who eat them. Indeed, blood banks in other nations refuse to take blood from people who were residing in Britain during those cavalier times.

Perhaps the bovine disease had resulted from feeding meaty diets to these herbivorous beasts, or perhaps from a combination of excessive manganese in their feed lots together with back-lining them with pesticides; to this day no one knows. But what was known was that the deadly neurological disease was caused by prions, mere fragments of proteins.

Notwithstanding, British government authorities refused to accept that the disease could be passed on to beef-eating, gelatine-eating humans. Not until March 1999, nine years after the outbreak of the disease, did they ban human consumption of infected cows.[42] Since the English tend to understate the severity of disasters, let's just say that that was a scientific and political mistake. Understandably, no one in Britain today could be persuaded that a BSE cow is substantially equivalent to a non-BSE cow.

Primed to be suspicious of any tampering with their foods, the British public simply didn't buy the lie of 'substantial equivalence'. Once they realised Frankenstein foods were being sold in shops, their outrage propelled many supermarkets into banning them from their shelves. Food manufacturers in turn got the message and banished GE ingredients from their products.

Fuelling the outrage was a political hot potato from the Rowett Institute of Nutrition and Health in Aberdeen, Scotland. Arpad Pusztai, a biochemist at the Institute, had disclosed in 1998 that young rats, fed on two transgenic lines of potatoes, had suffered immune system defects and stunted growth.[43] The Royal Society, after reviewing some of Pusztai's research, condemned it as flawed. *The Lancet* in turn ran an editorial accusing the Royal Society of 'breathtaking impertinence' and condemning the US FDA and the British Government for allowing GE products to enter the food chain without rigorous tests for effects on health.[44]

The British Medical Association, which represents 115,000 members, then entered the fray. In 1999 it called for a moratorium on GE foods and crops, stating that it was scientifically incorrect to classify these foods as 'substantially equivalent' to non-GE foods, and cited the possibility of unforeseen processes and proteins resulting from gene interactions.[45] Remember, the same warning had been issued by FDA scientists.

Thousands of scientists world-wide, many of them leaders in microbiology, genetics and epidemiology, didn't buy the lie either. Hundreds of them, from 55 countries, had signed an open letter, warning governments of the potential dangers to the environment, to human and animal health, and of the social implications of biopiracy.[46] Further, they urged governments to halt the genetic engineering of all life forms.

Chilling warnings

A central concern amongst those against genetic engineering has been the potential for horizontal gene transfer: the ability of genes to jump from GE crops and foods into the genes of bacteria, animals and people. That this does happen has now been confirmed. Professor Heinrich Kaatz at Jena University in Germany identified GE genes in bacteria and fungi in bee larvae.[47,48] How did they get there? The adult bees had supped on GE canola pollen, then fed the brood; and the engineered genes had then infiltrated the gut microbes of the baby bees. Another German study had also found GE genes in soil bacteria. How did they get there? From GE sugar beet growing nearby.[49]

Epidemiologists have also been worried that in the absence of long-term safety tests, GE foods could be damaging people's health. Hence the claim that the world's greatest feeding trial is currently being conducted on US and Canadian citizens. But they are not the only experimental guinea pigs for GE foods. The Organisation for Economic Co-operation and Development (OECD) estimates that 'up to 60 per cent of processed foods in many developed countries contain some GE materials, even if only in very limited amounts'.[50]

In Australia and New Zealand, for instance, despite mandatory labelling laws for processed foods, people there have unknowingly been eating foods containing GE materials since 1996: the labelling laws enacted in 2001 do not apply to foods from restaurants, hotels and take-aways; there is no requirement to label oils or foods containing oils derived from GE soy, corn, canola, or cotton seed—in many products such oils are disguised under the label 'vegetable oil'; GE flavours are excluded from labelling requirements, as are processing aids and food additives; and processed foods containing derivatives of GE soy, corn, canola, cotton seed, potatoes, rice or sugarbeet have been approved for the Australasian diet—derivatives can include lecithin, maltodextrin, dextrin, glucose, ascorbic acid, tocopherols (vitamin E), and xanthum gum.[51–53]

If animal studies are anything to go by, then a recent Russian study, conducted by Dr Irina Ermakova at the Russian Academy of Sciences in Moscow, is warning enough. After two years of research, Ermakova had found that when rats were fed GE soy, 36 per cent of their pups were severely stunted, and over half died within three weeks of birth—a death rate six to eight times higher than that for the progeny of rats fed on non-GE soy. Equally worrisome was the finding that of those that did survive, all were sterile.[54]

One GE food had already killed. Because of a corporate and governmental cover-up, most people, however, have never heard of it. In 1989, 37 Americans died and 1,500 were permanently disabled, suffering from eosinophilia myalgia syndrome, after ingesting L-tryptophan. The Japanese manufacturer, Showa Denko K.K., had switched to using a GE bacterium to produce the amino acid, without labelling the product as such.[37] Never before had tryptophan caused health problems. Nevertheless the FDA banned it in the United States. But not once has the FDA acknowledged that the tryptophan was made by a living GE organism. And Showa Denko K.K. destroyed all biological evidence and some potentially incriminating records of the manufacturing process.[37,55–58]

There has also been scientific concern about the dangers of creating virulent micro-organisms. Perhaps the best example of this is cited in a report published in *New Scientist*.[59] Australian scientists in Canberra, while attempting to genetically engineer a contraceptive vaccine for mice, accidentally created a deadly virus. To penetrate the mouse cell with the genes for sterility, they used the relatively harmless mousepox virus. But the GE version was lethal. Ominously, the mousepox virus is related to the human smallpox virus. But for the vigilance of the scientists involved, the environmental release of this micro-organism would have been catastrophic. Nevertheless, when scientists play God, sooner or later human error is bound to occur.

Equally chilling has been the creation and environmental release of suicide genes. Crops with genes that make the seeds of the GE plants sterile had been trialled in the US, Europe and Australia. Two forms of terminator technology exist: one is a genetic sequence that codes for a universal poison that kills all cells; the other produces an enzyme, such as barnase, that scrambles the gene sequence and destroys through chaos.[60] Should just one of those genes jump into a domesticated or wild variety of the same species, or should it completely jump species, phyla or kingdoms, those life forms would be exterminated. This would be the ultimate act of genocide. Fifteen patents for terminator technology exist. The co-owner of these patents is the US government.

Twenty years before GE foods began to flood onto supermarket shelves, George Wald, Nobel Laureate in Medicine or Physiology in 1967, and Professor of Biology at Harvard University, had warned his colleagues against tampering with genes. In his essay, 'The Case against Genetic Engineering' he had warned: 'Recombinant DNA technology [genetic engineering] faces our society with problems unprecedented not only in the history of science, but of life on the Earth. It places in human hands the capacity to redesign living organisms, the products of some three billion years of evolution.[61]

'Such intervention must not be confused with previous intrusions upon the natural order of living organisms; animal and plant breeding, for example, or the artificial induction of mutations, as with X-rays. All such earlier procedures worked within single or closely related species. The nub of the new technology is to move genes back and forth, not only across species lines, but across any boundaries that now divide living organisms. The results will be essentially new organisms. Self-perpetuating and hence permanent. Once created, they cannot be recalled.

'Up to now, living organisms have evolved very slowly, and new forms have had plenty of time to settle in. Now whole proteins will be transposed overnight into wholly new associations, with consequences no one can foretell, either for the host organism, or their neighbors.

'It is all too big and is happening too fast. So this, the central problem, remains almost unconsidered. It presents probably the largest ethical problem that science has ever had to face. Our morality up to now has been to go ahead without restriction to learn all that we can about nature. Reconstructing nature was not part of the bargain. For going ahead in this direction may not only be unwise but dangerous. Potentially, it could breed new animal and plant diseases, new sources of cancer, novel epidemics.'[61]

George Ward's warning that 'it is all too big and is happening too fast' remains pertinent even to this very day for, just as this book was about to go to press, the world's media, on 21 May, 2010, announced with great fanfare a technological breakthrough they claimed would rival that of the splitting of the atom nearly a hundred years ago: an entrepreneurial American scientist and billionaire, Craig Venter, and his team have created the first synthetic life form.[62] By mapping the genes of a bacterium with the aid of a computer, they assembled a completely artificial DNA sequence of over a billion base pairs, and inserted it into a cell after first removing the bacterium's existing DNA. In essence they created the first cell that is totally controlled by a synthetic chromosome built from four bottles of chemicals, one for each of the four nucleotides that make up DNA. Next on his agenda, according to Venter, is the creation of a cell created from scratch.

So, playing God has now become a reality.

Hogwash for the hungry

Given the worldwide opposition to GE foods, America—which has always refused to segregate GE from non-GE produce and hence makes identification of the unwanted produce impossible—lost much of its corn and soy market, particularly in Europe. And despite US government efforts to palm off the unwanted produce as food aid, many nations, including Zimbabwe and Kosovo, slammed their gates on this Trojan horse. Consequently, US citizens are paying $20 billion dollars each year to subsidise crops no one outside the US wants.

Undeterred, the seed barons devised a plan: use the time-tested ploy of stealth; infiltrate the food chain; contaminate ordinary crops with corporate genes through field trials; blur the differences between traditional plant and animal breeding practices and genetic engineering by describing both as 'biotechnology'; lobby governments into supporting them by warning of the economic consequences of failing to jump on the gene train.

And that is the state of affairs today. Well, almost. The barons had yet two more cards up their sleeves.

The first: push the line that GE foods will help feed the world's starving people. What hogwash! Even the conservative United Nations World Food Programme has declared that the world is producing one-and-a-half times the food needed to provide everyone in the world with an adequate and nutritional diet, the deficiencies in micronutrients cited above notwithstanding.[63]

The reason that one-seventh of the world's population are suffering from hunger is poverty, not lack of food. They simply don't have the money to buy food. In political parlance, there's an unequal distribution of food in the world. And who are starving? Many of the very farmers whose communities disintegrated thanks to the Green Revolution.

The second: spin the tale that GE foods will be our salvation during this time of global climate meltdown; that the new technology will help us survive the mess generated by an earlier technology; that where nature, or God, has failed, where not one of the planet's 35,000 edible plants will suffice, Frankenstein Inc can create new drought-resistant, flood-resistant, chaos-immune crops. Ho hum.

Nuking foods, and nanotech nonsense

Irresponsible irradiation

Tampering with foods, alas, is a never-ending story. Given that ours is a nuclear age, it's understandable that governments are now endorsing a nuclear attack on our foods: blitzing them with gamma radiation, or with X-rays or electron beams. Depending on a government's mandated dose for each food, the radiation is equivalent to between 5 and 6 million chest X-rays at the very least, and typically up to the equivalent of 330 million chest X-rays. And for some foods, as high as 2.3 billion chest X-rays. And the reason? To kill all living organisms, (insect, microbial, and plant seeds) all in the name sterility, longer shelf-life, transport-life, and pest extermination. Though the US is the leader in this, hot on its heels are China, India, Pakistan, Iran, the Philippines, Thailand, Mexico, South Africa, and Brazil.[64]

The Europeans, however, are far more cautious, for the only foods the European Parliament has approved for irradiation since 1999 are dried aromatic herbs, spices and vegetable seasonings. Admittedly, some nations of the European Union (EU), notably Belgium, France, the Czech Republic, the Netherlands, Italy, Poland and the United Kingdom, had received prior authorisation for the irradiation of some foods, including fish, shellfish, poultry, pototoes, garlic, onions, vegetables, pulses, fruit and cereals.[65] To comply with EU law, such foods, and any food containing irradiated ingredients, must be labelled 'irradiated' to ensure that consumers can make an informed choice.

But in 2002 the European Parliament imposed a ban on any further approvals because of safety concerns and public outrage at yet another attempt to tamper with foods. Nevertheless, because of trade with countries that do irradiate food—notably the US, China, Singapore and South Korea—unlabelled, irradiated foods, and irradiated herbal supplements, such as alfalfa, aloe vera, garlic, guarana, Korean and Siberian ginseng, saw palmetto, and turmeric are illegally appearing on European supermarket shelves.[66–68]

In the US, the FDA approves the irradiation of a vast range of foods: beef, chicken, lamb, pork, turkey, eggs, fruits, vegetables, sprouting seeds, juices, molluscan shellfish (oysters, clams, mussels and scallops), dozens of herbs, spices and seasonings, including herbal teas, as well as wheat flour, and all pet foods.[69] The radiation dose limit in the US is the equivalent of up to 1 billion chest X-rays.[64] The approval even extends to meat purchased by the National School Lunch Program. And the FDA is considering the approval of ready-to-eat foods (frozen dinners, luncheon meat, nuts, baby food, pre-cut salads and snack foods); and crustacean shellfish (crabs, shrimp and lobsters). Current US labelling laws exist only to alert the first purchaser of irradiated food. Hence consumers of irradiated foods prepared in restaurants, hotels and hospitals, and take-away bars, or those prepared for schools and airlines never know that they're eating nuked foods.

In Australia and New Zealand, regulatory authorities approve the irradiation of imported herbs, spices and herbal teas, other therapeutic goods, as well as tropical fruit, including breadfruit, carambola (starfruit), custard apples, lychees, longans, mangoes, mangosteen, papaya and rambutan.[70] Irradiation of pet food and grain fed to animals has also been approved. And, as with the EU laws on labelling, Australasian laws require labelling of any food containing any irradiated ingredient; but the Australasian labelling laws do not apply to animal feed or pet food.

So, what danger do irradiated foods pose to our health? None whatsoever, say US regulatory watchdogs. Unlike their precautionary-principled European counterparts, the US watchdogs are so confident about irradiated foods, and so cavalier about their citizens' health, that since 2002 they've even been toying with the idea, originating from Big Business and driven by Congress, of changing the current labelling laws to be rid of the word 'irradiated'. The reason? Many consumers don't want irradiated foods in their diets, and by disguising the process and calling it 'electronic pasteurisation', or 'cold pasteurisation', government, in cahoots with Big Business, will keep the public clueless to what they are eating.

Despite US government watchdog reassurances, there is plenty of evidence to suggest that irradiated foods are potentially dangerous to human health. The high energy gamma rays emitted by the radioactive isotopes Cobalt-60 and Caesium-137, the latter a waste product of the nuclear industry, knock electrons from their atomic orbits, and split chemical bonds apart, thereby creating unstable molecules. In essence irradiation creates free radicals, indeed new molecules.

That ionising radiation causes malformed embryos, genetic damage and cancer had been well documented following the US nuclear attack on the people of Hiroshima and Nagasaki in 1945, and amongst the people affected by the fallout from the Chernobyl nuclear reactor meltdown in Ukraine in 1986. It had also been documented following fallout from the 67 US atmospheric nuclear tests in the Marshall Islands between 1946 and 1958, the total yield of which was equivalent to over 7,000 Hiroshima bombs; and following the British nuclear tests at five sites on the Australian mainland and territories between 1952 and 1963, the most notorious being the site at Maralinga in South Australia—not only were hundreds of British and Australian servicemen deliberately exposed to radiation to test the effects of radiation on people, so were the Aboriginal people in the region; and, after the Kite Test on 11th October, 1956, the people in the cities of Adelaide and Melbourne could also be added to the large group of guinea pigs, since both cities were heavily contaminated. But, as with all things nuclear, that had been kept secret. Of course, all these effects were the result of irradiating people directly.

But what about foods? Irradiation damages vitamins, chemically degrades carbohydrates, and chemically changes proteins. Another identified danger is the damage to oils, or in biochemical jargon, lipids. And specifically, damage to the fatty acid component of lipids, such as palmitic acid, oleic acid, stearic acid, linolenic acid, myristic acid, and so on. Each lipid is made up of a molecule of alcohol and a long chain of one of these fatty acids. Lipids reside in plentiful amounts not only in animal fatty tissue, but also, as phospholipids, in all cell walls, and as sterols in such compounds as cholesterol and sex hormones. So as you read further you should realise, unlike our regulatory guardians of food safety, that there are health implications from eating nuked foods.

Back in 1971, two food researchers from the University of Massachusetts discovered that irradiation stews up a new class of chemicals—called cyclobutanones—that have never been found in any food. In fact, they have never been found in any substance.[71,72]

Then, during the 1990s, two researchers at Queen's University, Belfast, identified two specific cyclobutanones in irradiated chicken, pork, beef, lamb and eggs: 2-DCB (2-dodecylcyclobutanone), the irradiated by-product of palmitic acid, and 2-TCB (2-tetradecylcyclobutanone), the irradiated by-product of stearic acid.[73-78] According to the researchers, the greater the magnitude of radiation, measured in kiloGrays (kGy), the greater the levels of these hitherto unknown chemicals.[74,77] (When undergoing a chest X-ray, a person is exposed to about 0.0000004 kGy).

These cyclobutanones were detectable even when food was irradiated at 0.5 kGy,[78] equivalent to 16 million chest X-rays (depending on the food, the US legal limit ranges from 3 to 4.5 kGy, and the Codex Alimentarius Committee—a joint programme of the World Health Organisation (WHO) and the United Nation's Food and Agriculture Organisation (FAO) to establish international food standards—currently approves a cap of 10 kGy, although it is aiming for 60 kGy, the equivalent of 2 billion chest X-rays). The cyclobutanones were even detectable in a sample of chicken 13 years after it had been irradiated.[74]

Other researchers, both from Northern Ireland and Germany, have also identified 2-DCB and 2-TCB in irradiated mangoes, papayas, salmon, Camembert cheese, duck, peanuts, pistachios and instant soup mix.[79,80] A third cyclobutanone, 2-TDCB (2-tetradecylcyclobutanone), a by-product of irradiated oleic acid, was also identified in irradiated mangoes and papaya.[79] The scientific community has since identified the irradiated by-products of linoleic and myristic acid.

Meanwhile, German government researchers at the Federal Research Centre for Nutrition and Food in Karlsruhe—who, since the 1970s had been investigating the potential toxicity of cyclobutanones—were directed by a UN committee to identify specific dangers from human exposure to these chemicals. They discovered that 2-DCB does indeed damage both rat and human cells; the higher the radiation, the greater the damage.[81,82] They also found that both 2-DCB and 2-TDCB cause slight but significant chromosome breakage in human bowel cells.[83] Their research continues.

Ever since the 1950s, researchers had been documenting the harmful effects of irradiated foods on experimental animals. They had found: premature death, mutations and chromosomal damage, foetal death and other reproductive problems, immune system disorders, fatal internal bleeding, organ damage, tumours, (and the increased frequency of tumours), stunted growth, nutritional deficiencies and the formation in food of carcinogens, as well as the formation of mutant bacteria.[84-109]

Indian researchers had even discovered that, when undernourished children were fed irradiated wheat, they showed elevated levels of abnormal chromosomes in their lymphocytes (white blood cells).[98]

Despite all this evidence, what did the representative of the joint FAO/IAEA (International Atomic Energy Agency) International Consultation Group on Food Irradiation, at the March 2001 meeting, state about cyclobutanones? 'Preliminary results were negative with regard to genotoxicity [damage to genes] and cytotoxicity [damage to cells].'[110] Another lie; this was another ploy to support the needs of industry, and another betrayal of human health needs.

From the early 1960s the WHO and the FAO, two organisations that purport to have the interests of global health at heart, had teamed up with the International Atomic Energy Agency (IAEA)—an organisation that represents the interests of the nuclear industry—to investigate the safety of irradiated foods. But, as the Washington-based consumer-protection group, Public Citizen, has revealed, the WHO and the FAO by and large ceded power to the IAEA, the result being that research about the damaging effects of irradiated food was either misrepresented or ignored.[84] And from the 1970s onwards the focus of this consortium has been to encourage the legalisation, commercialisation and trade of irradiated foods among world governments, and to control the dissemination of news about irradiated foods so that the public would be none the wiser.

Hence in 1980 the statement from an FAO/IAEA/WHO 'Expert Committee' read: ' … the irradiation of any food commodity up to an overall dose of 10 kGy presents no toxicological hazard; hence toxicological testing of foods as treated is no longer required.'[111]

And in 1999, the statement from an FAO/IAEA/WHO 'Study Group', obviously having taken a leaf out of the GE lobby group's book, read: 'Irradiated foods are, from a nutritional viewpoint, substantially equivalent or superior to thermally sterilized foods.'[112] Yet another lie.

But, as they say, the proof of the pudding is in the eating; and it was something scores of cat owners in Australia learned the hard way. In 2008 about 30 cats died and at least 90 were neurologically damaged because they'd eaten a Canadian brand of dried cat food that had been irradiated.[113–115] The Canadian manufacturer had exported the pet food to 49 other countries, none of which irradiate imported pet food, and there had been no reports of any health problems there.

But the Australian Quarantine and Inspection Service had demanded that the dried cat food be irradiated—any imported pet food not cooked over a specified temperature must be bombarded with 50 kiloGrays of gamma radiation; that dose is equivalent to 1.6 billion X-rays, and is 12,000 times the dose that will kill a human, let alone any other organism. Because Australian law exempts irradiated pet food from being labelled as such, pet owners were flummoxed by the harm to their cats. But for the skills of an astute Sydney veterinary neurologist, Dr Georgina Child, who had first noticed the neurological syndrome, which includes paralysis and brain damage, and had linked it to irradiation of the cat food, no one would be any the wiser. Tony Burke, the Australian Government's Minister for Agriculture, Fisheries and Forestry, did at least acknowledge the danger of irradiated foods, if not to all pets and humans then at least to cats, and subsequently banned the irradiation of cat food.

Nanoed be thy name

If we were magnanimous and could ignore corporate greed, we might say that the Green Revolution invigorated Earth's bountiful harvest, that the Grocery Revolution boosted consumers' food choices, that the Biotech Revolution put new life into foods. And, in the same vein, at the dawning of the Revolution in Nanotechnology, we could say that no matter what, new matter is at hand; where nature has failed, we will create new molecules to build new toys, new foods, a new kingdom on Earth. Praise be.

So what is nanotechnology? It's the manipulation of matter at the atomic level, making new molecules by reconfiguring their atomic building blocks. Down in this shadowy world, the diameter of an atom is a mere tenth to half a billionth of a metre, or nanometre; the smallest molecules, the colloids, range from one to 100 nanometres. To fathom the infinitesimal size of the world into which scientists are delving, consider this: the particles that jiggle and jostle down there are 80,000 times smaller than the width of a hair on your head.

The first inkling we had that the nanoworld would be the next frontier of human conquest came in 1959, in a speech presented by American physicist Richard Feynman to fellow scientists entitled 'There's plenty of room at the bottom.'[116] Feynman envisaged a time when the 24 volumes of the *Encyclopaedia Britannica* would be reduced in size to fit on a pinhead; when printed volumes would be transformed into codes to fit on a disk; when room-size computers would be reduced to the size of the computers inside our skulls; when doctors would employ miniature probes and scanning devices, and surgeons would operate with miniature scalpels; when scientists would be able to see and explore and manipulate the infinitesimal world, and rearrange atoms to create new matter.

As you can gather, Feynman's vision has become our reality. Compact discs, DVDs, laptop computers, CT scans, magnetic resonance imaging and microscopic surgery are centre stage in our world, thanks to nanotechnology. By means of scanning tunnelling microscopes, scientists can now see the shadowy world of atoms and molecules. Indeed they created their first nanoparticle, carbon-60, a so-called buckyball, in 1985. Since then they've managed to create a playbox of other buckyballs, as well as nanotubes, nanospheres, nanoshells and quantum dots, each with unique chemical, electrical, physical and optical qualities.

All industry sectors have in turn begun to incorporate man-made nanoparticles into their products. According the US-based Woodrow Wilson International Center for Scholars, 580 nanotechnology-based products, manufactured by 300 companies in 20 countries, were in the global marketplace in October 2006.[117] In just a year-and-a-half after May 2004, the number of nanotech products had grown by 175 per cent, proving that nanotechnology was on a roll. The greatest growth has been in health and fitness products, especially personal care products, cosmetics and clothing. But also represented are computers and electrical goods and sports equipment. And yes, food was well represented, having about 70 nanotech delights from which to choose.

There's no problem with that; or so we hope, for no government has bothered to regulate nanotechnology, nor to legislate for the labelling of such products. Not one has bothered to consider that products made from man-made nanoparticles may be different to other products. Hence, few scientists have bothered to find out how each unique nanoparticle affects human health, let alone the environment.[118,119]

From the limited studies that have been conducted, evidence suggests that some nanoparticles, when inhaled, lodge in animals' airways, and that some make their way along nerves to animals' brains.[120,121]

But no one has a clue about the health effects of the man-made nanoparticles that are absorbed through the skin from suncreams and cosmetics (for it is known that particles up to 1,000 nanometres are readily absorbed through the skin) or about the effects of those that are absorbed through our guts from the food products we eat.

Of course, we've lived with nanoparticles since time began. The air we breathe, the food we eat, the water we drink, and many of the substances we slap on our skin, are composed of nature's nanoparticles. We, like every other living organism, are geared to living on nanoparticles, absorbing nanoparticles, incorporating them into cellular tissues and processes.

But our bodies are not geared to absorbing man-made nanoparticles. Ever since the industrial revolution, particularly since the advent of the internal combustion engine, we've been churning out man-made nanoparticles inadvertently, as by-products of burning fossil fuels—on a busy city street we inhale about 25 million nanoparticles in each breath we take.[122] And, as we well know, inhaling hydrocarbon nanoparticles, inadvertently or not, can cause various cancers and damage the heart and blood vessels.

But now we're beginning to add new nanoparticles to the mix. And we're doing it intentionally. For this foolhardy adventure to begin, all that was needed was a cavalier attitude, gung-ho energy, corporate greed, compliant governments, no public discussion, and a public that is readily duped by high-tech promises.

Yes, the ingredients are already in place for mass production to begin. Today about 200 transnational food companies—including Nestlé, Kraft Foods, Unilever, PepsiCo, Cargill, ConAgra Foods, General Mills, Sara Lee, H.J. Heinz, Campbell Soup, McCain Foods and Goodman Fielder—are heavily investing in nanotech research and development.[123] Agrochemical companies, including Syngenta, BASF, Bayer CropScience and Monsanto, are doing so too.[124] And they're all racing to patent their nanotech delights. In the pipeline are nanotech packaging, food colours, flavours and nutrients; nanotech herbicides and pesticides; nanotech fertilisers; and of course nanotech seeds. And they'll be unlabelled, so you won't have a clue what you're eating. But be assured, they won't be morsels we are adapted to eating, or drinking, or breathing.

Welcome to the world of atomically modified foods! Nanoed be thy name. Amen.

Who Speaks for Life?

Since time immemorial, life has been the domain of everyone. Plants in particular have pervaded every aspect of human society, in gardens and buildings, in rituals and religion, for health and nourishment, and as medicines. They impact on every facet of life on this planet. Most spiritual traditions uphold the belief that there is a sacred trust under which human beings accept stewardship of the Earth. And most people accept that there are bounds to the balance, order and harmony of Mother Nature.

But by treating life as a laboratory, a commodity, a patentable item that can be manipulated, scientists, biotechnologists and politicians are smashing those limits. And all of us, like it or not, are the experimental guinea pigs.

Given that we're also experimental guinea pigs for the pharmaceutical, chemical, electromagnetic and nuclear industries, is it any wonder that many of us, as well as the planet, are ailing?

But all is not gloom and doom. We do have choices. Individually we can change our lives for the better. And collectively we can heal the world. The clue resides in the human continuum, in those lifestyles that sustained our kind since time immemorial. This very thing is the topic that we'll explore in Volume 2.

References

PART ONE—SICK SOCIETY, AILING MEDICINE

INTRODUCTION

1. The National Heart Foundation of Australia. *The Shifting Burden of Cardiovascular Disease in Australia*, Report by Access Economics Pty Ltd, Barton, ACT, Australia, 2005.
2. Personal telephone conversation with Professor Andrew Tonkin, Chief Medical Adviser to the National Heart Foundation of Australia, May 2005.
3. Cancer Council of SA. "Graphical presentation of cancer trends in South Australia and comparison countries": *Statistics all cancers*, 2006; Eastwood, South Australia, Australia. [Online, accessed 6th July, 2009]. URL:http://www.cancersa.org.au
4. Cancer Council of SA, ibid reference 3: *Statistics colon cancer (excludes rectal cancers)*, 2006.
5. Cancer Council of SA, ibid reference 3: *South Australian Cancer Statistics, Monograph 5: Lymphomas, Myelomas and Leukaemias*, 2006.
6. Cancer Council of SA, ibid reference 3: *Statistics female breast cancer*, 2006.
7. Cancer Council of SA, ibid reference 3: *Statistics non-Hodgkin lymphoma*, 2006.
8. International Agency for Research on Cancer (IARC). Parkin DM, Whelan SL, Ferlay J, Teppo L, and Thomas DB (editors). *Cancer Epidemiology: Cancer Incidence in Five Continents, Volume VIII*. IARC publication no. 155, Lyon, France, 2002.
9. International Union Against Cancer. *Childhood cancer: Rising to the challenge*. Geneva, Switzerland, 2006; p. 10.
10. Cancer Council of SA, ibid reference 3: *Statistics brain cancer*, 2006.
11. International Diabetes Institute. Dunstan D, Zimmet P, Welborn T, Sicree R, Armstrong T, Atkins R, Cameron A, Shaw J, and Chadban S, on behalf of AusDiab Steering Committee. *Diabesity and Associated Disorders in Australia, 2000: the Accelerating Epidemic. The Australian Diabetes, Obesity and Lifestyle Study (AusDiab)*, Melbourne, Victoria, Australia, 2001.
12. International Diabetes Institute. Barr ELM, Mogliano DJ, Zimmet PZ, Polkinghorne KR, Atkins RC, Dunstan DW, Murray SG, and Shaw JE. *AusDiab 2005, the Australian Diabetes, Obesity and Lifestyle Study, Tracking the Accelerating Epidemic: Its Causes and Outcomes*, Melbourne Victoria, Australia, 2006.
13. Arthritis Australia. *Arthritis, the Bottom Line: the Economic Impact of Arthritis in Australia*. Report published by Access Economics Pty Ltd for Arthritis Australia, Forest Lodge, NSW, Australia, 2005.
14. Heimer, H. "Outer causes of inner conflicts: environment and autoimmunity". *Environmental Health Perspectives*, 1999; 107 (10): 504–509.
15. The Autoimmune Diseases Coordinating Committee, US National Institutes of Health. *Progress in Autoimmune Diseases Research*, Report to Congress, Bethesda, Maryland, USA, 2005.
16. American Autoimmune Related Diseases Association. [Online, accessed 8th July, 2009]. URL:http://www.aarda.org
17. Cooper GS, and Stroehla BC. "The epidemiology of autoimmune diseases." *Autoimmunity Reviews*, 2003; 2 (3): 119–125.
18. Onkamo P, Vaananen S, Karvonen M, and Tuomilehto J. "Worldwide increase of Type 1

diabetes: the analysis of the data on published incidence trends." *Diabetologia*, 1999; 42 (12): 1395–1403.

19. Australian Institute of Health and Welfare. *Incidence of Type 1 Diabetes in Australia 2000–2006: First Results*. Diabetes Series No. 9, Cat. no. CVD 42, Canberra, ACT, Australia, 2008.
20. International Diabetes Federation. *IDF Diabetes Atlas*, 4th edition, "Country summary", Brussels, Belgium, 2009.
21. Diabetes UK. *Diabetes in the UK 2004: A Report from Diabetes UK, October 2004*. London, UK, 2004.
    [Online, accessed 8th July, 2009]. URL:http://diabetes.org.uk.
    Citing Barnett T. (editor), *The Insulin Treatment of Diabetes. A Practical Guide*. E-MAP Healthcare, London, UK, 1998.
22. Barnett MH, Williams DB, Day S, Macaskill P, and McLeod JG. "Progressive increase in incidence and prevalence of multiple sclerosis in Newcastle, Australia: a 35-year study." *Journal of the Neurological Sciences*, 2003; 213 (1–2): 1–6.
23. Australian Centre for Asthma Monitoring. *Asthma in Australia 2003*, Australian Institute of Health and Welfare, Asthma Series No. 1, Cat no. 1, Canberra, ACT, Australia, 2003.
24. Australian Centre for Asthma Monitoring. *Asthma in Australia 2008*, Australian Institute of Health and Welfare, Asthma Series No. 3, Cat no. ACM 14, Canberra, ACT, Australia, 2003.
25. Australasian Society of Clinical Immunology and Allergy (ASCIA). *The Economic Impact of Allergic Disease in Australia: Not To Be Sneezed At*. Report published by Access Economics Pty Ltd for ASCIA, Balgowlah, NSW, Australia, 2007.
26. Boseley S. "Allergy epidemic looms for children." *The Guardian Weekly*, Thursday, February 19th–Wednesday, Feb 24th, 2004; 170, (9): 19.
27. Kanner L. "Autistic disturbances of affective contact." *Nervous Child*, 1943; 2: 217–250.
28. Coulter HL. *The Medical Assault on the American Brain: Vaccination, Social Violence, and Criminality*, North Atlantic Books, Berkeley, California, USA, 1990.
29. Lotter V. "Epidemiology of autistic conditions in young children." *Social Psychiatry and Psychiatric Epidemiology*, 1967; 1 (4): 163–173.
30. Brask BH. *A Prevalence Investigation of Childhood Psychoses*, Paper presented at the 16th Scandinavian Congress of Psychiatry, Aarhus University, Aarhus, Denmark, 1–4 July, 1970.
31. Fombonne E. "Epidemiology of autistic disorder and other pervasive developmental disorders." *Journal of Clinical Psychiatry*, 2005; 66 (Supplement 10): 3–8.
32. Fombonne E. "Epidemiological surveys of autism and other pervasive developmental disorders: an update." *Journal of Autism and Developmental Disorders*, 2003; 33 (4): 365–382.
33. MacDermott S, Williams K, Ridley G, Glasson E, and Wray J. *The Prevalence of Autism in Australia: Can it be Established from Existing Data?* A report prepared for Australian Advisory Board on Autism Spectrum Disorders, Frenchs Forest, NSW, Australia, 2006.
34. Centers for Disease Control and Prevention. "Prevalence of autism spectrum disorders: Autism and Developmental Disabilities Monitoring Network, six sites, United States, 2000." *Morbidity and Mortality Weekly Report*, 2007; 56 (SS01): 1–11.
35. Carlsen E, Giwercman A, Kelding N, and Skakkebaek NE. "Evidence for decreasing quality of semen during past 50 years." *British Medical Journal*, 1992; 305 (6854): 609–613.
36. Krausz C, and Forti G. "Clinical aspects of male infertility." In: K McElreavey, *The Genetic Basis of Male Infertility: Results and Problems in Cell Differentiation*, Springer, Berlin, Germany, 2001; p. 1.

37. Australian Bureau of Statistics. *Mental Health and Wellbeing: Profile of Adults, Australia*. Cat no. 4326.0, Canberra, ACT, Australia, 1998.
38. Sawyer MG, Arney FM, Baghurst PA, Clark JJ, Graetz BW, Kosky RJ, Nurcombe B, Patton GC, Prior MR, Raphael B, Rey J, Whaites LC, and Zubrick SR. *Child and Adolescent Component of the National Survey of Mental Health and Well-Being: Mental Health of Young People in Australia*, Commonwealth Department of Health and Aged Care, Canberra, ACT, Australia, 2000.
39. Australian Bureau of Statistics. *National Health Survey: Mental Health, Australia*, 2001. Cat no. 4811.0, Canberra, ACT, Australia, 2003.
40. Australian Bureau of Statistics. *2007 National Survey of Mental Health and Wellbeing*. Cat no. 4326.0, Canberra, ACT, Australia, 2007.
41. Charlton, B., *Psychiatry and the Human Condition*, Radcliffe Medical Press, Oxford, UK, 2000; pp. 1–2.
42. Zinn C, Karcher H, Dolley M, Rochal J, Yamauchi M, Rhein R, Sheldon T, Dorozynski A, and Kingman S. "Suicide". *British Medical Journal*, 1994; 308 (6920): 7–11.
43. Australian Institute of Health and Welfare. *Australian Long-term Trends in Mortality Workbooks*, GRIM Books, Canberra, ACT, Australia, 2005.
44. Australian Bureau of Statistics. *National Health Survey, 2001*. Cat. no. 4363.0.55.001, Canberra, ACT, Australia, 2001.
45. Organisation of Economic Co-operation and Development (OECD). *A Disease-based Comparison of Health Systems: What is Best and at What Cost?* OECD Publication Series, Paris, France, 2003, pp. 324–326.
46. Australian Government Department of Health and Aging. National Surveillance Case Definitions for the Australian *National Notifiable Diseases Surveillance System*. [Online, accessed 11th November, 2009]. URL:http://www.health.gov.au/internet/main/publishing/nsf/Content/cdna-casedefinitions.htm
47. Yusuf S, Reddy S, Ounpuu S, and Anand S. "Global burden of cardiovascular diseases: Part 1: General considerations, the epidemiologic transition, risk factors, and impact of urbanization." *Circulation* (Journal of the American Heart Foundation), 2001; 104: 2746–2753.
48. Lindeberg S, Berntorp E, Nilsson-Ehle P, Terent A, and Vessby B. "Age relations of cardiovascular risk factors in a traditional Melanesian society: the Kitava study." *American Journal of Clinical Nutrition*, 1997; 66 (4): 845–852.
49. Latto C. "Medical Safaris—Food for Thought." *International Journal of Environmental Studies*, 1978; 12: 9–12.
50. Newby JA, and Howard V. "Environmental influences in cancer aetiology." *Journal of Nutritional and Environmental Medicine*, 2005; 15 (2–3): 56–114.
51. Stefansson V. *Cancer: Disease of Civilization? An Anthropological and Historical Survey*. Hall and Wang, New York, NY, USA, 1960.
52. Price WA. Report of an interview with Dr Joseph Herman Romig. In: "Primitive and modernized North American Indians." *Nutrition and Physical Degeneration: A Comparison of Primitive and Modern Diets and Their Effects*, Paul B Hoeber, Inc, Medical Book Department of Harper and Brothers, New York, NY, USA, 1939. Cited in Stefansson V, ibid reference 51.
53. Bulkley JL. "Cancer among primitive tribes." *Cancer*, 1927; 4 (4): 289–295. Cited in Stefansson V, ibid reference 51.
54. Bainbridge WS. *The Cancer Problem*, The Macmillan Company, London, UK, 1914. Cited in

Stefansson V, reference 51.

55. McCarrison R. "Introduction" to: *Studies in Deficiency Disease*. H Frowde and Hodder & Stoughton, London, UK, 1921.
56. Tipper EH. *The Cradle of the World and Cancer: A Disease of Civilization*, Charles Murray, London, UK, 1927.
57. Renner W. "Cancer and the Creoles of Sierra Leone." *British Medical Journal*, 1911; 1: 110–111.
58. Hearsey H. "Cancer in the Colonies." *British Medical Journal*, 1906; 1: 1562–1563.
59. Berglas A. *Cancer: Nature, Cause and Cure*. Institute Pasteur, Paris, 1957. Cited in Stefansson V, ibid reference 51.
60. Hoffman FL. *Cancer and Civilization*. Speech presented to Belgian National Cancer Congress at Brussels, Belgium, 1923. Cited in Stefansson V, ibid reference 51.
61. Eaton SB, Konner M, Shostak M. "Stone agers in the fast lane: chronic degenerative diseases in evolutionary perspective." *American Journal of Medicine*, 1988; 84 (4): 739–749.
62. Riveros M. "First observation of cancer among the Pampido Indians of the Paraguayan Chaco." *International Surgery*, 1970; 53 (1): 51–55.
63. Schaeffer O. "When the Eskimo comes to town." *Nutrition Today*, 1971; 6: 8–16.
64. O'Dea K, Patel M, Kubisch D, Hopper J, and Traianedes K. "Obesity, diabetes and hyperlipidaemia in a Central Australian Aboriginal community with a long history of acculturation." *Diabetes Care*, 1993; 16: 1004–1010.
65. O'Keefe JH Jr, and Cordain L. "Cardiovascular disease resulting from a diet and lifestyle at odds with our Paleolithic genome: how to become a 21st- century hunter-gatherer." *Mayo Clinic Proceedings*, 2004; 79 (1): 101–108.
66. Jonsson T, Olsson S, Ahren B, Bog-Hansen TC, Dole A, and Lindeberg S. "Agrarian diet and diseases of affluence: do evolutionary novel dietary lectins cause leptin resistance?" *BMC Endocrine Disorders*, 2005.
67. Cordain L, Eaton SB, Miller JB, Mann N, and Hill K. "The paradoxical nature of hunter-gatherer diets: meat based, yet non-atherogenic." *European Journal of Clinical Nutrition*, 2002; 56 (Supplement 1): 42–52.
68. Cordain L, Eaton SB, and Sebastian A, Mann N, Lindeberg S, Watkins BA, O'Keefe JH, and Brand-Miller J. "Origins and evolution of the Western diet: health implications for the 21st century." *American Journal of Clinical Nutrition*, 2005; 81 (2): 341–354.
69. Editorial: "Multiple sclerosis in South Africa." *South African Medical Journal*, 1966; 40 (20): 453.
70. Bird AV, and Kerrich JE. "Multiple sclerosis in South Africa." *South African Medical Journal*, 1969; 43 (33): 1031–1033.
71. Bhigjee A. "Multiple sclerosis in a black patient." *South African Journal of Medicine*, 1987; 72 (12): 873–875.
72. Ames FR, and Louw S. "Multiple sclerosis in Coloured South Africans." *Journal of Neurology, Neurosurgery and Psychiatry*, 1977; 40 (8): 729–735.
73. Adam AM. "Multiple sclerosis: epidemic in Kenya". *East African Medical Journal*. 1989; 66 (8): 503–506.
74. Dean G, Bhigjee AI, Bill PL, Chikanza IC, Thomas JE, Levy LF, and Saffer D. "Multiple sclerosis in black South Africans and Zimbabweans." *Journal of Neurology, Neurosurgery and Psychiatry*, 1994; 57 (9): 1064–1069.
75. Kioy PG. "Emerging picture of multiple sclerosis in Kenya". *East African Medical Journal*, 2001; 78 (2): 93–96.

76. Bhigjee AI, Moodley K, and Ramkisson K. "Multiple sclerosis in KwaZulu Natal, South Africa: an epidemiological and clinical study." *Multiple Sclerosis*, 2007; 13 (9): 1095–1099.
77. Anderson HR. "The epidemiological and allergic features of asthma in the New Guinea Highlands." *Clinical Allergy*, 1974; 4 (2): 171–183.
78. Woolcock AJ, Dowse GK, Temple K, Stanley H, Alpers MP, and Turner KJ. "The prevalence of asthma in the South-Fore people of Papua New Guinea. A method for field studies of bronchial reactivity." *European Journal of Respiratory Diseases*, 1983; 64 (8): 571–581.
79. Rios-Dalenz J, Correa P, and Haenszel W. "Human cancer morbidity from cancer in La Paz, Bolivia." *International Journal of Cancer*, 1981; 28 (3): 307–314.
80. Koifman S, and Koifman RJ. "Environment and cancer in Brazil: an overview from a public health perspective." *Mutation Research*, 2003; 544 (2–3): 305–311.
81. Acosta O, Sierra G, and Gomez NA. "Cancer in Ecuador." *ASCO (American Society of Clinical Oncology) News and Forum*, April 2009.
[Online, accessed 8th July, 2009]. URL:http: www.asco.org/anf/News
82. Hurtig A-K, and San Sebastian M. "Geographical differences in cancer incidence in the Amazon basin of Ecuador in relation to residence near oil fields." *International Journal of Epidemiology*, 2002; 31: 1021–1027.
83. San Sebastian M, and Hurtig A-K. "Cancer among indigenous people in the Amazon basin of Ecuador, 1985–2000." *Pan American Journal of Public Health*, 16 (5): 328–333.
84. Catlin, G. *Letters and Notes on the Manners, Customs and Conditions of the North American Indians, written during eight years' travel amongst the wildest tribes of Indians in North America*. Willis P. Hazard, Philadelphia, Pennsylvania, USA, 1857.
85. Catlin G. *North American Indians, Volume 2: Being Letters and Notes on their Manners, Customs and Conditions, written during eight years' travel amongst the wildest tribes of Indians in North America, 1932–1839*. Leary, Stuart and Co., Philadelphia, Pennsylvania, USA, 1913.
86. Sheppard DF. *Maori Land: Maori Health*, Eighth National Rural Health Conference, Alice Springs, Northern Territory, Australia, 10–13th March, 2005.
87. Hawkesworth J (Editor). *An Account of Voyages Undertaken by Order of His Present Magesty for Making Discoveries in the Southern Hemisphere, And successively performed by Commodore Byron, Captain Wallis, Captain Carteret, and Captain Cook, in the Dolphin, the Swallow, and the Endeavour: drawn up from the Journals which were kept by several Commanders. And from Papers of Joseph Banks, Esq*. Printed for W Strahan and T Cadell, London, UK, 1773; volumes 2 and 3: pp. 136 and 357.
88. Elkin AP. *Aboriginal Men of High Degree*, 1st edition: 1945; 2nd edition: University of Queensland Press, St Lucia, Queensland, Australia, 1977.
89. Reid J, and Trompf P. (Editors). *The Health of Aboriginal Australia*, Harcourt Brace Jovanovich Publishers, Sydney, NSW, Australia, 1991, pp. 1–3.
90. Abbie AA. *The Original Australians*, AH and AW Reed, Sydney, NSW, Australia, 1970.
91. Cowlishaw G. 1978. "Infanticide in Aboriginal Australia", *Oceania*, 1978; 48 (4): 262–283.
92. Anderson W. "The colonial medicine of settler states: comparing histories of indigenous health." *Health and History*, 2007; 9 (2): 144–154.
93. New Zealand Ministry of Health. *Taking the Pulse: the 1996/97 New Zealand Health Survey*, Wellington, New Zealand; Chapter 7: Diabetes, pp. 99–109.
94. US National Institutes of Health, and National Institute of Diabetes and Digestive and Kidney Diseases. *Diabetes in America*, 2nd Edition, National Diabetes Information

Clearing House, Bethesda, Maryland, USA. Publication no. 95–1468; Chapter 34: "Diabetes in North American Indians and Alaska Natives," 1995, pp. 683–701.

95. Public Health Agency of Canada. *Diabetes in Canada: Facts and Figures*, National Diabetes Fact Sheets, Ottawa, Ontario, Canada, 2008.

96. Knowler WC, Bennett PH, Hamman RF, and Miller M. "Diabetes incidence and prevalence in Pima Indians: a 19-fold greater incidence than in Rochester, Minnesota." *American Journal of Epidemiology*, 1978; 108 (6): 497–505.

97. Australian Bureau of Statistics. *The Health and Welfare of Australia's Aboriginal and Torres Strait Islander Peoples, 2008*. Cat no. 4704.0, Canberra, ACT, Australia, 2008.

98. Australian Institute for Health and Welfare (AIHW). *Chronic Kidney Disease in Australia*, AIHW Cat. no. PHE 68, Canberra, ACT, Australia, 2005. pp. 90–93.

99. O'Dea K. "Marked improvement in carbohydrate and lipid metabolism in diabetic Australian Aborigines after temporary reversion to traditional lifestyle." *Diabetes*, 1984; 33 (6): 593–603.

100. Australian Department of Health and Aging. *Pharmaceutical Benefits Scheme: History, 1948–49 to 2007–08*.
 [Online, accessed 10th July, 2009].
 URL:http://www.health.gov.au/internet/main/publishing.nsf/Content/053BB36E2A4173AACA2575910012F753/$File/BookPage19-21.pdf

101. Australian Department of Health and Aging. *Expenditure and Prescriptions Twelve Months to 30 June 2008*, Pharmaceutical Policy and Analysis Branch, Canberra, ACT, Australia, 2007. [Online, accessed 10th July, 2009].
 URL:http://www.health.gov.au/internet/wcms/publishing.nsf/Content/pbs_expenditure_prescriptions_copy 1

102. Personal correspondence with Kevin Norton, Professor of Exercise Science at the University of South Australia, May, 2005.

103. Department of Health and Aged Care, and the Australian Institute of Health and Welfare (AIHW). *National Health Priority Area Report on Cancer Control, 1997*. Department of Health and Family Services, and AIHW, AIHW Cat. no. PHE 4, Canberra, ACT, Australia, 1998, p. 5.

104. The Honorable Nicola Roxon MP, (Australian) Minister for Health and Aging. Media Release: *New PBS Medicines Listed*. February 1, 2009.
 [Online, accessed 11th November, 2009].
 URL:http://www.health.gov.au/internet/ministers/publishing.nsf/Content/mr-yr09-nr-nr014.htm

105. Andersen HC. *The Stories of Hans Christian Andersen: A New Translation from the Danish*, DC Frank and J Frank (editors), Duke University Press, Durham, North Carolina, USA. First published in *Fairy Tales for Children*, CA Reitzel, Copenhagen, Denmark, 1837

CHAPTER 1—Death by Doctoring

Quote of Marcel Proust: from *À la Recherche du Temps Perdu*, Volume 3, 'The Guermantes' Way', 1920.

1. Taylor RB. *White Coat Tales: Medicine's Heroes, Heritage and Misadventures*, Springer, London, UK, 2007, pp. 121–122.

2. Gellhorn A. "Medical ethics—so what's the story?" *In Vitro Cellular and Developmental*

Biology-Plant, 1977; 13 (10): 588–594.
3. Reich WT (editor). *Encyclopedia of Bioethics*, revised edition, volume 5, Simon and Schuster MacMillan, New York, NY, USA, 1995.
4. Buckman R, and Sabbagh K. *Magic or Medicine? An Investigation of Healing and Healers*, Macmillan, London, UK, 1993.
5. Griggs B. *Green Pharmacy: A History of Herbal Medicine*. J. Norman and Hobhouse, London, UK, 1981.
6. Moser C. "Diseases of Medical Progress." *The New England Journal of Medicine*, 1956; 255 (13): 606–614.
7. Moser RH. *Diseases of Medical Progress: A Survey of Diseases and Syndromes Unintentionally Induced as the Result of Properly Indicated, Widely Accepted Therapeutic Procedures*, Charles C Thomas, Publisher, Springfield, Illinois, USA, 1959.
8. Illich I. *Limits to Medicine: Medical Nemesis, the Expropriation of Health*, Marion Boyars, London, UK, 1976.
9. Mendelsohn RS. *Confessions of a Medical Heretic*, Warner Books Inc, New York, NY, USA, 1979.
10. Mendelsohn RS, Crile G, Epstein S, Heimlich H, Levin AS, Pinckney ER, Spodick R, Moscowitz R, and White G. *Dissent in Medicine: Nine Doctors Speak Out*, Contemporary Books, Chicago, Illinois, USA, 1985.
11. Jackson DM and Soothill R. *Is the Medicine Making You Ill?* Angus and Robertson, North Ryde, NSW, Australia, 1989.
12. Reusch H. *Naked Empress or the Great Medical Fraud*, CIVIS, Zurich, Switzerland, 1982.
13. Goldacre B. *Bad Science*, Fourth Estate, London, UK, 2008.
14. Swan N. Australian Broadcasting Corporation, *Health Report*, date of broadcast unknown but content of it confirmed by Dr Norman Swan via e-mail on 14/7/2009.
15. Shimmel EM. "The hazards of hospitalization." *Annals of Internal Medicine*, 1964; 60 (1): 100–110.
16. Brennan TA, Leape LL, Laird NM, Hebert L, Localio AR, Lawthers AG, Newhouse JP, Weiler PC, and Hiatt HH. "Incidence of adverse events and negligence in hospitalized patients: results of the Harvard Medical Practice Study I." *The New England Journal of Medicine*, 1991; 324 (6): 370–376.
17. Leape LL, Brennan TA, Laird N. Lawthers AG, Localio AR, Barnes BA, Hebert L, Newhousse JP, Weiler PC, and Hiatt H. "The nature of adverse events in hospitalized patients: results of the Harvard Medical Practice Study II." *The New England Journal of Medicine*, 1991; 324 (6): 377–384.
18. Kohn LT, Corrigan JM, and Donaldson MS. (editors). *To Err is Human: Building a Safer Health System*, Institute of Medicine, National Academy of Sciences, Washington, D.C. USA, 1999.
19. Thomas EJ, Studdert DM, Burstin HR, Orav EJ, Zeena T, and Williams EJ. "Incidence and types of adverse events and negligence care in Utah and Colorado." *Medical Care*, 2000, 38 (3): 261–271.
20. Leape LL. "Error in medicine." *Journal of the American Medical Association*, 1994; Dec. 21; 272 (23): 1851-7.
21. Wilson RM, Runciman WB, Gibberd RW, Harrison BT, Newby L, and Hamilton JD. "The Quality in Australian Health Care Study." *Medical Journal of Australia*, 1995; 163 (9): 458–471.
22. Weingart SN, Wilson RM, Gibberd W, and Harrison B. "Epidemiology of medical error." *British Medical Journal*, 2000; 320 (17237): 774–777.

23. Rose G. *Compulsory Vaccination: A Statement of Concern from the Health Care Reform Group*, Glebe, NSW, Australia, 1991, p. 13.
24. Williams D, and Feely J. "Underreporting of adverse drug reactions: attitudes of Irish doctors." *Irish Journal of Medical Science*, 1999; 168 (4): 257-261.
25. Holland EG, and Degruy FV. "Drug-induced disorders." *American Family Physician*, 1997; 56 (7): 1781–1788, 1791–1792.
26. Manasse HR Jr. "Medication use in an imperfect world: drug misadventuring as an issue of public policy, Part 1." *American Journal of Hospital Pharmacy*, 1989; 46 (5) :929–44.
27. RR Porter. "The contribution of the biological and medical sciences for human welfare." Presidential Address to the British Association for the Advancement of Science, Swansea Meeting, 1971 (London, UK: The Association, 1972) pp. 95–97.
28. Lamour I, Dolphin RG, Baxter H, Morrison S, Hooke DH, McGrath BP. "A prospective study of hospital admissions due to drug reactions." *Australian Journal of Hospital Pharmacy*, 1991; 21 (2): 90–95.
29. Australian Government Public Health Service. Adverse Drug Reaction Advisory Committee. *The New Epidemic: A Collection of Case-studies by ADRAC, between 1975 and March 1981, Including Cases Portrayed in the ADRAC Film "The New Epidemic"*. Canberra, ACT, Australia, 1987; Cat. no. 8216021.
30. Gold J. "A crisis of confidence." *Australian Penthouse*, April 1983, p. 39.
31. Mann RD. *Modern Drug Use: An Enquiry on Historical Principles*, MTP Press, Lancaster, UK, 1984.
32. Rath M. *Death by Medicine*. Dr Rath Health Organization, Santa Clara, California, USA, 2009.
    [Online, accessed 11th July, 2009].
    URL:http://www4.dr-rath-foundation.org/features/death_by_medicine.html
33. Zhan C, and Miller MR. "Excess length of stay, charges and mortality attributable to medical injuries during hospitalization." *Journal of the American Medical Association*, 2003; 290 (14): 1868–1874.
34. HCUPnet, Healthcare Cost and Utilization Project for the Agency for Healthcare Research and Quality. Cited by Rath M, ibid reference 32.
    [Online, accessed 11th July, 2009]. URL:http://hcup.ahrq.gov/HCUPnet.asp
35. Weinstein RA. "Nosocomial infection update." *Emerging Infectious Diseases*, 1998; 4 (3): 416–420.
36. Lazarou J, Pomeranz BH, and Corey PN. "Incidence of adverse drug reactions in hospitalized patients: a meta-analysis of prospective studies." *Journal of the American Medical Association*, 1998; 279 (15): 1200–1205.
37. Suh DC, Woodall BS, Shin SK, and Hermes-De Santis ER. "Clinical and economic impact of adverse drug reactions in hospitalized patients." *The Annals of Pharmcotherapy*, 2000; 34 (12): 1373–1379.
38. Starfield B. "Is US health really the best in the world?" *Journal of the American Medical Association*, 2000; 284 (4): 483–485.
39. Leape L. National Patient Safety Foundation Press Release. *Nationwide Poll on Patient Safety, 100 Million Americans See Medical Mistakes Directly Touching Them*. National Patient Safety Foundation, October 9, 1997.
    [Online, accessed 19th July, 2009]. URL:http://www.npsf.org/pr/pressrel/finalgen.htm
40. Orr RD, Pang N, Pellegrino ED, and Siegler M. "Use of the Hippocratic Oath: a review of twentieth century practice and a content analysis of oaths administered in medical schools in the U.S. and Canada in 1993." *Journal of Clinical Ethics*, 1997; 8 (4): 377–388.

41. Pellegrino ED. "Professional codes." In: J Sugarman and DP Sulmasy (editors). *Methods in Medical Ethics*, Georgetown University Press, Washington, D.C., USA, 2001, pp. 80–87.
42. McNeill PM, and Dowton SB. "Declarations made by graduating medical students in Australia and New Zealand." *Medical Journal of Australia*, 2002; 176 (3): 123–125.
43. Mills S. "What does the Hippocratic oath mean?" *Irish Medical Times*, Opinion, April 24, 2009.
[Online, accessed 19th November, 2009].
URL:http://www.imt.ie/opinion/2009/04/what_does_the_hippocratic_oath.html
44. Graham D. "Revisiting Hippocrates: does an oath really matter?" *Journal of the American Medical Association*, 2000; 284 (22): 2841–2842.
45. Editor's choice: "Facing up to medical error." *British Medical Journal*, 2000; 320 (7237): 0.

CHAPTER 2—Tools of Medicine

Quote from Susan Love MD: from *Overdosed America: The Broken Promise of American Medicine*, John Abramson.

1. Farnsworth NR, Akerele O, Bingel AS, Soejarto DD, and Guo Z. "Medicinal plants in therapy, Update." *Bulletin of the World Health Organization*, 1985; 63 (6): 965–981.
2. Huffman MA, Gotoh S, Izutsu D, Koishimizu K, and Kalunde MS. "Further observations on the use of the medicinal plant *Vernonia amygdalina (Del)* by a wild chimpanzee, its possible effect on parasite load, and its phytochemistry." *African Study Monographs*, 1993; 14 (4): 227–240.
3. Spinney L. "I know what's good for me." *The Independent*, London, UK, August 3, 2005.
4. Leroi-Gourhan A. "The flowers found with Shanidar IV, a Neanderthal burial in Iraq." *Science*, 1975; 190 (4214): 562–564.
5. Solecki RS. "Shanidar IV, a Neanderthal flower burial in northern Iraq." *Science*, 1975; 190 (4217): 880–881.
6. Griggs B. *Green Pharmacy: A History of Herbal Medicine*. J. Norman and Hobhouse, London, UK, 1981.
7. Capra F. *The Turning Point: Science, Society and the Rising Culture*, Fontana Paperbacks, Glasgow, UK, 1982, pp. 40–41.
8. Bacon F. *Novum Organum: Or True Directions Concerning the Interpretation of Nature*, 1620. B Montague (editor and translator), *The Works*, 3 volumes, Parry and MacMillan, Philadelphia, Pennsylvania, USA, 1854. Online: Hanover Historical Texts Project, 2001. Online, accessed 20th July, 2009].
URL:http://history.hanover.edu/texts/Bacon/novorg.html
9. Brown WM. "Polymorphism in mitochondrial DNA of humans as revealed by restriction endonuclease analysis." *Proceedings of the National Academy of Sciences of the United States of America*, 1980; 77 (6): 3605–3609.
10. Jones JS, and Rouhani S. "How small was the bottleneck?" *Nature*, 1986; 319 (6053): 449–450.
11. Cann RL, Stoneking M, and Wilson AC. "Mitochondrial DNA and human evolution." *Nature*, 1987; 325 (6099): 31–36.
12. Rouhani S. "Molecular genetics and the pattern of human evolution: plausible and implausible models." In: P Mellars, and C Stringer (editors), *The Human Revolution: Behavioral and Biological Perspectives in the Origins of Modern Humans*, Princeton University Press, Princeton, New Jersey, USA, 1989, pp. 47–61.

13. Butzer KW, Beaumont PB, and Vogel JC. "Lithostratigraphy of Border Cave, KwaZulu, South Africa: a Middle Stone Age sequence beginning c. 195,000 b.p." *Journal of Archaeological Science*, 1978; 5 (4): 317–341.
14. Rightmire GP, and Deacon HJ. "Comparative studies of late Pleistocene human remains from Klasies River mouth, South Africa." *Journal of Human Evolution*, 1991; 20 (2): 131–156.
15. Rightmire GP. "Out of Africa: Modern human origins special feature: Middle and later Pleistocene hominins in Africa and Southwest Asia." *Proceedings of the National Academy of Sciences of the United States of America*, 2009; 106 (38): 16046–16050.
16. Walter RC, Buffler RT, Bruggemann JH, Guillaume MMM, Berhe SM, Negassi B, Libsekal Y, Cheng H, Edwards RL, von Cosel R, Neraudeau D, and Gagnon M. "Early human occupation of the Red Sea coast of Eritrea during the last interglacial." *Nature* (Letters), 2000; 405 (6782): 65–69.
17. McDougall I, Brown FH, and Fleagle JG. "Stratigraphic placement and age of modern humans from Kibish, Ethiopia." *Nature* (Letters), 2004; 433 (7027): 733–736.
18. *Appalachian State University News*, Boone, North Carolina, USA. "Appalachian geologist investigates Homo sapiens' oldest known trackways." September 15, 2009.
[Online, accessed 29th November, 2009].
URL:http://www.news.appstate.edu/2009/09/15/geologist-homo-sapiens/
19. Tiner JH. *Louis Pasteur: Founder of Modern Medicine* (Sower Series). Mott Media, Milford, Michigan, USA, 1990.
20. Goldberg JG (editor). *Psychotherapeutic Treatment of Cancer Patients*, Transaction Publishers, New Brunswick, New Jersey, USA, 1990, "Introduction", p. x.
21. Rosenthaler L. *The Chemical Investigation of Plants*, Monographs on Modern Chemistry, J Kendall, and J Read (editors), G Bell and Sons Ltd, London, UK, 1930, pp. 1–12.
22. Liebenau J. *Medical Science and Medical Industry: The Formation of the American Pharmaceutical Industry*, John Hopkins University Press, Baltimore, Maryland, USA, 1987.
23. World Trade Organization. *Uruguay Round General Agreement on Tariffs and Trade* (GATT), Uruguay, 1994. *Agreement of Trade-Related Aspects of Intellectual Property Rights* (TRIPS), Part II–"Standards concerning the availability, scope and use of Intellectual Property Rights", Section 5, Article 27.1 and Article 33.
[Online, accessed 29th November, 2009].
URL:http://www.wto.org/english/docs_e/legal_e/27-trips_04c_e.htm
24. *New Internationalist*. "Big Pharma: the Facts." 2003; 362: 18–19.
25. Sellers GJ (editor). "Special Report: Fourth Annual 50." *Pharmaceutical Executive*, May, 2003.
26. Robinson J. *Prescription Games: Money, EGO, and Power Inside the Global Pharmceutical Industry*, Simon and Schuster, New York, NY, USA, 2001.
27. Kegley CW Jr, and Wittkopf WR. *World Politics: Trend and Transformation*, Bedford/St. Martins, New York, NY, USA, 2001, p 231.
28. Public Citizen Congress Watch. *Rx R&D Myths: The Case Against the Drug Industry's R&D "Scare Card"*, 12th November, 2001.
[Online, accessed 15th July, 2009].
URL:http://www.citizen.org.publications/release.cfm?ID=7065&secID=1078&catID=126
29. Families USA Foundation. *Profiting from Pain: Where Prescription Drug Dollars Go*, July 2002.
[Online, accessed 14th July, 2009]. URL:http://www.familiesusa.org
30. Angell M. *The Truth About the Drug Companies: How They Deceive Us and What to Do About It*, Random House, New York, NY, USA, 2004.

31. Public Citizen Congress Watch. *The Other Drug War: Big Pharma's 625 Washington Lobbyists*, 23rd July, 2001. [Online, accessed 15th July, 2009]. URL:http://citizen.org/publications/release.cfm?ID=7077&secID=1078&catID=126
32. Cohen R. "An epidemic of neglect: neglected diseases and the health burden in poor countries." *Multinational Monitor*, 2002; 23 (6): 9–13.
33. *IMS World Review 2003*, [Online, accessed 15th July, 2009]. URL:http://www.IMS-global.com.
34. Moynihan R. "Sweetening the pill." *The Age, Good Weekend*, Melbourne, Australia, 31 May, 2003, pp. 16–21
35. O'Reilly D. "Drug doctors under fire." *The Bulletin*, Australia, 24 March, 1992, pp. 21,22.
36. Fortune. *The 2002 Fortune 500*. [Online, accessed 15th July, 2009]. URL:http://www.fortune.com

CHAPTER 3—Why Modern Medicine May Be Harming You

1. Personal correspondence with Kevin Norton, Professor of Exercise Science at the University of South Australia, May, 2005.
2. Television advertisement for Codral, by Johnson & Johnson.
3. Gigaldi M. *Biopharmaceutics and Clinical Pharmacokinetics*, 2nd Edition, Lea and Febiger, Philadelphia, Pennsylvania, USA, 1977.
4.. Saunders L. *The Absorption and Distribution of Drugs*, Balliere Tindall, London, UK, 1974.
5. Smith SE, Rawlins MD. *Variability in Human Drug Response*, Butterworths, London, UK, 1973.
6. Editorial. "Pharmacogenetics—expectations and reality: drug response and toxicity depend on genes, environment, and behaviour." *British Medical Journal*, 2004; 329: 4–6.
7. Holland EG, and Degruy FV. "Drug-induced disorders." *American Family Physician*, 1997; 56 (7): 1–7.
8. *There Was an Old Lady Who Swallowed a Fly*. Written by Alan Mills, lyrics by Rose Bonne, sung by Burle Ives, Brunswick Records, White Plains, NY, USA, 1953.
9. Gurwitz JH, and Avorn J. "The ambiguous relation between aging and adverse drug reactions." *Annals of Internal Medicine*, 1991; 114 (11): 956–966.
10. Fugh-Berman A. "Herb-drug interactions." *The Lancet*, 2000; 355 (9208): 134–138.
11. Editorial. "Drug industry situation uncertain but hopeful." *Journal of the American Medical Association*, 1964; 187 (11): 35. Quoting a speech made by James D Gallagher, director of Medical Research at Lederle Laboratories, at a conference presented by the American College of Neuropsychopharmacology in Washington, DC, on January 16, 1964.
12. Schardein JL. *Drugs as Teratogens*, CRC Press, Cleveland, Ohio, USA, 1976.
13. Smithells RW. "Drug teratogenicity." In: WHW Inman (editor), *Monitoring for Drug Safety*, MTP Press, Lancaster, England, UK, 1986; pp. 383–390.
14. Bross I. "Animals in cancer research: a multi-million dollar fraud", *Fundamental and Applied Toxicology*, 6 November, 1982.
15. Hawkins DF (editor). *Drugs and Pregnancy: Human Teratogenesis and Related Problems*, D.F. Hawkins (editor), Churchill Livingstone, New York, NY, USA, 1983.
16. Lorke D. "A new approach to acute toxicity testing." *Archives of Toxicology*, 1983; 54: 275–287.
17. McLachlan JA, Pratt RM, and Markert CL. *Developmental Toxicology: Mechanisms and Risks*

(The Banbury Report), Cold Spring Harbor Laboratory, Cold Spring Harbor, NY, USA, 1987; p. 313.
18. Sharpe R. *The Cruel Deception: The Use of Animals in Medical Research*, Thorsons Publishing Group, Wellingborough, Northamptonshire, UK, 1988.
19. Croce P. *Vivisection or Science–A Choice to Make*, CIVIS (International Centre of Scientific Information on Vivisection) Publications, Lugano, Switzerland, 1991.
20. Reusch H. *Naked Empress or the Great Medical Fraud*, CIVIS, Zurich, Switzerland, 1982.
21. Brent RL. "Utilization of animal studies to determine the effects and human risks of environmental toxicants (drugs, chemicals, and physical agents)." *Pediatrics*, 2004; 113 (4): 984–995.
22. Bailey J, Knight A, and Balcombe J. "The future of teratology research is in vitro." *Biogenic Amines*, 2005; 19 (2): 97–146.
23. Knight A, Bailey J, and Balcombe J. "Animal experiments harm human health." *American Chronicle* [Online newspaper], 8 October 2005.
[Online, accessed 15th July, 2009].
URL:http://www.americanchronicle.com/articles/viewArticle.asp?artcleID=2819
24. Balcombe J, Barnard N, and Sandusky C. "Laboratory routines cause animal stress." *Contemporary Topics in Laboratory Animal Science*, 2004; 43 (6): 42–51.
25. Yusuf S, Collins R, and Peto R. "Why do we need some large and simple randomized trials?" *Statistical Medicine*, 1984; 3: 409–420.
26. Altman DG. "Size of clincal trials." *British Medical Journal* (Clinical Research Edition), 1983; 286 (6381): 1842–1843.
27. Van Spall HGC, Toren A, Kiss A, and Fowler RA. "Eligibility criteria of randomized controlled trials published in high-impact general medical journals." *Journal of the American Medical Association*, 2007; 297 (11): 1233–1240.
28. Relman AS, and Angell M. "America's other drug problem: how the drug industry distorts medicines and politics." *The New Republic*, December 16, 2002, pp. 27–41.
29. Angell M. *The Truth about the Drug Companies: How They Deceive Us and What to Do About It*, Random House, New York, NY, USA, 2004.
30. Angell M. "Drug companies and doctors: a story of corruption." *The New York Review of Books*, January 15, 2009; 56 (1): 8–12.
31. Angell M. Ibid reference 29, p. 30.
32. Angell M. "The body hunters." *The New York Review of Books*, October 6, 2005; 52 (15): 23–25.
33. Angell M. "The ethics of clinical research in the third world." *The New England Journal of Medicine*, 1997; 337 (12): 847–849.
34. Shah S. *The Body Hunters: Testing New Drugs on the World's Poor*, The New Press, New York, NY, USA, 2006.
35. Demicheli V, Jefferson T, Rivetti A, and Price D. "Vaccines for measles, mumps and rubella in children." *Cochrane Database of Systematic Reviews*, 2005; 4 (CD004407).
36. Jefferson T, Rivetti A. Harnden AR. Di Pietrantonj C, and Demicheli V. "Vaccines for preventing influenza in healthy children." *Cochrane Database of Systematic Reviews*, 2008; 2 (CD0048979).
37. Macartney K, and McIntyre P. "Vaccines for post-exposure prophylaxis against varicella (chicken pox) in children and adults." *Cochrane Database of Systematic Reviews*, 2008; 3 (CD001833).
38. Soares-Weiser K, Goldberg E, Tamimi G, Leibovici L, and Pitan F. "Rotavirus vaccine for preventing diarrhoea." *Cochrane Database of Systematic Reviews*, 2004; 1 (CD002848).

39. *Physicians' Desk Prescriber*, 61st Edition, Thomson, Montvale, New Jersey, USA, 2007; pp. 819, 1405, 1426, 1452, 1457, 1478, 1550, 1596, 1902, 1915, 1930, 1986, 2007, 2020, 2032, 2037, 2065, 2073, 2076, 2098, 2102, 2111, 2947, 2951, 2956, 3427, and 3467.
40. US Centers for Disease Control and Prevention. "Prevalence of autism spectrum disorders; Autism and Developmental Disabilities Monitoring Network, United States, 2006." *Morbidity and Mortality Weekly Report*, December 18, 2009; 58 (SS10): 1–20.
41. Kogan MD, Blumberg SJ, Schieve LA, Boyle CA, Perrin JM, Ghandour RM, Singh GK, Strickland BB, Trevathan E, and Van Dyck PC. "Prevalence of parent-reported diagnosis of autism spectrum disorder among children in the US, 2007." *Pediatrics*, 2009; 124 (9): 1395–1404.
42. Smith PJ, Chu SY, and Barker LE. "Children who have received no vaccines: who are they and where do they live?" *Pediatrics*, 2004; 114 (1): 187–195.
43. Olmsted D. "The age of autism: the Amish anomaly." United Press International, April 18, 2005.
    [Online, accessed 11th January, 2010].
    URL:http://www.upi.com/Science_News/2005/04/19/The-Age-of-Autism-The-Amish-anomaly/UPI-95661113911795/
44. Olmsted D. "The age of autism: Julia." United Press International, April 19, 2005.
    [Online, accessed 11th January, 2010].
    URL:http://www.upi.com/Science_News/2005/04/19/The-Age-of-Autism-Julia/UPI-55491113918060/
45. Olmstead D. "The age of autism: absence of evidence." United Press International, May 9, 2005.
    [Online, accessed 11th January, 2010].
    URL:http://www.upi.com/Science_News/2005/05/09/The-Age-of-Autism-Absence-of-evidence/UPI-50051115667435/
46. Olmstead D. "The age of autism: witness." United Press International, May 10, 2005.
    [Online, accessed 11th January, 2010].
    URL:http://www.upi.com/Science_News/2005/05/10/The-Age-of-Autism-Witness/UPI-36431115734474/
47. Olmstead D. "The age of autism: one in 15,000 Amish." United Press International, June 8, 2005.
    [Online, accessed 11th January, 2010].
    URL:http://www.upi.com/Science_News/2005/06/08/The-Age-of-Autism-One-in-15000-Amish/UPI-74721118251747/
48. Olmstead D. "The age of autism: 'a pretty big secret". United Press International, December 7, 2005. [Online, accessed 11th January, 2010].
    URL:http://www.upi.com/Health_News/2005/12/07/The-Age-of-Autism-A-pretty-big-secret/UPI-68291133982531/
49. Olmstead D. "The age of autism: Amish ways." United Press International, June 6, 2005.
    [Online, accessed 11th January, 2010].
    URL:http://www.upi.com/Science_News/2005/06/The-Age-of-Autism-Amish-ways/UPI-80061118082873/
50. Olmsted D. "The age of autism: 'Amish bill' introduced." United Press International, July 28, 2006.
    [Online, accessed 11th January, 2010].
    URL:http://www.upi.com/Health_News/2006/07/28/The-Age-of-Autism-Amish-bill-introduced/UPI-35321154110819/

51. Olmstead D. "The age of autism: the last word." United Press International, July 18, 2007.
    [Online, accessed 11th January, 2010].
    URL:http://www.upi.com/Health_News/2007/07/18/The-Age-of-Autism-The-last-word/UPI-57611184777255/
52. Generation Rescue/SurveyUSA. *Cal-Oregon Vaccinated vs. Unvaccinated Survey*, Generation Rescue, Sherman Oaks, California, USA, and SurveyUSA, Verona, New Jersey, USA. Press release: Portland, Oregon, September 25, 2007.
    [Online, accessed 11th January, 2010].
    URL:http://www.GenerationRescue.org/survey.html
53. US Centers for Disease Control and Prevention. "Mental health in the United States: prevalence of diagnosis and medication treatment for attention-deficiency/hyperactivity disorder; United States, 2003." *Morbidity and Mortality Weekly Report*, September, 2005; 54 (34): 842–847.

CHAPTER 4—Drug Hype

Quote of Dr Oliver Wendell Holmes Sr: from *Currents and Counter-Currents in Medical Science with Other Addresses and Essays*, 1861.

1. Landymore-Lim L. *Poisonous Prescriptions*, PODD, Subiaco, Western Australia, Australia, 1996, p. 115.
2. The Wellcome Museum of the History of Medicine. Exhibition Case S1, Science Museum, London, UK, 1992. Cited in Landymore-Lim L, ibid reference 1.
3. Riley CR. *Rising Life Expectancy: A Global History*, Cambridge University Press, Cambridge, England, UK, 2001: pp. 2 and 21.
4. Hawkes K. "Grandmothers and the evolution of human longevity." *American Journal of Human Biology*, 2003; 15 (3): 380–400.
5. Gurven M, and Kaplan H. "Longevity among hunter-gatherers: a cross cultural examination." *Population and Development Review*, 2007; 33 (2): 321–365.
6. Petrie CC. *Tom Petrie's Reminiscences of Early Queensland (Dating from 1937)*, first published by Watson & Ferguson, Brisbane, Queensland, 1904. Re-published by University of Queensland Press Paperbacks, St Lucia, Queensland, Australia, 1992.
7. McCloy P. "Becoming an elder." *Manzine*, Issue 1, 23 June, 2001.
    [Online, accessed 14th January, 2010].
    URL:http://www.manhood.com.au/manhood.nsf/8178b1c14b1e9b6b8525624f0062fe9f/0551d6316ec5001f4a256a740043263a!OpenDocument
8. Ship SJ, and Tarbell R. *Our Nations' Elders Speak: Ageing and Cultural Diversity, A Cross-Cultural Approach*, published by the National Indian and Inuit Community Health Representatives Organization (NIICHRO), Kahnawake, Quebec, Canada, 1997.
    [Online accessed 14th January, 2010].
    URL:http://www.niichro.com/Elders/Elders7.html
9. McNamara R. "Mortality Trends. 1. Historical Trends." In: JA Ross (editor), *International Encyclopedia of Population, Vol 2*, The Free Press, New York, NY, USA, 1982, pp. 459–461.
10. Westminster Abbey, London, UK. "The Library and Archives, People Buried or Commemorated, Thomas Parr."
    [Online, accessed 16th July, 2009].
    URL:http://www.westminster-abbey.org/our-history/people/thomas-parr
11. Dubos R. *Mirage of Health: Utopias, Progress and Biological Change*, Harper & Row, New

York, NY, USA, 1959, pp. 88-89.
12. Illich I. *Limits to Medicine: Medical Nemesis, the Expropriation of Health*, Marion Boyars, London, UK, 1976, pp. 23–30.
13. McKeown T. *The Role of Medicine: Dream, Mirage or Nemesis*, Princeton University Press, Princeton, New Jersey, USA, 1979, pp. 29–44.
14. Mc Keown T. *The Modern Rise of Population*, Edward Arnold, London, UK, 1976.
15. McKeown T, Brown RG, and Record RG. "An Interpretation of the Modern Rise of Population in Europe." *Population Studies*, 1972; 26 (3): 345–82.
16. RR Porter. "The contribution of the biological and medical sciences for human welfare." Presidential Address to the British Association for the Advancement of Science, Swansea Meeting, 1971 (London, UK: The Association, 1972) pp. 95–97.
17. Pollard JH. "Morbidity and Longevity." In: Ross JA (editor), *International Encyclopedia of Population, Vol 2*, The Free Press, New York, NY, USA, 1982, pp. 452–459.
18. Coulter HL. *The Medical Assault on the American Brain: Vaccination, Social Violence, and Criminality*, North Atlantic Books, Berkeley, California, USA, 990, pp. 83 and 101.
19. Rutstein SO. "Factors associated with trends in infant and child mortality in developing countries during the 1990s." *Bulletin of the World Health Organization*, 2000; 78 (10): 1256–1270.
20. Riley CR, ibid reference 3; p. 1.
21. Gavrilova NS, Kushnareva YE, Gavrilov LA, Semyonova VG, Gavrilova AL, Evdokushkina NN, and Lapshin EV. "Human longevity: past, present and future." A.N. Belozersky Institute, Moscow State University, Russia. In: *Longevity Report 52*, (Truro, Cornwall, UK), 1995: 9 (52): 3–4.
[Online, accessed 16th July, 2009].
URL:http://www.quantium.plus.com/lr/lr52.htm#Human%20Longevity

CHAPTER 5—To Vaccinate or Not to Vaccinate

1. *Rogers v. Whitaker*, the High Court of Australia 1992, 175 CLR 479; 19th November, 1992.
2. Posfay-Barbe KM, Heininger U, Aebi C, Desgrandchamps D, Vaudaux B, and Siegrist C-A. "How do physicians immunize their own children? Differences between pediatricians and nonpediatricians." *Pediatrics*, 2005; 116 (5): 623–633.
3. Katz-Sidlow RJ, and Sidlow R. "A look at the pediatrician as parent: experiences with the introduction of Varicella vaccine." *Clinical Pediatrics*, 2003; 42 (7): 635–640.
4. Diekema DS, and the Committee of Immunization of Children. "Responding to parental refusals of immunization of children." *Pediatrics*, 2005; 115 (5): 1428–1431.
5. Dionne M, Boulianne N, Duval B, Lavoie F, Laflamme N, Carsley J, Valiquette L, Gagnon S, Rochette L, and De Serres G. "Lack of conviction about vaccination in certain Quebec vaccinators." *Canadian Journal of Public Health*, 2000; 92 (2): 100–104.
6. Kinnersley P. "Attitudes of general practitioners towards their vaccination against hepatitis B." *British Medical Journal*, 1990; 300 (6719): 238.
7. Gerety RJ. "Hepatitis B transmission between dental and medical workers and patients." *Annals of Internal Medicine*, 1981; 95 (2): 229–231.
8. Preblud SR, and Hinman AR. "Rubella vaccination of hospital employees." *Journal of the American Medical Association*, 1981; 245 (7): 736–737.
9. Orenstein WA, Heseltine PN, LeGagnoux SJ and Portnoy B. "Rubella vaccine and susceptible hospital employees. Poor physician participation." *Journal of the American*

Medical Association, 1981; 245 (7): 711–713.
10. Bishburg E, Shah M, and Mathis AS. "Influenza vaccination among residents in a teaching hospital." *Infection Control and Hospital Epidemiology*, 2008; 29: 89–91.
11. Saluja I, Theakston KD, and Kaczorowski J. "Influenza vaccination rate among emergency department personnel: a survey of four teaching hospitals." *Canadian Journal of Emergency Medical Care*, 2005; 7 (1): 17–21.
12. Ohrt CK, and McKinney WP. "Achieving compliance with influenza immunization of medical house staff and students. A randomized controlled trial." *Journal of the American Medical Association*, 1992; 267 (10): 1377–1386.
13. Dole L. *The Blood Poisoners*, Gateway Book Company, Croydon, Surrey, UK, 1965; chapter 2.
14. Kenneth R, and Wear A, *The Medical Revolution of the Seventeenth Century*, Cambridge University Press, Cambridge, UK, 1989; p. 178. Citing K. Dewhurt, *Dr Thomas Sydenham (1624–1689): His Life and Original Writings*, University of California Press, Berkeley, California, USA, 1966; p. 163.
15. Wohl AS. *Endangered Lives: Public Health in Victorian Britain*, JM Dent and Sons Ltd, London, UK, 1983; p. 133.
16. Editorial: *The Lancet*, July 15, 1871.
17. Hadwen, W.S. "Sanitation v. vaccination–the origin of smallpox." *Truth*, January 17, 1923.
18. Wallace WR. *The Wonderful Century: It's Successes and Its Failures*, Swan Sonnenschein and Co, London, UK, 1898; In chapter entitled "Vaccination a Delusion."
19. Wallace WR. *To Members of Parliament and Others: Forty-five Years of Registration Statistics, Proving Vaccination to be Both Useless and Dangerous (S374: 1885)*. Reprinted in Wallace WR, ibid reference 18.
20. Ruata C. "Vaccination in Italy." *New York Medical Journal*, July 22, 1899. Cited in Dr JW Hodge, *The Vaccination Superstition*, Niagara Falls, NY, USA, 1901 (Read before the Western New York Homeopathic Medical Society in Buffalo) April 11, 1902; pp. 6–7.
21. Briggs JT. *Leicester: Sanitation versus Vaccination*. Anti-Vaccination League, London, UK, 1912; chapter 103.
22. Slotten RA. *The Heretic in Darwin's Court: The Life of Alfred Russel Wallace*, Columbia University Press, New York, USA, 2004; pp. 422–436.
23. Scheibner V. *Vaccination: 100 Years of Orthodox Research shows that Vaccines Represent a Medical Assault on the Immune System*, published by Viera Scheibner, Blackheath, NSW, Australia, 1993; pp. 205–223.
24. Report of the Philippines Health Service by Dr V. de Jesus, 1920. Cited in Koch WF. *Survival Factor in Neoplastic and Viral Diseases, An Introduction to Carbonyl and Free Radical Therapy*, Natural Immunity Series, 1961; chapter 2.
[Online, accessed 7th September, 2009]. URL:http://www.williamkoch.com
25. Kalokerinos A, and Dettman G. "Viral vaccines vital or vulnerable." *The Australasian Nurses Journal*, 1980; 9 (9): 27–32.
26. "Smallpox in vaccinated and re-vaccinated Japan." *The Vaccination Inquirer*, May 1, 1908; 30: 28. "Smallpox in Japan", ibid., July 1, 1908; 30: 62. And "The argument from Japan." ibid., October 1, 1909, 31: 141–143.
27. Hodge JW. "The failure of vaccination to protect from smallpox in re-vaccinated Japan." *The Twentieth Century Magazine*, 1910; 2 (12): 508–522.
28. Pitcairn J. "The fallacy of vaccination." *Ladies Home Journal*, May, 1910.
29. McCormick WJ. "The changing incidence and mortality of infectious disease in relation to changed trends in nutrition." *Medical Record*, Medical Journal and Record Publishing

Company Inc, September, 1947. Reprinted by the Lee Foundation for Nutritional Research, Milwaukee, Wisconsin, USA; reprint no. 5a.

30. Dubos R. *Mirage of Health: Utopias, Progress and Biological Change*, Rutgers University Press, Brunswick, New Jersey, USA, 1959.
31. Illich I. *Limits to Medicine: Medical Nemesis–The Expropriation of Health*, Marion Boyars, London, UK, 1976.
32. McKeown T. *The Role of Medicine: Dream, Mirage or Nemesis?* Nuffield Provincial Hospital Trust, London, UK, 1976.
33. McKinlay JB, and McKinlay SM. "The questionable contribution of medical measures to the decline of mortality in the United States in the twentieth century." *Milbank Memorial Fund Quarterly*, Summer, 1977; 55 (3): 405–428.
34. Obomsawin R. *Universal Immunization: Medical Miracle or Masterful Mirage*, Health Action Network Society, Burnaby, British Columbia, Canada, 1996; Section 1: "WHO Smallpox Eradication Success Re-Considered."
35. Baratosy P. *Vaccination: It's Your Informed Choice*, published by Peter Bararatosy, Adelaide, South Australia, Australia, 2004; pp. 12–13.
36. McBean E. *The Poisoned Needle: Suppressed Facts about Vaccination*. Health Research Books, Pomeroy, California, USA, 1959; Chapter IV: "The history of vaccinations".
37. Galazka A, and Tomaszunas-Blaszczyk J. "Why do adults contract diphtheria." *Eurosurveillance*, 1997; 2 (8): 60–63.
38. Winslow CEA. "Who killed Cock Robin?" *American Journal of Public Health*, 1944; 34: 658–659.
39. McBean E. Ibid reference 36, Chapter II: "Smallpox Declined Before Vaccination was Enforced."
40. Biggs JT. *Leicester: Sanitation versus Vaccination*, Part 13, Chapter 107: "London Evidence Against Anti-Toxin", National Anti-Vaccination League, London, UK, 1912.
41. Loat L. *The Truth about Vaccination and Immunization*. Health For All Publishing Company, London, England, UK, 1951; Part II.
42. Kater MH. *Doctors under Hitler*, University of North Carolina Press, Chapel Hill, North Carolina, USA, 2000; pp. 40–41.
43. Stowman K. "Diphtheria rebounds." *Epidemiological Information Bulletin*, UN Refugee and Relief Agency, Health Division, Washington, DC, USA, 15th February, 1945; 1: 157–168.
44. Crowley, T. Letter published in the *South Yorkshire Times*, March 11th, 1938. In: Beddow-Bayly M. *The "Schick" Inoculation for Immunisation Against Diphtheria: An Exposure of its Dangers and Fallacies*. Second Edition, The National Anti-Vaccination League, London, UK, 1939. Section 5: "Shick Immunisation," No. 18.
45. Dole L. *The Blood Poisoners*, Gateway Book Company, Croydon, Surrey, UK; 1965.
46. Editorial: "Diphtheria incidence and trends in relation to artificial immunization, with some comparative data for scarlet fever." *Public Health Reports*, 15th February, 1946; 61 (7): 203–237.
47. Stowan K. "The epidemic outlook in Europe." *Epidemiological Information Bulletin*, UN Refugee and Relief Agency, Health Division, Washington, DC, USA, February 15, 1945; 1: 101–111.
48. Liebow AA, and Bumstead JH. "Cutaneous and other aspects of diphtheria." In: Lieutenant General LD Heaton, Colonel JB Coates Jr., and WP Havens Jr. (editors), *Internal Medicine in World War II*, Volume II, Infectious Diseases; Office of the Surgeon General, Department of the Army, Washington, DC, USA, 1963; pp. 275–279.
49. Mendelsohn R. "The truth about immunization." *The People's Doctor*, April, 1978; p. 1.

50. Galazka AM, and Robertson SE. "Diphtheria: patterns in the developing world and the industrialized world." *European Journal of Epidemiology*, 1995; 11 (1): 107–117.
51. Edsall G. *Some Unsolved Problems in Diphtheria*, World Health Organisation, WHO/BAG/75.2, July 4, 1975.
52. Schneerson R. "Similarities between the pathogenesis of and immunity to diphtheria and pertussis: the complex nature of serum antitoxin-induced immunity to these two diseases." *Clinical Infectious Diseases*, 1999; 28: 136–139.
53. Hedrich A. *Epidemic Studies: The Monthly Variation of Measles Susceptibles in Baltimore, Maryland from 1901 to 1928*. Thesis, John Hopkins University, Baltimore, Maryland, USA, 1933.
54. Vitek CR, and Wharton M. "Diphtheria in the former Soviet Union: reemergence of a pandemic epidemic." *Emerging Infectious Diseases*, 1998; 4 (4): 539–550.
55. Robbins JB, Schneerson R, Trolifors B. "Pertussis in developed countries." *The Lancet*, 2002; 360 (9334): 657–658.
56. Editorial: "Diphtheria in the 1990s–do we have all the answers?" *Eurosurveillance*, 1997; 2 (8): Article 1.
57. Vitek CR, Brisgalov SP, Bragina VY, Zhilyakov AM, Bisgard KM, Brennan M, Kravtsova ON, Lushniak BD, Lyerla R, Markina SS, and Strebel PM. "Epidemiology of epidemic diphtheria in three regions, Russia, 1994–1996." *European Journal of Epidemiology*, 1999; 15 (1): 75–83.
58. Holt LE Jr., and McIntosh R. *Molt's Diseases of Infancy and Childhood*, 11th edition, D. Appleton-Century, New York, USA, 1940; p. 1083.
59. Pruitt BA, and Pruitt JH. "History of trauma care." In: ME Moore, DV Feliciano, and KL Mattox (editors). *Trauma*, Edition 5, McGraw-Hill Professional, New York, USA, 2003, pp. 13–16.
60. Boyd J. "Tetanus in Two World Wars." In: "Section of Epidemiology and Preventive Medicine", *Proceedings of the Royal Society of Medicine*, 1958; 52 (2): 109–110.
61. Murray CK, Hinkle MK, and Yun HC. "History of infections associated with combat-related injuries." *The Journal of Trauma*, 2008; 64 (3): S221–S231.
62. Bollet AJ. "The major infectious epidemic diseases of Civil War soldiers." *Infectious Disease Clinics of North America*, 2004; 18 (2): 293–309.
63. Noon G. "The treatment of casualties in the Great War." In: P Griffith (editor), *British Fighting Methods in the Great War*. Routledge, New York, USA, 1998; p. 95–97.
64. Furste WA. "A golden opportunity." *The Journal of Trauma*, 1998; 44 (6): 1110–1112.
65. Adams EB, Laurence DR, Smith JWG. *Tetanus*. Blackwell Scientific, Oxford, UK, 1969; p. 745.
66. MacLennan JD. "Anaerobic infections of war wounds in the Middle East." *The Lancet*, 1943; 2: 63–66, 94–99, 123–126.
67. Wahdan H. "Causes of the antimicrobial activity of honey." *Infection*, 1998; 26 (1): 26–31.
68. Long AP, and Sartwell PE, "Tetanus in the U.S. Army in World War II. *Bulletin of the US Army Medical Department*, 1947; 7: 371–385.
69. Glen F. "Tetanus–a preventable disease: including an experience with civilian casualties in the Battle for Manila (1945)." *Annals of Surgery*, 1946; 124 (6): 1030–1040.
70. Noon D. Ibid reference 63, p. 96.
71. Conybeare ET. "Tetanus in the civilian population of England and Wales." In: "Section of Epidemiology and Preventive Medicine", *Proceedings of the Royal Society of Medicine*, 1958; 52 (2): 112–114.

72. Fraser DW. "Tetanus in the United States, 1900–1969: analysis by cohorts." *American Journal of Epidemiology*, 1972; 96 (4): 306–312.
73. Boyd JSK. "Tetanus in the African and European theatres of war, 1939–1945." *The Lancet*, 1946; 1: 113–119.
74. Hall WW. "The U.S. Navy's war record with tetanus toxoid." *Annals of Internal Medicine*, 1948; 28 (2): 298–308.
75. Boyer JK, Corre-Hurst L, Sapin-Jalouste H, and Tissier M. "Le tetanos en milieu urbain: conditions d'apparition-deduction a prophylactiques." [In French], [Tetanus in urban conditions: conditions under which it appears and preventive measures.] *La Presse Medicale*, 1953; 61 (34): 701–703.
76. Hedrick EC. "Tetanus: two cases in immunized persons." *California Medicine*, 1953; 79 (1): 49–50.
77. Long AP. "Immunization to tetanus." *Industrial Medicine and Surgery*, 1954; 23 (6): 275–277.
78. Moss GW, Waters GG, and Brown MH. "The efficacy of tetanus toxoid." *Canadian Journal of Public Health*, 1955; 46 (4): 142–147.
79. Christensen NA, And Thurber DL. "Clinical experience with tetanus: 91 cases." *Proceedings of the Staff Meetings, Mayo Clinic*; 1957; 32 (7): 146–158.
80. Edsall G. "Specific prophylaxis of tetanus." *Journal of the American Medical Association*, 1959; 171: 417–427.
81. Peterson HI. "A case of tetanus in spite of active toxoid prophylaxis." *Acta Chirurgia Scandinavica*, 1965; 129: 235–237.
82. National Communicable Disease Center. *Tetanus Surveillance Report No. 1*, Atlanta, Georgia, USA, Bureau of Disease Prevention and Environmental Control, United States Public Health Service, February 1, 1968.
83. Peebles TC, Levine L, Eldred MC, and Edsall G. "Tetanus-toxoid emergency boosters: a reappraisal." *The New England Journal of Medicine*, 1969; 280 (11): 575–581.
84. Goulon M, Girard O, Grosbuis S, Desormeau JP, and Capponi MF. "Les anticorps antitetaniques: titrage avant seroanatoxinotherapie chez 64 tetanique." [In French] ["Antitetanus antibodies: assay before anatoxinotherapy in 64 tetanus patients."] *La Nouvelle Presse Medicale*, 1972; 1 (45): 3049–3050.
85. Spittle BJ. Pollock M. and O'Donnell TV. "Tetanus occurring in spite of active immunisation." *New Zealand Medical Journal*, 1973; 77 (491): 250–251.
86. Berger SA, Cherubin CE, Nelson S, and Levine L. "Tetanus despite preexisting antitetanus antibody." *Journal of the American Medical Association*, 1978; 240 (8): 769–770.
87. Dittman S. *Atypische Verlaeute nach Schutzimpfungen*. Johan Ambrosius Barth, Leipzig, Germany, 1981; p. 156.
88. Baptist EC. "Tetanus in a partially immunized infant with burns." *Pediatric Infectious Disease*, 1984; 3 (5): 487–488.
89. Vieira BI, Dunne JW, and Summers, Q. "Cephalic tetanus in an immunized patient." *Medical Journal of Australia*, 1986; 145: 156–157.
90. Passen EL, and Andersen B. "Clinical tetanus despite a protective level of toxin-neutralising antibody." *Journal of the American Medical Association*, 1988; 255 (9): 1171–1173.
91. Crone NE, and Reder AT. "Severe tetanus in immunized patients with high anti-tetanus titers." *Neurology*, 1992; 42: 761–764.
92. Luisto M, and Iivanainen M. "Tetanus of immunized children." *Developmental Medicine and Child Neurology*, 1993; 35 (4): 351–355.
93. Pryor T, Onarecker C, and Coniglione T. "Elevated abitoxin titers in a man with

generalized tetanus." *The Journal of Family Practice*, 1997; 44: 299–303.
94. Shimoni Z, Dobrousin A, Cohen J, and Pilik S. "Tetanus in an immunised patient." *British Medical Journal*, 1999; 319: 1049.
95. Vinson DR. "Immunisation does not rule out tetanus." *British Medical Journal*, Letters, 2000; 320: 383.
96. Abramanian FM. "Fatal tetanus in a drug abuser with "protective" anti- tetanus antibodies." *The Journal of Emergency Medicine*, 2000, 18 (2): 189–193.
97. Atabek ME, and Pirgon O. "Tetanus in a fully immunized child." *Journal of Emergency Medicine*, 2005; 29 (3): 345–346.
98. Maselle SY, Matre R, Mbise R, and Hofstad T. "Neonatal tetanus despite protective serum antitoxin concentration." *FEMS Microbiology Letters*, 2006; 76 (3): 171–176.
99. Koenig K, Ringe H, Dorner BG, Diers A, Uhlenberg B, Mueller D, Varnholt V, and Gaedicke G. "Atypical tetanus in a completely immunized 14-year-old boy." *Pediatrics*, 2007; 120 (5): 1355–1358.
100. Galazka AM. *The Immunological Basis of Immunization Series Module 3: Tetanus*. World Health Organisation, Geneva, Switzerland, 1993 (WHO/EPI/Gen 93.13); p. 6.
101. Pascual FB. McGinley EL, Zanardi LR, Cortese MM, and Murphy TV. "Tetanus Surveillance: United States, 1998–2000." *Morbidity and Mortality Weekly Report*, 3003; 52 (SS03): 1–8.
102. Lopez RE and Holle RL. "Demographics of lightning casualties." *Seminars in Neurology*, 1995; 15: 286–295.
103. Coulter HL, and Fisher BL. *A Shot in the Dark*, Harcourt Brace Jovanovich, New York, 1985.
104. Fisher BL. *Vaccines, Autism and Chronic Inflammation*, National Vaccination Information Center, Vienna, Virginia, USA, 2008.
105. Bernard S, Enayati A, Redwood L, Roger H, and Binstock T. "Autism: a novel form of mercury poisoning." *Medical Hypotheses*, 2001; 56 (4): 462–471.
106. Colman E. "Mercury in infants given vaccines containing thiomersal." *The Lancet*, Correspondence, 2003; 361 (9358): 699.
107. Hornig M, Chian D, and Lipkin WI. "Neurotoxic effects of postnatal thimerosal are mouse strain dependent." *Molecular Psychiatry*, 2004; 9: 833–845.
108. Westphal GA, Asgari S, Schutz TG, Buenger J, Mueller M, and Hallier E. "Thimerosal induces micronuclei in the cytochalasin B block micronucleus test with human lymphocytes." *Archives of Toxicology*, 2003 77 (1): 50–55.
109. Geier MR, and Geier DA. "Neurodevelopmental disorders after thimerosal-containing vaccines: a brief communication." *Experimental Biological Medicine*, 2003 228 (6): 660–664.
110. DeLong G. "Can vaccines trigger autism?" *Social Science Research Network*, 2008; Abstract no. 1207850.
111. Centers for Disease Control and Prevention. "Prevalence of autism spectrum disorders–autism and developmental disabilities monitoring network, six cities, United States, 2000." *Morbidity and Mortality Weekly Report*, 2007; 56 (SS-1): 1–40.
112. Walton, J. "Absorption of aluminium and its effects on brain cells." In: *Aluminium: Report of an International Meeting, 20–21 April 1995, Brisbane*. National Environmental Health Health Monographs: Metal Series No. 1; P Imray, MR Moore, PW Callan, and W Lock (editors); Department of Human Services, Australia: pp. 22–34.
113. Walton J, Hams G, and Wilcox D. "Bioavailability of aluminium from drinking water: co-exposure with foods and beverages." *Research Report No. 83*, Melbourne, Victoria, Australia; Urban Water Research Association of Australia; 1994. Cited in Walton, ibid

reference 112.
114. Perl DP. "Relationship of aluminum to Alzheimer's disease." *Environmental Health Perspectives*, 1985; 63: 149–153.
115. Alfrey AC, LeGendre GR, and Kaehny WD. "The dialysis encephalopathy syndrome: possible aluminum intoxication." *The New England Journal of Medicine*, 1976; 294: 184–188.
116. Klatzo I, Wisniewski H, and Streicher E. "Experimental production of neurofibrillary degeneration: I Light microscopic observations." *Journal of Neuropathology and Experimental Neurology*, 1965; 24: 187–199.
117. Terry RD and Pena C. "Experimental production of neurofibrillary degeneration. 2. Electron microscopy, phosphatase histochemistry and electron probe analysis." *Journal of Neuropathology and Experimental Neurology*, 1965; 24: 200–210.
118. Crapper DR, Krishnan SS, and Dalton AJ. "Brain aluminum distribution in Alzheimer's disease and experimental neurofibrillary degeneration." *Science*, 1973; 180 (4083): 511–513.
119. Uemura E. "Intranuclear aluminum accumulation in chronic animals with experimental neurofibrillary changes." *Experimental Neurology*, 1984; 85 (1): 10–18.
120. Hollosi M. "Stable intrachain and intrachain complexes of neurofilament peptides: a putative link between aluminium and Alzheimer disease." *Proceedings of the National Academy of Sciences*, 1994; 91: 4902–4906.
121. Bilkei-Gorzo A. "Neurotoxic effect of enteral aluminum." *Food and Chemical Toxicology*, 1993; 31 (5): 357–361.
122. Crapper DR, Krishnan SS, and Quirrkat S. "Aluminum, neurofibrillary degeneration and Alzheimer's disease." *Brain*, 1976; 99: 67–80.
123. Perl DP, and Brody AR. "Alzheimer's disease: x-ray spectrometric evidence of aluminum accumulation in neurofibrillary tangle-bearing neurons." *Science*, 1980; 208: 297–299.
124. Perl, DP. "Aluminum and Alzheimer's disease: intraneuronal x-ray studies." *Banbury Report 15: Biological Aspects of Alzheimer's Disease*. Cold Spring Harbor Laboratory, Cold Spring Harbor, NY, USA, 1983; pp. 425–431. Cited in Perl DP, ibid reference 114.
125. Walton J, Tuniz C, Fink D, Jacobsen G, and Wilcox D. "Uptake of trace elements of aluminum into the brain from drinking water." *Neurotoxicology*, 1995; 16 (1): 187–190.
126. Becaria A, Campbell A, and Bondy SC. "Alumium as a toxicant." *Toxicology and Industrial Health*, 2002; 18 (7): 309–320.
127. Clauberg, M. and Joshi, JG. "Regulation of serine protease activity by aluminum: implications for Alzheimer disease."*Proceedings of the National Academy of Sciences*, 1993; 90: 1009–1012.
128. Evans P. "Free radicals in brain metabolism and pathology." *British Medical Bulletin*, 1993; 49: 577–587.
129. Wisniewski HM, Sturman JA, Shek JW, "Aluminum chloride induced neurofibrillary changes in the developing rabbit, a chronic animal model." *Annals of Neurology*, 1980; 8 (5): 479–490.
130. Varner JA, Jensen KF, Horvath W, and Isaacson RL. "Chronic administration of aluminum-fluoride and sodium-fluoride to rats in drinking water: alterations in neuronal and cerebrovascular integrity." *Brain Research*, 1998; 784: 284–298.
131. Vogt T. "Water quality and health: study of a possible relationship between aluminum in drinking water and dementia." *Sosiale og Okonomiske Studier* (Central Bureau of Statistics), Oslo, Norway, 1986; 61: 1–99.
132. Flaten TP. "Geographic associations between aluminium in drinking water and death rates with dementi al (including Alzheimer's disease), Parkinson's disease and amylotrophic lateral sclerosis in Norway." *Environmental Geochemistry and Health*, 1990;

12: 152–167.
133. Flaten TP. "Aluminum as a risk factor in Alzheimer's disease, with emphasis on drinking water." *Brain Research Bulletin*, 2001; 55 (2): 187–196.
134. McLachlan DRC, Bergeron C, Smith JE, Boomer D, and Rifat SL. "Risk for neuropathologically confirmed Alzheimer's disease and residual aluminum in muncipal drinking water employing weighted residential histories." *Neurology*, 1996; 46 (2): 401–405.
135. Martyn CN, Barker DJ, Osmond C, Harris EC, Edwardson JA, and Lacey RF. "Geographic relation between Alzheimer's disease and aluminum in drinking water." *The Lancet*, 1989; 1 (8629): 59–62.
136. Rondeau V, Commenges D, Jacqmin-Gadda H, and Dartigues JF. "Relation between aluminum in concentrations in drinking water and Alzheimer's disease: an 8-year follow-up study." *American Journal of Epidemiology*, 2000; 152 (1): 59–66.
137. Jacqmin H, Commenges D, Letenneur L, Barberger-Gateau P, and Dartigues J-F. "Components of drinking water and the risk of cognitive impairment in the elderly." *American Journal of Epidemiology*, 1994; 139 (1): 48–57.
138. Rondeau V, Jacqmin-Gadda H, Commenges D, and Dartigues J-F. "Aluminum in drinking water and cognitive decline in elderly subjects: the Paquid Cohort." *American Journal of Epidemiology*, 2001; 154 (3): 288–290.
139. Jacqmin-Gadda H, Commenges D, Letenneur L, and Dartigues JF. "Silica and aluminum in drinking water and cognitive impairment in the elderly." *Epidemiology*, 1996; 7 (3): 281–285.
140. Gillette-Guyonnet S, Andrieu S, and Vellas B. "The potential influence of silica present in drinking water on Alzheimer's disease and associated disorders." *The Journal of Nutrition, Health and Aging*, 2007: 11 (2): 119–123.
141. Gajdusek DC, and Salazar AM. "Amylotrophic lateral sclerosis and Parkinsonism syndromes in high incidence among the Auyu and Jakai people of West New Guinea." *Neurology*, 1982; 32: 107–126. Cited in Perl DP, ibid reference 114.
142. Gajdusek DC. "Foci of motor neuron disease in high incidence in isolated populations of East Asia and the Western Pacific." In: *Human Motor Neuron Diseases, Advances in Neurology*, LP Rowland (editor), Raven Press, New York, USA, 1982; volume 36, pp. 363–394. Cited in Perl DP, ibid reference 114.
143. Sharaki H, and Yase H. "Amylotrophic lateral sclerosis in Japan." In: *Handbookd of Clinical Neurology*, PJ Vinken and GW Bruyn (editors), North Holland, Amsterdam, The Netherlands, 1975; volume 22, pp. 353–419.
144. Crapper McLachlarf DR, McLachlan CD, Krishnan B, Krishan SS, Dalton AJ and Steele JC. "Aluminium and calcium in soil and food from Guam, Palau and Jamaica: implications for amylotrophic lateral sclerosis and Parkinsonism-dementia syndromes of Guam." *Environmental Geochemistry and Health*, 1989; 112 (2): 45–53.
145. Perl DP and Good PF. "The association of aluminum, Alzheimer's disease, and neurofibrillary tangles." *Journal of Neural Transmission*, Supplementum, 1987; 24: 205–211.
146. Lindegarde B. "Aluminum and Alzheimer's disease." *The Lancet*, 1989; 267–268.
147. Yase Y. "Pathogenesis of amylotrophic lateral sclerosis." *The Lancet*, 1972; 2: 292–296.
148. Yase Y. "Environmental contribution to the ALS process." In: Serratrice Gea (editor), *Neuromuscular Diseases*, Raven Press, New York, USA, 1984, pp. 335–339.
149. McLachlan D. "Intramuscular desferioxamine in patients with Alzheimer's disease." *The Lancet*, 1991; 337: 1304.
150. US Alzheimer's Association. "2009 Alzheimer's Disease Facts and Figures." *Alzheimer's*

and Dementia, 2009; 5 (3).
151. Bassili WR, and Stewart GT. "Epidemiological evaluation of immunisation and other factors in the control of whooping cough." *The Lancet*, 1976; 1 (7957): 471–474.
152. Ditchburn RK. "Whooping cough after stopping pertussis immunisation." *British Medical Journal*, 1979; 2 (6183), (Correspondence): 207–208.
153. Ditchburn RK. "Whooping cough after stopping pertussis immunisation." *British Medical Journal*, 1979; 1 (6178): 1601–1603.
154. Stewart GT. "Whooping cough in relation to other childhood infections in 1977–9 in the United Kingdom." *Journal of Epidemiology and Community Health*, 1981; 35 (2): 139–145.
155. Stewart GT. "Vaccination against whooping cough: efficacy versus risks." *The Lancet*, 1977; 1 (8005): 234–237.
156. Stewart GT. "Toxicity of pertussis vaccine: frequency and probability of reactions." *Journal of Epidemiology and Community Health*, 1979; 33 (2): 150–156.
157. Stewart GT. "Whooping cough and pertussis vaccine: a comparison of risks and benefits in Britain during the period 1968–83." *Developments in Biological Standardization*, 1985; 61: 395–405.
158. Shelton T. "Dutch whooping cough epidemic puzzles scientists." *British Medical Journal*, 1998; 316 (7125): 91–94.
159. de Melker HE, Schellekens JFP, Neepelenbroek, SE, Mooi FR, Rumke HC, and Conyn-van Spaendonck MAE. "Reemergence of pertussis in the highly accinated population of the Netherlands: observations on surveillance data." *Emerging Infectious Diseases*, 2000; 6 (7): 348–355.
160. Hutchins SS, Cochi SL, Brink EW, Patriarca PA, Wassilak SG, Rovira EZ, and Hinman AR. "Current epidemiology of pertussis in the United States." *The Tokai Journal of Clinical Medicine*, 1988; 13 (Supplement): 103–109.
161. Centers for Disease Control and Prevention. "Resurgence of pertussis–United States, 1993." *Morbidity and Mortality Weekly Report*, 1993; 42 (49): 945–968.
162. National Centre for Immunization Research and Surveillance of Vaccine Preventable Diseases, and the Australian Institute of Health and Welfare, Australian Government of Health and Aging. "Vaccine Preventable Disease and Vaccine Coverage in Australia, 2003 to 2005." In: *Communicable Diseases Intelligence*, 2007; 31, Supplement: 49–54.
163. Cordova SP, Gilles MT, and Beers MY. "The outbreak that had to happen: Bordetella pertussis in north-west Western Australia in 1999." *Communicable Diseases Intelligence*, 2000; 24 (12): 375–379.
164. Kenyon TA, Izurieta H, Shulman ST, Rosenfeld E, Miller M, Daum R, Strebel PM. "Large outbreak of pertussis among young children in Chicago, 1993: investigation of potential contributing factors and estimation of vaccine effectiveness." *Pediatric Infectious Diseases*, 1996; 15 (8): 655–661.
165. Christie C, Marx ML, Marchant CD, and Reising SF. "The 1993 epidemic of pertussis in Cincinnati: resurgence of disease in a highly immunized population of children." *The New England Journal of Medicine*, July 1994; 331 (1): 16–21.
166. Strebel P, Hussey G, Metcalf C, Hanslo D, and Simpson J. "An outbreak of whooping cough in a highly vaccinated community." *Journal of Tropical Pediatrics*, 1991; 37 (2): 71–76.
167. Mulholland K. "Measles and pertussis in developing countries with good vaccine coverage." *The Lancet*, 1995; 345 (8945): 305–307.
168. Trollfors B, and Rabo E. "Whooping cough in adults." *British Medical Journal (Clinical Research Edition)*, 1981; 283 (6293): 696–697.
169. Mink CA, Sirota NM, and Nugent S. "Outbreak of pertussis in a fully immunized

adolescent and adult population." *Archives of Pediatrics and Adolescent Medicine*, 1994; 148 (2): 153–157.

170. Crowcroft NS, Andrews N, Rooney C, Brisson M, and Miller E. "Deaths from pertussis are underestimated in England." *Archives of Disease in Childhood*, 2002; 86 336–338.

171. Matthias RG "Whooping cough in spite of immunization." *Canadian Journal of Public Health*, 1978; 69 (2): 130–132.

172. Bennett NM. "Whooping cough in Melbourne." *Medical Journal of Australia*, 1973; 2 (10): 481–487.

173. Blakely T, Mansoor O, and Baker M. "The 1996 pertussis epidemic in New Zealand: descriptive epidemiology." *New Zealand Medical Journal*, 1999; 112 (1081): 30–33.

174. Van Loo IH, and Mooi FR. "Changes in the Dutch Bordetella pertussis population in the first 20 years after the introduction of whole-cell vaccines." *Microbiology*, 2002; 148 (7): 2011–2018.

175. Mannerstedt G. "Pertussis in adults." *Journal of Pediatrics*, 1934; 5 (5): 596–600.

176. Srugo I, Benilevi D, Madeb R, Shapiro S, Shohat T, Somekh E, Rimmar Y, Gershtein V, Gershtein R, Marva E, and Lahat N. "Pertussis infection in fully vaccinated children in day-care centers, Israel." *Emerging Infectious Diseases*, 2000; 6 (5): 526–529.

177. Frost WH, Frobisher M, Van Volkenburgh VA, and Levin ML. "Diphtheria in Baltimore: a comparative study of morbidity, carrier prevalence and antitoxin immunity in 1921–1924 and 1933–1936." *American Journal of Hygiene*, 1936, 24: 568–586.

178. Pannum PL. *Observations Made During the Epidemic of Measles on the Faroe Islands in the Year 1846*. Delta Omega Society, New York, USA, 1940.

179. Christensen PE, Schmidt H, Bang HO, Andersen V, Jordal B, and Jensen O. "An epidemic of measles in Southern Greenland, 1951: measles in virgin soil, I." *Acta Medica Scandinavica*, 1953; 144: 313.

180. Arroyo M, Alia JM, Mateos ML, Carrasco JL, Ballesteros F, and Lardinois R. "Natural immunity to measles, rubella and mumps among Spanish children in the pre-vaccination era." *International Journal of Epidemiology*, 1986; 15 ((1): 95–100.

181. Fields B, Knipe DM, Howley PM, and Griffin DE. *Field's Virology*. Lippincott Williams and Wilkins, Hagerstown, Maryland, USA, 2006; p. 1538.

182. Horstmann DM, Schuedersberg A, Emmons JE, Evans BK, Randolph MF, and Andiman WA. "Persistence of vaccine-induced immune responses to rubella: comparison with natural infection." *Review of Infectious Diseases*, 1985; 7 (Supplement 1): 80–85.

183. Buxbaum S, Doerr HW, and Allwinn R. "Epidemiological analysis of immunity against vaccine-preventable diseases" rubella, measles, mumps and chickenpox." *Deutsche Medizinische Wochenschrift* [In German], 2001; 126 (46): 1289–1293.

184. Horwitz G, Grunfeld K, Lysgaard-Hansen B, and Kjeldsen K. "The epidemiology and natural history of measles in Denmark. " *American Journal of Epidemiology*, 1974; 100 (2): 136–149.

185. Office of National Statistics.*Twentieth Century Mortality*, CD-Rom, Her Magesty's Stationery Office (HMSO), London, UK, 2001.

186. Veeder BS. "The morbidity and mortality of pertussis and measles with particular reference to age." In: *American Association for Study and Prevention of Infant Mortality: Transactions of the Seventh Annual Meeting, Milwaukee, October 19–21, 1916*. Franklin Printing Company, Baltimore, Maryland, USA, 1917; p. 98.

187. Halsey NA, Modlin JF, and Jabbour JT; US Centers for Disease Control and Prevention. *Measles Suveillance Report No. 11, 1977–1981*. September 1982; 6–89.

188. Baratta RO, Ginter MC, Price MA, Walker JW, Skinner RG, Prather EC, and David JK.

"Measles (rubeola) in previously immunized children." *Pediatrics*, 1970; 46 (3): 397–402.

189. Wyll SA, and Witte JJ. "Measles in previously vaccinated children: an epidemiological study." *Journal of the American Medical Association*, 1971; 216 (8): 1306–1310.

190. Lerman SJ, and Gold E. "Measles in children previously vaccinated against measles." *Journal of the American Medical Association*, 1971; 216 (8): 1311–1314.

191. Currier RW, Hardy GE Jr., and Conrad JL. "Measles in previously vaccinated children: evaluation of an outbreak." *American Journal of Diseases of Children*, 1972; 124 (6): 854–857.

192. Linnemann CC Jr., Rotte TC, Schiff GM, and Youtsey JL. "A seroepidemiologic study of a measles epidemic in a highly immunized population." *American Journal of Epidemiology*, 1972; 95 (3): 238–246.

193. Schluederberg A, Lamm SH, Landrigan PJ, and Black FL. "Measles immunity in children vaccinated before one year of age." *American Journal of Epidemiology*, 1973; 97 (6): 402–409.

194. Cherry JD, Feigin RD, Lobes LA Jr., Hinthorn DR, Shackelford PG, Shirley RH, Lins RD and Choi SC. "Urban measles in the vaccine era: a clinical, epidemiologic, and serologic study." *Journal of Pediatrics*, 1972; 81 (2): 217–230.

195. Weiner LB, Corwin RM, Nieburg PI, and Feldman HA. "A measles outbreak among adolescents." *The Journal of Pediatrics*, 1977; 90 (1): 17–20.

196. Shasby DM, Shope TC, Downs H, Herrmann KL, and Polkowski J. "Epidemic measles in a highly vaccinated population." *The New England Journal of Medicine*, 1987; 296 (11): 585–589.

197. Krause PJ, Cherry JD, Deseda-Tous J, Champion JG, Strassburg M, Sullivan C, Spencer MJ, Bryson YJ, Welliver RC, and Boyer KM. "Epidemic measles in young adults." *Annals of Internal Medicine*, 1979; 90 (6): 873–876.

198. Judelsohn RG, Fleissner ML, O'Mara DJ. "School-based measles outbreaks: correlation of age at immunization with risk of disease." *American Journal of Public Health*, 1980; 70 (11): 1162–1165.

199. McKinlay JB, and McKinlay SM. "The questionable contribution of medical measures to the decline of mortality in the United States in the Twentieth Century." *The Millbank Memorial Fund Quarterly: Health and Society*, 1977; 55 (3): 405–428.

200. McKinlay JB, and McKinlay SM. Ibid reference 199; pp. 421–425.

201. Wittke JJ, and Axnick NW, "The benefits from ten years of measles immunization in the United States." *Public Health Reports*, 1975; 90 (3): 205–207.

202. Centers for Disease Control and Prevention. "Recommendations of the Immunization Practices Advisory Committee Measles Prevention: Supplementary Statement." *Morbidity and Mortality Weekly Report*, January 13, 1989; 38 (1): 11–14.

203. Wassilak SGF, Orenstein WA, Strickland PL, Butler CA, and Bart KJ. "Continuing measles transmission in students despite a school-based outbreak control program." *American Journal of Epidemiology*, 1985; 122 (2): 208–217.

204. Centres for Disease Control and Prevention. "Measles outbreak among vaccinated high school students: Illinois." *Morbidity and Mortality Weekly Report*, 1984; 33 (24): 349–351.

205. Gustafson TL, Lievens AW, Brunell PA, Moellenberg RG, Buttery CM, and Sehulster LM. "Measles outbreak in a fully immunized secondary school population." *The New England Journal of Medicine*, 1987; 316 (13): 771–774.

206. Davis RM, Whitman ED, Orenstein WA, Preblud SR, Markowitz LE, and Hinman AR. "A persistent outbreak of measles despite appropriate prevention and control measures." *American Journal of Epidemiology*, 1987; 126 (3): 438–439.

207. Markowitz LE, Preblud SR, Orenstein WA, Rovira EZ, Adams NC, Hawkins CE, and Hinman AR. "Patterns of transmission in measles outbreaks in the United States, 1985–

1986." *The New England Journal of Medicine*, 320 (2): 75–81.
208. Nkowane BM, Bart SW, Orenstein WA, and Baltier M. "Measles outbreak in a vaccinated school population: epidemiology, chains of transmission and the role of vaccine failures." *American Journal of Public Health*, 1987; 77 (4): 434–438.
209. Rullan JV, Pozo F, Gamble WB Jr., Jackson K, and Parker RL." Measles in a highly vaccinated South Carolina school population." In: *Proceedings of the 36th Annual Conference of the Epidemic Intelligence Service, April 6–10, 1987*, US Centers for Disease Control and Prevention, Atlanta, Georgia, USA, 1987; p. 24.
210. Hersh BS, Markowitz LE, Hoffman RE, Hoff DR, Doran MJ, Fleishman JC, Preblud SR, and Orenstein WA. "A measles outbreak at a college with a prematriculation immunization requirement." *American Journal of Public Health*, 1991; 81 (3): 360–364.
211. Hutchins S, Markowitz L, Atkinson W, Swint E, Hadler S. "Measles outbreaks in the United States, 1987 through 1990." *The Pediatric Infectious Disease Journal*, 1996; 15 (1): 31–38.
212. Brunell PA. "Measles one more time." *Pediatrics*, 1990; 86 (3): 474–478.
213. Centers for Disease Control and Prevention. "Measles: United States, first 26 weeks, 1989." *Morbidity and Mortality Weekly Report*, 1989; 38 (50): 863–866, 871–872.
214. Centers for Disease Control and Prevention. "Health objectives for the nation public health burden of vaccine-preventable diseases among adults: standards for adult immunization practice." *Morbidity and Mortality Weekly Report*, 1990; 39 (41): 725–729.
215. Chen RT, Goldbaum GM, Wassilak SB, Markowitz LE, and Orenstein WA. "An explosive point-source measles outbreak in a highly vaccinated population. Modes of transmission and risk factors for disease." *American Journal of Epidemiology*, 1989; 129 (1): 173–182.
216. Centers for Disease Control and Prevention. "Public-sector vaccination efforts in response to the resurgence of measles among preschool-aged children: United States, 1989–1991." *Morbidity and Mortality Weekly Report*, 1992; 41 (29): 522–525.
217. Edmonson MB, Addiss DG, McPherson JT, Berg JL, Circo SR, and Davis JP. "Mild measles and secondary vaccine failure during a sustained outbreak in a highly vaccinated population." *Journal of the American Medical Association*, 1990; 263 (18): 2467–2471.
218. Matson DO, Byington C, Canfield M, Albrecht P, Feigin RD. "Investigation of a measles outbreak in a fully vaccinated school population including serum studies before and after revaccination." *The Pediatric Infectious Disease Journal*, 1993; 12 (4): 292–299.
219. St Geme JW Jr., George BL, Bush BM. "Exaggerated natural measles following attenuated virus immunization." *Pediatrics*, 1976; 57 (1): 148–149.
220. Davis SF, Strebel PM, Atkinson WL, Markowitz LE, Sutter RW, Scanlon KS, Friedman S, and Hadler SC. "Reporting efficiency during a measles outbreak in New York City, 1991." *American Journal of Public Health*, 1993; 83 (7): 1011–1015.
221. Poland GA, and Jacobson RM. "Failure to reach the goal of measles elimination: apparent paradox of measles infections in immunized persons." *Archives of Internal Medicine*, 1994; 154 (16): 1815–1820.
222. Centers for Disease Control and Prevention. "Rubella and congenital rubella syndrome: United States, January 1, 1991–May 7, 1994." *Morbidity and Mortality Weekly Report*, 1994; 43 (21): 397–401.
223. Centers for Disease Control and Prevention. "Measles at an international gymnastics competition: Indiana, 1991." *Morbidity and Mortality Weekly Report*, 1992; 41 (07): 109–111.
224. Ammari LK, Bell LM, and Hodinka RL. "Secondary measles vaccine failure in healthcare workers exposed to infected patients." *Infection Control and Hospital Epidemiology*, 1993; 14 (2): 81–86.

225. Centers for Disease Control and Prevention. "Measles–United States, 1996, and the interruption of indigenous transmission." *Morbidity and Mortality Weekly Report*, 1997; 46 (11): 242–246.
226. Centers for Disease Control and Prevention. "Measles: United States, 1997." *Morbidity and Mortality Weekly Report*, 1998; 47 (14): 273–276.
227. Centers for Disease Control and Prevention. "Measles: United States, 1999." *Morbidity and Mortality Weekly Report*, 2000; 49 (25): 557–560.
228. Centers for Disease Control and Prevention. "Import-associated measles outbreak: Indiana, May–June 2005." *Morbidity and Mortality Weekly Report*, 2005; 54 (42): 1073–1075.
229. Centers for Disease Control and Prevention. "Preventable measles among U.S. residents, 2001–2004." *Morbidity and Mortality Weekly Report*, 2005; 54 (33): 817–820.
230. Centers for Disease Control and Prevention. "Measles: United States, 2005." *Morbidity and Mortality Weekly Report*, 2006; 55 (50): 1348–1351.
231. Centers for Disease Control and Prevention. "Update: Measles—United States, January–July, 2008." *Morbidity and Mortality Weekly Report*, 2008; 57 (33): 893–896.
232. Centers for Disease Control and Prevention. "Transmission of measles among a highly vaccinated school population–Anchorage, Alaska, 1998." *Morbidity and Mortality Weekly Report*, 1999; 47 (51, 52): 1109–1111.
233. Katz SL, and Hinman AR. "Summary and conclusions: measles elimination meeting, 16–17 March." *Journal of Infectious Disease*, 2004; 189 (Supplement 1): 43–47.
234. Rawls WE, Rawls ML, and Chernesky MA. "Analysis of a measles epidemic: possible role of vaccine failures." *Canadian Medical Association Journal*; 1975; 113 (10): 941–944.
235. Yuan L. "Measles outbreak in 31 schools: risk factors for vaccine failure and evaluation of a selective revaccination strategy." *Canadian Medical Association Journal*; 1994; 150 (7): 1093–1098.
236. Sekla L, Stackiw W, Eibisch G, Johnson I. "An evaluation of measles serodiagnosis during an outbreak in a vaccinated community." *Clinical and Investigative Medicine*, 1988; 11 (4): 304–309.
237. Boulianne N, De Serres G, Duval B, Joly JR, Meyer F, Dery P, Alary M, Le Henaff D, and Theriault N. "Major measles epidemic in the region of Quebec despite a 99% vaccine coverage." *Canadian Journal of Public Health*, 1991; 82 (3): 189–190.
238. Centers for Disease Control and Prevention. "Measles: Quebec." *Morbidity and Mortality Weekly Report*, 1989; 38 (18): 329–330.
239. Ozanne G, and D'Halewyn M-A. "Secondary immune response in a vaccinated population during a large measles epidemic." *Journal of Clinical Microbiology*, 1992; 30 (7): 1778–1782.
240. Hull HF, Montes JM, Hays PC, and Lucero RL. "Risk factors for measles vaccine failure among immunized students." *Pediatrics*, 1985; 76 (4): 518–523.
241. de Oliveira SA, Soares WN, Dalston MO, de Almeida MT, and Costa AJ. "Clinical and epidemiological findings during a measles outbreak occurring in a population with a high vaccination coverage." [In Portuguese]. *Revista da Sociedade Brasilera de Medicina Tropical*, 1995; 28 (4): 339–343.
242. Miller CL. "Deaths from measles in England and Wales, 1970–83." *British Medical Journal*, (Clinical Research Edition), 1985; 290 (6466): 443–444.
243. Warin JF, Harker P, and Mayon-White RT. "Measles in vaccinated children in Oxford." *The Lancet*, 1972; 2 (7781): 810–812.
244. Hicks NR. "Misplaced loss of confidence in measles vaccination: an investigation in a primary school." *Journal of the Royal College of General Practitioners*, 1989; 39: 151–152.

245. Carter H, and Gorman D. "Measles outbreak in Fife: which MMR policy?" *Public Health*, 1993; 107 (1): 25–30.
246. Hidaka Y, Aoki T, Akeda H, Miyazaki C, and Ueda K. "Serological and clinical characteristics of measles vaccine failure in Japan." *Scandinavian Journal of Infectious Diseases*, 1994; 26 (6): 725–730.
247. Kawamoto A, Honda T, Ishida K, Ozeki T, Hayashibara H, Shiraki K, and Hino S. "Two independent outbreaks of measles in partially vaccinated junior high schools in Tottori, Japan." *Archives of Virology*, 1995; 140 (2): 349–354.
248. Hirose M, Hidaka Y, Miyazaki C, Ueda K, Yoshikawa H. "Five cases of measles secondary vaccine failure with confirmed seroconversion after live measles vaccination." *Scandinavian Journal of Infectious Diseases*, 1997; 29 (2): 187–190.
249. Ong G, Hoon HB, Ong A, Chua LT, Kai CS, and Tai GK. "A 24-year review on the epidemiology and control of measles in Singapore, 1981–2004." *Southeast Asian Journal of Tropical Medicine and Public Health*, 2006; 37 (1): 96–101.
250. Albonico H-U. "Arguments against routine mumps immunization." [In German]. *Sozial und Praventivmedizin*, 1995; 40 (2): 116–123.
251. Williams P, and Hull H. "Status of measles in The Gambia, 1981." *Reviews of Infectious Diseases*, 1983; 5 (3): 391–394.
252. Commey JO, and Richardson JE. "Measles in Ghana: 1973–1982." *Annals of Tropical Paediatrics*, 1984; 4 (3): 189–194.
253. Kenya PR. "Measles and mathematics: control or eradication." *East African Medical Journal*, 1990; 67 (12): 856–863.
254. Dabis F, Sow A, Waldman RJ, Bikakouri P, Senga J, Madzou G, and Jones TS. "The epidemiology of measles in a partially vaccinated population in an African city: implications for immunizing programs." *American Journal of Epidemiology*, 1988; 127 (1): 171–178.
255. Whittle HC, Aaby P, Samb B, Jensen H, Bennett J, Simondon R. "Effect of subclinical infection on maintaining immunity against measles in vaccinated children in West Africa." *The Lancet*, 1999; 353 (9147): 98–102.
256. Adu FD, Ikusika A, and Omotade O. "Measles outbreak in Ibadan: serological and virological identification of affected children in selected hospitals." *The Journal of Infection*, 1997; 35 (3): 241–245.
257. Lagunju IA, Orimadegun AE, Oyedemi DG. "Measles in Ibadan: a continuous scourge." *African Journal of Medicine and Medical Sciences*, 2005; 34 (4): 383–387.
258. Ekanem EE. "A 10-year review of morbidity from childhood preventable diseases in Nigeria." *Journal of Tropical Pediatrics*, 1988; 34: 325.
259. Coetzee N, Hussey GD, Visser G, Barron P, and Keen A. "The 1992 measles epidemic in Cape Town: a changing epidemiological pattern." *South African Medical Journal*, 1994; 84 (3): 145–149.
260. Murray M, and Rasmussen Z. "Measles outbreak in a northern Pakistani village: epidemiology and vaccine effectiveness." *American Journal of Epidemiology*, 2000; 151 (8): 811–819.
261. Puvimanasinghe JP, Arambepola CK, Abeysinghe NM, Rajapaksa LC, and Kulatilaka TA. "Measles outbreak in Sri Lanka, 1999–2000." *The Journal of Infectious Diseases*, 187 (Supplement 1): 241–245.
262. Atrasheuskaya AV, Kulak MV, Neverov AA, Rubin S, Ignatyev GM. "Measles cases in highly vaccinated population of Novosibirsk, Russia, 2000–2005." *Vaccine*, 2008; 26 (17): 2111–2118.

263. Paunio M, Peltola H, Valle M, Davidkin I, Virtanen M, and Heinonen OP. "Explosive school-based measles outbreak." *American Journal of Epidemiology*, 1998; 148 (11): 1103–1110.
264. Paunio M, Hedman K, Davidkin I, Valle M, Heinonen OP, Leinikki P, Salmi A, and Peltola H. "Secondary measles vaccine failures identified by measurement of IgG avidity: high occurrence among teenagers vaccinated at a young age." *Epidemiology and Infection*, 2000; 124 (2): 263–271.
265. Nagy G, Kosa S, Takatsy S, and Koller M. "The use of IgM tests for analysis of the causes of measles vaccine failures: experience gained in a epidemic in Hungary in 1980-1981." *Journal of Medical Virology*, 1984; 13 (1): 93–103.
266. Agocs MM, Markowitz LE, Straub I, and Domok I. "The 1988–1989 measles epidemic in Hungary: assessment of vaccine failure." *International Journal of Epidemiology*, 1992; 21 (5): 1007–1013.
267. Centers for Disease Control and Prevention. "Measles outbreak: Romania, 1997." *Morbidity and Mortality Weekly Report*, 1997; 46 (49): 1159–1163.
268. Hellenbrand W, Siedler A, Tischer A, Meyer C, Reiter S, Rasch G, Teichmann D, Santibanez S, Altmann D, Claus H, and Kramer M. "Progress towards measles elimination in Germany." *The Journal of Infectious Diseases*, 2003; 187 (Supplement 1): 208–216.
269. Pedersen IR, Mordhorst CH, Glikmann G, and Von Magnus H. "Subclinical measles infection in vaccinated seropositive individuals in arctic Greenland." *Vaccine*, 1989; 7 (4): 345–348.
270. Herceg A, Passaris I, and Mead C. "An outbreak of measles in a highly immunised population: immunisation status and vaccine efficacy." *Australian Journal of Public Health*, 1994; 18 (3): 249–252.
271. McDonnell LF, Jorm LR, Patel MS. "Measles outbreak in Western Sydney. Vaccine failure or failure to vaccinated?" *Medical Journal of Australia*, 1995; 162 (9): 471–475.
272. Cullen RM, and Walker WJ. "Measles epidemics 1949–91: the impact of mass immunisation in New Zealand." *New Zealand Medical Journal*, 1996; 109 (1032): 400–402.
273. Hardy IR, Lennon DR, and Mitchell EA. "Measles epidemic in Auckland 1984–85." *New Zealand Medical Journal*, 1987; 100 (823): 273–275.
274. Harrison GP, and Durham GA. "The 1991 measles epidemic: how effective is the vaccine?" *New Zealand Medical Journal*, 1992; 105 (938): 280–282.
275. Ceyhan M, Kanra G, Vargel S, Isikcelik Y. "The evaluation of vaccination against measles at nine months of age (report of an epidemic)." *Turkish Journal of Pediatrics*, 1992; 34 (3): 127–133.
276. Yu X, Wang S, Guan J, Mahemuti P, Gou A, Liu Q, Jin X, and Ghildyal R. "Analysis of the cause of increased measles incidence in Xinjiang, China in 2004." *The Pediatric Infectious Disease Journal*, 2007; 26 (6): 513–518.
277. Muscat M, Bang H, and Glismann S. "Measles is still a cause for concern in Europe." *Eurosurveillance*, 2008; 13 (4): Article 18837.
278. Moss WJ, and Griffin DE. "Global measles elimination." *Nature Reviews Microbiology*, 2006; 4: 900–908.
279. Weibel RE, Sokes J Jr, Buynak EB, Whitman JE Jr, and Hilleman MR. "Live, attenuated mumps-virus vaccine: 3. Clinical and serological aspects in a field situation." *The New England Journal of Medicine*, 1967; 276 (5): 245–251.
280. Centers for Disease Control and Prevention. "Current trends mumps: United States, 1985–1988. *Morbidity and Mortality Weekly Report*, 1989; 38 (7): 101-1-5.

281. Wharton M, Cochi SL, Hutcheson RH, Bistowish JM, and Shaffner W. "A large outbreak of mumps in the postvaccine era." *Journal of Infectious Diseases*, 1988; 158 (6)" 1253–1260.
282. Hersh BS, Fine PE, Kent WK, Cochi SL, Kahn LH, Zell ER, Hays PL, and Wood CL. "Mumps outbreak in a highly vaccinated population." *Journal of Pediatrics*, 1991; 119 (2): 187–193.
283. Centers for Disease Control and Prevention. "Brief report: update: mumps activity— United States, January 1–October 7, 2006." *Morbidity and Mortality Weekly Report*, 2006; 55 (42): 1152–1153.
284. Briss PA, Fehrs LJ, Parker RA, Wright PF, Sannella EC, Hutcheson RH, and Schaffner W. "Sustained transmission of mumps in a highly vaccinated population: assessment of primary vaccine failure and waning vaccine-induced immunity." *Journal of Infectious Diseases*, 1994; 169 (1): 77–82.
285. Cheek JE, Baron R, Atlas H, Wilson DL, and Crider RD Jr. "Mumps outbreak in a highly vaccinated school population. Evidence for large-scale vaccination failure." *Archives of Pediatrics and Adolescent Medicine*, 1995; 149 (7): 774–778.
286. Anderson LJ, and Seward JF. "Mumps epidemiology and immunity: the anatomy of a modern epidemic." *The Pediatric Infectious Disease Journal*, 2008; 27 (10): 75–79.
287. Schaffzin JK, Pollock L, Schulte C, Henry K, Dayan G, Blog D, and Smith P. "Effectiveness of previous mumps vaccination during a summer camp outbreak." *Pediatrics*, 2007; 120 (4): 862–868.
288. Centers for Disease Control and Prevention. "Update: multistate outbreak of mumps: United States, January 1–May 2, 2006. *Morbidity and Mortality Weekly Report*, 2006; 55 (20); 559–563.
289. Centers for Disease Control and Prevention. "Brief report: update: mumps activity— United States, January 1–October 7, 2006." *Morbidity and Mortality Weekly Report*, 2006; 55 (42): 1152–1153.
290. Bitsko RH, Cortese MM, Dayan GH, Rota PA, Lowe L, Iversen SC, and Bellini WJ. "Detectiion of RNA of mumps virus during an outbreak in a population with a high level of measles, mumps, and rubella vaccine coverage." *Journal of Clinical Microbiology*, 2008; 46 (3): 1101–1103.
291. Kancheria VS, and Hanson IC. "Mumps resurgence in the United States." *Journal of Allergy and Clinical Immunology*, 2006; 118 (4): 938–941.
292. Dayan GH, Quinlisk MP, Parker AA, Barskey AE, Harris Ml, Schwarz JM, Hunt K, Finley CG, Leschinsky DP, O'Keefe Al, Clayton J, Kightlinger LK, Dietie EG, Berg J, Kenyon CL, Goldstein ST, Stokely SK, Redd SB, Rota PA, Rota J, Bi D, Roush SW, Bridges CB, Santibanez TA, Parashar U, Bellini WJ, and Seward JF. "Recent resurgence of mumps in the United States." *The New England Journal of Medicine*, 2008; 358 (15): 1580–1589.
293. Public Health Agency of Canada. "Outbreak of mumps, Montreal, October 1998 to March 1999–with a particular focus on a school." *Canada Communicable Disease Report*, 2000; 25-08.
294. Watson-Creed G, Saunders A, Scott J, Lowe L, Pettipas J, and Hatchette TF. "Two successive outbreaks of mumps in Nova Scotia among vaccinated adolescents and young adults." *Canadian Medical Association Journal*, 2006; 175 (5): 483–488.
295. Matter HC, Cloetta J, and Zimmermann H; Sentinella Arbeitsgemeinschaft. "Measles, mumps, and rubella: monitoring in Switzerland through a sentinel network, 1986–94." *Journal of Epidemiology and Community Health*, 1995; 49 (Supplement 1): 4–8.
296. Shlegel M, Osterwalder JJ, Galeazzi RL, and Vernazza PL. "Comparative efficacy of three mumps vaccines during disease outbreak in eastern Switzerland: cohort study." *British*

Medical Journal, 1999; 319 (7206): 352–353.
297. Germann D, Stroehle A, Eggenberger K, Steiner CA, and Matter L. "An outbreak of mumps in a population partially vaccinated with the Rubini strain." *Scandinavian Journal of Infectious Diseases*, 1996; 28 (3): 235–238.
298. Richard Jl, Zwahlen M, Feuz M , and Matter HC; Swiss Sentinel Surveillance Network. "Comparison of the effectiveness of two mumps vaccines during an outbreak in Switzerland in 1999 and 2000: a case-cohort study." *European Journal of Epidemiology*, 2003; 18 (6): 569–577.
299. Gabutti G, Rota MC, Salmaso S, Bruzzone BM, Bella A, and Crovari P; Serological Study Group. "Epidemiology of measles, mumps and rubella in Italy." *Epidemiology and Infection*, 2002; 129 (3): 543–550.
300. Pons C, Pelayo T, Pachon I, Galmes A, Gonzalez L, Sanchez C, and Martinez F. "Two outbreaks of mumps in children vaccinated with the Rubini strain in Spain indicate low vaccine efficacy." *Eurosurveillance*, 2000; 5 (7): Article 14.
301. Cardenosa N, Dominguez A, Camps N, Martinez A, Torner N, Navas E, and Salleras L. "Non-preventable mumps outbreaks in school children in Catalonia." *Scandinavian Journal of Infectious Diseases*, 2006; 38 (8): 671–674.
302. Goncalves G, de Araujo A, and Monteiro Cardoso ML. "Outbreak of mumps associated with poor vaccine efficacy–Oporto, Portugal, 1996." *Eurosurveillance*, 1998; 3 (12): Article 2.
303. Dias JA, Cordeiro M, Afzal MA, Freitas MG, Morgado MR, Silva JL, Nunes LM, Lima MG, and Avilez F. "Mumps epidemic in Portugal despite high vaccine coverage: preliminary report." *Eurosurveillance*, 1996; 1 (4): Article 2.
304. Kumar V. "Measles outbreak in Gibraltar, August–October 2008: a preliminary report." *Eurosurveillance*, 2008; 13 (45): Article 19034.
305. Parent du Chatelet I , Floret D, Antona D, and Levy-Bruhl D. "Measles resurgence in France in 2008, a preliminary report." *Eurosurveillance*, 2009; 14 (6): Article 19118.
306. Vandermeulen C, Roelants M, Vermoere M, Roseeuw K, Goubau P, and Hoppenbrouwers K. "Outbreak of mumps in a vaccinated child population: a question of vaccine failure." *Vaccine*, 2004; 22 (21–22): 2713–2716.
307. Kaaijk P, van der Zeijst BA, Boog MC, and Hoitink CW. "Increased mumps incidence in the Netherlands: review on the possible role of vaccine strain and genotype." *Eurosurveillance*, 2008; 13 (26): Article 18914.
308. Wehner H, Morris R, Logan M, Hunt D, Jin L, Stuart J, and Cartwright K. "A secondary school outbreak of mumps following the childhood immunization programme in England and Wales." *Epidemiology and Infection*, 2000; 124: 131–136.
309. Reaney EA, Tohani VK, Devine MJ, Smithson RD, and Smyth B. "Mumps outbreak among young people in Northern Ireland." *Communicable Disease and Public Health*, 2001: 4 (4): 311–315.
310. Donaghy M, Cameron JC, and Friedrichs V. "Increasing incidence of mumps in Scotland: options for reducing transmission." *Journal of Clinical Virology*, 2006; 35 (2): 121–129.
311. van den Bosch CA, Cohen B, Walters T, and Jin L. "Mumps outbreak confined to a religious community." *Eurosurveillance*, 2000; 5 ((5): Article 15.
312. Pugh RN, Akinosi B, Pooransingh S, Kumar J, Grant S, Livesley E, Linnane J, and Ramaiah S. "An outbreak of mumps in the metropolitan area of Walsall, UK." *International Journal of Infectious Disease*, 2002; 6 (4): 283–187.
313. Centers for Disease Control and Prevention. "Mumps epidemic—United Kingdom, 2004–2005." *Morbidity and Mortality Weekly Report*, 2006; 55 (7): 173–175.

314. Cohen C, White JM, Savage EJ, Glynn JR, Choi Y, Andrews N, Brown D, and Ramsay ME. "Vaccine effectiveness estimates, 2004–2005 mumps outbreak, England." *Emerging Infectious Diseases*, 2007; 13 (1): 12–17.
315. Roberts C, Porter-Jones B, Crocker J, and Hart J. "Mumps outbreak on the Island of Anglesey, North Wales, December 2008–January 2009." *Eurosurveillance*, 2009; 14 (5): Article 19109.
316. Gee S, O'Flanagan D, Fitzgerald M, and Cotter S. "Mumps in Ireland, 2004–2008." *Eurosurveillance*, 2008; 13 (18): Article 18857.
317. Whyte D, O'Dea F, McDonnell C, O'Connell NH, Callinan S, Brosnan E, Powell J, Monahan R, Fitzgerald R, Mannix M, Greally T, Dee A, and O'Sullivan P. "Mumps epidemiology in the mid-west of Ireland 2004–2008: increasing disease burden in the university/college setting." *Eurosurveillance*, 2009; 14 (16): Article 19182.
318. Kubinyiova M, Benes C, Prikazsky V, Roubalova K, and Castkova J. "Mumps vaccination in the Czech Republic." *Eurosurveillance*, 2008; 13 (27): Article 18920.
319. Bernard H, Schwarz NG, Melnic A, Bucov V, Caterinciuc N, Pebody RG, Mulders M, Aidyralieva C, and Hahne S. "Mumps outbreak ongoing since October 2007 in the Republic of Moldova." *Eurosurveillance*, 2008; 13 (13): Article 8070.
320. Atrasheuskaya AV, Blatun EM, Kulak MV, Atrasheuskaya A, Karpov IA, Rubin S, and Ignatyev GM. "Investigation of mumps vaccine failures in Minsk, Belarus, 2001–2003. *Vaccine*, 2007; 25 (24): 4651–4658.
321. Pogorzelska M, Oldak E, Sulik A. "Mumps: still actual epidemiological problem in Poland." *Przeglad Epidemiologiczny* [In Polish], 2005; 59 (4): 841–849.
322. Stefanoff P, and Rogalska J. "Mumps in Poland in 2006." *Przeglad Epidemiologiczny* [In Polish], 2008; 62 (2): 225–228.
323. Oda K, Kato H, Konishi A. "The outbreak of mumps in a small island in Japan." *Acta Paediatrica Japonica* (Overseas Edition), 1996; 38 (3): 224–228.
324. Lee JY, Na BK, Kim JH, Lee JS, Park JW, Shin GC, Cho HW, Lee HD, Gou UY, Yang Bk, Kim J, Kang C, and Kim WJ. "Regional outbreak of mumps due to genotype H in Korea in 1999." *Journal of Medical Virology*, 2004; 73 (1): 85–90.
325. Centers for Disease Control and Prevention. "Rubella Outbreak: Arkansas, 1999." *Morbidity and Mortality Weekly Report*, 2001; 50 (50): 1137–1139.
326. Gendrel D. "Measles and rubella." [In French]. *La Revue du Praticien*, 1997; 47 (13): 1434–1437.
327. Gilbert GL. *Infectious Disease in Pregnancy and the Newborn Infant*, Informa Health Care/Taylor and Francis Group, London, UK, 1991.
328. Krohn EF. "Epidemiological aspects of rubella in Europe." *International Journal of Epidemiology*, 1972; 1 (3): 267–270.
329. Chantler J, Wolinsky JS and Tingle A. "Rubella virus." In: Knipe DM, and Howley PM (editors), *Fields Virology*, 4th Edition, Lippincott Williams and Wilkins, Philadelphia, Pennsylvannia, USA; 2001: pp. 963–990.
330. Hughes DA, Darlington LG, and Bendich A (editors). *Diet and Human Immune Function*, Humana Press Inc, Totowa, New Jersey, USA; 2004.
331. Joncas JH. "Rubella immunization." *Canadian Medical Association Journal*, 1974; 111 (9): 907–911.
332. Fulginiti VA. "Controversies in current immunization policy and practices: one physician's viewpoint." *Current Problems in Pediatrics*, 1976; 6 (6): 3–25.
333. Welch JP. "Prevention of congenital rubella." *Canadian Medical Association Journal*, 1977; 117 (2): 151–156.

334. Colgrove J. "The ethics and politics of compulsory HPV vaccination." *The New England Journal of Medicine*, 2006; 355: 2389–2391.
335. Colgrove J. "Compulsory HPV vaccination." *The New England Journal of Medicine*, Correspondence, 2007; 356: 1074–1075.
336. Horstmann DM. "Controlling rubella: problems and perspectives." *Annals of Internal Medicine*, 1975; 83 (3): 412–417.
337. Honeyman MC, Forrest JM, and Dorman DC. "Cell-mediated immune response following natural rubella and rubella vaccination." *Clinical and Experimental Immunology*, 1975; 17 (4): 665–671.
338. Horstmann DM, Schluederberg A, Emmons JE, Evans BK, Randolph MF, and Andiman WA. "Persistence of vaccine-induced immune responses to rubella: comparison with natural infection." *Reviews of Infectious Diseases*, 1985; 7 (Supplement 1): 80–85.
339. Gilmore D, Robinson ET, Gilmour WH, and Urquhart GE. "Effect of rubella vaccination programme in schools on rubella immunity in a general practice population." *British Medical Journal* (Clinical Research Edition), 1982; 284 (6316): 628–630.
340. Stoffman JM, and Wolfish MG. "The susceptibility of adolescent girls to rubella." *Clinical Pediatrics*, 1976; 15 (7): 625–626.
341. Chappell JA, and Taylor MA. "Implications of rubella susceptibility in young adults." *American Journal of Public Health*, 1979; 69 (3): 279–281.
342. Tingle AJ, Chantler JK, Kettyls GD, Larke RP, and Schulzer M. "Failed rubella immunization in adults: association with immunologic and virological abnormalities." *Journal of Infectious Diseases*, 1985; 151 (2): 330–336.
343. Duclos P, Tepper ML, Weber J, and Marusyk RG. "Seroprevalence of measles-and rubella-specific antibodies among military recruits, Canada, 1991." *Canadian Journal of Public Health*, 1994; 85 (4): 278–281.
344. Evans PC and Reisinger KS. "Rubella susceptibility in Navajo women." *Journal of Reproductive Medicine*, 1975; 14 (2): 84–85.
345. Freis PC, Sussman EK, and Shearin R. "Sero-immunity screening of adolescent girls in a military population to determine susceptibility to the rubella virus." *Military Medicine*, 1976; 141: 684–685.
346. McKusick MJ. "Screening for rubella on a university campus." *Post Graduate Medicine*, 1976; 59: 202–205.
347. Lawless MR, Abramson JS, Harlan JE, and Kelsey DS. "Rubella susceptibility in sixth-graders: effectiveness of current immunization practice." *Pediatrics*, 1980; 65 (6): 1086–1089.
348. Schiff GM, Young BC, Stefanovic GM, Stamler EF, Knowlton DR, Grundy BJ, and Dorsett PH. "Challenge with rubella virus after loss of detectable vaccine-induced antibody." *Reviews of Infectious Diseases*, 1985; 7 (Supplement 1): 157–163.
349. Crowder M, Higgins HL, and Frost JJ. "Rubella susceptibility in young women of rural east Texas: 1980 and 1985." *Texas Medicine*, 1987; 83 (5): 43–47.
350. Johnson CE, Kumar ML, Whitwell JK, Staehle BO, Rome LP, Dinakar C, Hurni W, and Nalin DR. "Antibody persistence after primary measles-mumps-rubella vaccine and response to a second dose given at four to six vs. eleven to thirteen years." *The Pediatric Infectious Disease Journal*, 1996; 15 (8): 687–692.
351. van der Heijden OG, Conyn-van Spaendonck MA, Plantinga AD, and Kretzschmar ME. "A model-based evaluation of the national immunization programme against rubella infection and congenital rubella syndrome in The Netherlands." *Epidemiology and Infection*, 1998; 121 (3): 653–671.

352. Trier H, and Ronne T. "Duration of immunity and occurrence of secondary vaccine failure following vaccination against measles, mumps and rubella." [In Danish]. *Ugeskrift for Laeger*, 1992;154 (29): 2008–2013.

353. Just M, Just V, Berger R, Burkhardt F, and Schilt U. "Duration of immunity after rubella vaccination: a long-term study in Switzerland." *Reviews of Infectious Diseases*, 1985; 7 (Supplement 1): 91–94.

354. Davidkin I, Peltola H, Leinikki P, and Valle M. "Duration of rubella immunity induced by two-dose measles, mumps and rubella (MMR) vaccination. A 15-year follow-up in Finland." *Vaccine*, 2000; 18 (27): 3106–3112.

355. Allan B. "Rubella immunisation." *Australian Journal of Medical Technology*, 1973; 4: 26–27.

356. Horstmann DM, Liebhaber H, Le Bouvier GL, Rosenberg DA, and Halstead SB. "Rubella: reinfection of vaccinated and naturally immune persons exposed in an epidemic." *The New England Journal of Medicine*, 1970; 283 (15): 771–778.

357. Horstmann DM, Pajot TG, and Liebhaber H. "Epidemiology of rubella. Subclinical infection and occurrence of reinfection." *American Journal of Diseases in Children*, 1969; 118 (1): 133–136.

358. Wilkins J, Leedom JM, and Portnoy B, and Salvatore MA. "Reinfection with rubella virus despite live vaccine induced immunity. Trials of HPV-77 and HPV-80 live rubella virus vaccines and subsequent artificial and natural challenge studies." *American Journal of Disease in Children*, 1969; 118 (2): 275–294.

359. Abrutyn E, Hermann KL, Karchmer AW, Friedman JP, Page E, and Witte JJ. "Rubella vaccine comparative study. Nine-month follow up and serologic response to natural challenge." *American Journal of Disease in Children*, 1970; 120 (2): 129–133.

360. Chang TW, DesRosiers S, and Weinstein L. " Clinical and serologic studies of an outbreak of rubella in a vaccinated population." *The New England Journal of Medicine*, 1970; 283 (5): 246–248.

361. Forrest JM, Menser MA, Honeyman MC, Stout M, and Murphy AM. "Clinical rubella eleven months after vaccination." *The Lancet*, 1972; 300 (7774): 399–400.

362. Rachelefsky GS, and Herrmann KL. "Congenital rubella surveillance following epidemic rubella in a partially vaccinated community." *Journal of Pediatrics*, 1974; 84 (4): 474–478.

363. Kono R. "Rubella vaccination." *Bulletin of Pan American Organization*, 1976; 10 (3): 198–201.

364. Baba K, Yabuuchi H, Okuni H, Harima R, Minekawa Y, Taniuchi M, Otsuka T, Takahashi M, and Okuno Y. "Rubella epidemic in an institution: protective value of live rubella vaccine and serologicalbehavior of vaccinated, revaccinated and naturally immune groups." *Biken Journal*, 1978; 21 (1): 25–31.

365. Schiff GM, Rauh JL, Young B, Trimble S, Rotte T, and Schiff BE. "Rubella-vaccinated students. Follow-up in a public school system." *Journal of the American Medical Association*, 1978; 240 (24): 2635–2637.

366. Weibel, Buynak EB, McLean AA, and Hilleman MR. "Persistence of antibody after administration of monovalent and combined live attenuated measles, mumps, and rubella virus vaccines." *Pediatrics*, 1978; 61 (1): 5–11.

367. Weibel RE, Buynak EB, McLean AA, Roehm RR, and Hilleman MR. "Follow-up surveillance for antibody in human subjects following live attenuated measles, mumps and rubella virus vaccines." *Proceedings of the Society for Experimental Biology and Medicine*, 1979; 162 (2): 328–332.

368. Polk BF, White JA, De Girolami PC, and Modlin JF. "An outbreak of rubella among hospital personnel." *The New England Journal of Medicine*, 1980; 303 (10): 541–545.

369. Balfour HH Jr., Groth KE, Edelman CK, Amren DP, Best JM, and Banatvala JE. "Rubella

viraemia and antibody responses after rubella vaccination and reimmunisation." *The Lancet*, 1981; 317 (8229): 1078–1080.
370. Arbuckle TE, and Sherman GJ. "Is rubella syndrome a vanishing disease?" *Chronic Diseases in Canada*, Public Health Agency of Canada, 1992; 13 (21): 24–28.
371. Banatvala JE. "Rubella vaccines." In: AP Waterson (editor), *Recent Advances in Clinical Virology*, Churchill Livingstone, Edinburgh, 1977; pp. 171–190.
372. Lehane DE, Newburg NR, and Beam WE Jr. "Evaluation of rubella herd immunity during an epidemic." *Journal of the American Medical Association*, 1970; 213: 2236.
373. Klock LE, and Rachelefsky GS. "Failure of rubella herd immunity during an epidemic." *The New England Journal of Medicine*, 1973; 288 (2): 69–72.
374. Bart KJ, Orenstein WA, Preblud SR, and Hinman AR. "Universal immunization to interrupt rubella." *Review of Infectious Diseases*, 1985; 7 (Supplement 1): 177–184.
375. Weinstein L, and Chang TW. "Prevention of rubella." *Pediatrics*, 1975; 55 (1): 5–6.
376. Schoenbaum SC, Biano S, and Mack T. "The role of maternal parity. Epidemiology of congenital rubella syndrome." *Journal of the American Medical Association*, 1975; 2333 (2): 151–155.
377. Centers for Disease Control and Prevention. "Measles, rubella, and congenital rubella syndrome: United States and Mexico, 1997–1999." *Morbidity and Mortality Weekly Report*, 2000; 49 (46); 1048–1050, 1059.
378. Centers for Disease Control and Prevention. "Achievements in public health: elimination of rubella and congenital rubella syndrome–United States." *Morbidity and Mortality Weekly Report*, 2005; 54 (11): 279–282.
379. Strannegard O, Holm SE, Hermodsson S, Norrby R, and Lycke E. "Case of apparent reinfection with rubella." *The Lancet* (Letter), 1970; 1 (7640): 240–241.
380. Boue A, Nicolas A, and Montagnon B. "Reinfection with rubella in pregnant women." *The Lancet*, 1971; 1 (7712): 1251–1253.
381. Chin J. Ebbin AJ, Wilson MG, and Lennette EH. "Avoidance of rubella immunization of women during or shortly before pregnancy." *Journal of the American Medical Association*, 1971; 215 (4): 632–634.
382. Joncas J. "Immunization and related problems." [In French]. *L'Union Medicale du Canada*, 1971; 100 (6): 1124–1130.
383. Bott LM, and Eizenberg DH. "Congenital rubella after successful vaccination." *Medical Journal of Australia*, 1982; 1 (12): 514–515.
384. Forsgren M, and Soren L. "Subclinical rubella infection in vaccinated women with rubella-specific IgM response during pregnancy and transmission of virus to the fetus." *Scandinavian Journal of Infectious Diseases*, 1985; 17 (4): 337–341.
385. Morgan-Capner P, Hodgson J, Hambling MH, Dulake C, Coleman TJ, Boswell PA, Watkins RP, Booth J, Stern H, Best JM, and Banatvala JE. "Detection of rubella-specific IgM in subclinical rubella reinfection in pregnancy." *The Lancet*, 1985; 1 (8423): 244–246.
386. Kantoch M, and Imbs D. "Postinfection and postvaccination antirubella immunity." *Acta Virologica*, 1986; 30 (5): 381–389.
387. Miller CL, Miller E, and Waight PA. "Rubella susceptibility and the continuing risk of infection in pregnancy." *British Medical Journal* (Clinical Research Edition), 1987; 294: 1277–1278.
388. Robinson J, Lemay M, and Vaudry W. "Congenital rubella after anticipated maternal immunity: two cases and a review of the literature." *The Pediatric Disease Journal*, 1994; 13 (9): 812–815.
389. Aboudy Y, Fogel A, Barnea B, Mendelson E, Yosef L, Frank T, and Shalev E. "Subclinical

rubella infection during pregnancy followed by transmission of virus to fetus." *Journal of Infection*, 1997; 34 (3): 273–276.

390. Barfield W, Gardner R, Lett S, and Johnsen C. "Congenital rubella reinfection in a mother with anti-cardiolipin and anti-platelet antibodies." *The Pediatric Infectious Disease Journal*, 1997; 16 (2): 247–249.

391. Bott LM, Eizenberg DH. "Congenital rubella after successful vaccination." *Medical Journal of Australia*, 1982; 1 (12): 514–515.

392. Enders G, Calm A, and Schaub J. "Rubella embryopathy after previous maternal rubella vaccination." *Infection*, 1984; 12 (2): 96–98.

393. Saule H, Enders G, Zeller J, and Bernsau U. "Congenital rubella infection after previous immunity of the mother." *European Journal of Pediatrics*, 1988; 147 (2): 195–196.

394. Das BD, Lakhani P, Kurtz JB, Hunter N, Watson BE, Cartwright KA, Caul EO, and Roome AP. "Congenital rubella after previous maternal immunity." *Archives of Diseases in Children*, 1990; 65 (5): 545–546.

395. Miller E, Waight PA, Vurdien JE, White JM, Jones G, Miller BHR, Tookey PA, and Peckham CS. "Rubella surveillance to December 1990: A joint report from the PHLS and National Congenital Rubella Surveillance Programme." *Communicable Disease Review*, 1991; 1 (4): 33–37.

396. Miron D, On A. "Congenital rubella syndrome after maternal immunization." *Harefuah*, 1992; 122 (5): 291–293.

397. Serdula MK, Marks JS, Herrmann KL, Orenstein WA, Hall AD, and Bomgaars MR. "Therapeutic abortions following rubella infection in pregnancy: the potential impact on the incidence of congenital rubella syndrome." *American Journal of Public Health*, 1984; 74 (11): 1249–1251.

398. Public Health Agency of Canada. "Survey of congenital rubella syndrome, Montreal, Laval, and Monteregie, Quebec, 1985–1991." *Canada Communicable Disease Report*, 1996; 22 (5): F1–F2.

399. Public Health Agency of Canada. "Surveillance of congenital rubella syndrome and other rubella-associated adverse pregnancy outcomes." *Canada Communicable Disease Report*, 1996; 22 (5): F3–F4.

400. De Serres G, Dery P, Lebel M, et al. "Epidemiologie de la rubeole congenitale au Quebec de 1965 a 1994." [In French]. Presented at the V e Colloque quebecois sur les maladies infectieuses, Rimouski, Quebec, Canada, May, 1994. Cited in Public Health Agency, ibid reference 399.

401. Swartz TA, Praiss I, Isacson M, Nishmi M, Ben-Porath E, and Hornstein L. "Early results of an extensive rubella epidemic." *International Journal of Epidemiology*, 1975; 4 (4): 331–335.

402. Office of Population Censuses and Surveys, London. "Rubella-associated terminations of pregnancy." *OPCS Monitor*, February 5, 1980. Cited in Serdula et al, ibid reference 397.

403. Tobin JO, Sheppard S, Smithells RW, Milton A, Noah N, and Reid D. "Rubella in the United Kingdom, 1970–1983." *Reviews of Infectious Diseases*, 1985; 7 (Supplement 1): 47–52.

404. Kadoya R, Ueda K, Miyazaki C, Hidaka Y, and Tokugawa K. "Incidence of congenital rubella syndrome and influence of the rubella vaccination programme for schoolgirls in Japan, 1981–1989." *American Journal of Epidemiology*, 1998; 148 (3): 263–268.

405. Katow, S. "Rubella virus genome diagnosis during pregnancy and mechanism of congenital rubella." *Intervirology*, 1998; 41: 163–169.

406. Yellowlees H. "Incidence of congenital rubella." *British Medical Journal*, Correspondence, 1978; 2 (6151): 1569.

407. Miller E, Waight PA, Vurdien JE, Jones G, Tookey PA, and Peckham CS. "Rubella

surveillance to December 1992: second joint report from the PHLS and National Congenital Rubella Surveillance Programme." *Communicable Disease Report*, 1993; 3 (3): 35–39.

408. Plotkin SA, and Orenstein WA. *Vaccines*. Third Edition. WB Saunders Company, Philadelphia, Pennsylvania, USA, 1999; p. 410.

409. Lotter, V. "Epidemiology of autistic conditions in young children." *Social Psychiatry and Psychiatric Epidemiology*, 2004; 1 (3): 124–137.

410. Gardner SG, Bingley PJ, Sawtell PA, Weeks S and Gale EAM. "Rising incidence of insulin dependent diabetes in children aged under 5 years in the Oxford region: time trend analysis." *British Journal of Medicine*, 1997; 315 (7110): 713–717.

411. Bingley PJ, and Gale EAM "Rising incidence of IDDM in Europe." *Diabetes Care*, 1989; 12 (4): 289–295.

412. Diabetes Epidemiology Research International Group. Secular trends in incidence of childhood IDDM in 10 countries." *Diabetes*, 1990; 39 (7): 858–864.

413. Rahi JS, Dezateux C, and the British Congenital Cataract Interest Group. "Congenital and infantile cataract in the United Kingdom: underlying or associated factors." *Investigative Ophthalmology and Visual Science*, 2000; 41 (8): 2108–2114.

414. Cherry JD. "The 'new' epidemiology of measles and rubella." *Hospital Practice*, 1980; 15 (7): 49–57.

415. Centers for Disease Control and Prevention. "Current trends rubella and congenital rubella syndrome: United States, 1985–1988." *Morbidity and Mortality Weekly Report*, 1989; 38 (11): 173–178.

416. Centers for Disease Control and Prevention. "Current trends increase in rubella and congenital rubella syndrome: United States, 1988–1990." *Morbidity and Mortality Weekly Report*, 1991; 40 (6): 93–99.

417. Centers for Disease Control and Prevention. "Rubella and congenital rubella syndrome: United States, 1994–1997." *Morbidity and Mortality Weekly Report*, 1997; 46 (16): 350–354.

418. Vynncky E, Gay NJ, and Cutts FT. "The predicted impact of private sector MMR vaccination on the burden of congenital rubella syndrome." *Vaccine*, 2003; 21 (21–22): 2708–2719.

419. Centers for Disease Control and Prevention. "Progress toward elimination of rubella and congenital rubella syndrome: the Americas, 2003–2008." *Morbidity and Mortality Weekly Report*, 2008; 57 (43): 1176–1179.

420. Kelly H, Worth L, Karapanagiotidis T, and Riddell M. "Interruption of rubella virus transmission in Australia may require vaccination of adult males: evidence from a Victorian sero-survey." *Communicable Diseases Intelligence*, 2004; 28 (1): 69–73.

421. Briss PA, Fehrs LJ, Hutcheson RH, and Shaeffer W. "Rubella among the Amish: resurgent disease in a highly susceptible community." *The Pediatric Disease Journal*, 1992; 11 (11): 955–959.

422. Demicheli V, Jefferson T, Rivetti A, and Price D. "Vaccines for measles, mumps and rubella in children." *Cochrane Database of Systemic Reviews*, 2005; Issue 4, Article no: CD004407.

423. Cherry JD, Heininger U, Stehr K, and Christenson P. "The effect of investigator compliance (observer bias) on calculated efficacy in a pertussis vaccine trial." *Pediatrics*, 1998; 102 (4): 909–912.

424. Underwood M. *Treatise on the Diseases of Children: With General Directions for the Management of Infants from the Birth*, Published by T. Dobson, Philadelphia, Pennsylvania, USA, 1793. American Antiquarian Society database, first series 26291.

425. Paul JR. "Historical and geographical aspects of the epidemiology of poliomyelitis." *Yale Journal of Biology and Medicine*, 1954; 27 (2): 101–113.
426. Bell C. *The Nervous System of the Human Body As Explained in a Series of Papers, Read Before the Royal Society of London*, 3rd edition, London, UK, 1836, p. 434.
427. Badham J. *London Medical Gazette*, 1836; 17: 215.
428. Trevelyan B, Smallman-Raynor M, and Cliff AD. "The spatial dynamics of poliomyelitis in the United States: from epidemic emergence to vaccine-induced retreat, 1910–1971." *Annals of the Association of American Geographers*, 2005; 95 (2): 269–293.
429. Peters ST. *Epidemic: The Battle Against Polio*, Marshall Cavendish Corporation, Tarrytown, NY, USA, 2005; pp. 13–21.
430. Massachusetts State Board of Health. *Infantile Paralysis in Massachusetts, 1907–1912*, Wright and Potter Publishers, 1914. Published by Project Gutenberg Internet Library Archives, San Francisco, California, USA.
[Online, accessed 7th September, 2009]. URL:http://www.archive.org/details.infantile paraly00healgoog
431. Painter CF. "Infantile paralysis. An epidemic of thirty-eight cases." *The Journal of Bone and Joint Surgery*, 1902; s1-15: 414–433.
432. Caverly CS. *Infantile Paralysis in Vermont, 1894–1922*. Published and distributed by the Vermont State Department of Public Health, Burlington, Vermont, USA, 1924.
433. Roberts J. "Polio: the virus and the vaccine." *Ecologist*, May 2004, pp. 36–52.
434. Scobey RR. "The poison cause of poliomyelitis and obstructions to its investigation." *Archive of Pediatrics*, 1952; 69 (4): 172–193.
435. Van Sweeten G. *Aphorisms of Dr Herman Boerhaave*, Volume 10, 1765. Cited in Scobey, ibid reference 434.
436. Cooke J. *Treatise of Nervous Diseases*, 1824. Cited in Scobey, ibid reference 434.
437. Vulpian A. Quoted by Lovett RW, *Boston Medical and Surgical Journal*, 1908; 159: 131–138. Cited in Scobey, ibid reference 434.
438. Popow. Quoted by Mills CK, *Boston Medical and Surgical Journal*, 1883; 108: 248–250. Cited in Scobey, ibid reference 434.
439. Altman. *Australasian Medical Gazette*, July 3, 1897, p. 173. Quoted by LE Holt, and FH Bartlett. "Epidemiology of acute poliomyelitis: a study of thirty-five epidemics." *American Journal of the Medical Sciences*, 1908; 135 (5): 647–661. Cited in Scobey, ibid reference 434.
440. Vonderabe AR. *Archives of Neurology and Psychiatry*, 1931; 25: 29–43. Cited in Scobey, ibid reference 434.
441. Gringer RR. *Archives of Neurology and Psychiatry*, 1931; 25: 649–653. Cited in Scobey, ibid reference 434.
442. Onuff (1900). Quoted by RW Lovett, *Boston Medical and Surgical Journal*, 1908; 159: 131–138. Cited in Scobey, ibid reference 434.
443. Philippe and Gauthard (1903). Quoted by RW Lovett, *Boston Medical and Surgical Journal*, 1908; 159: 131–138. Cited in Scobey, ibid reference 434.
444. Obrastoff (1902). Quoted by RW Lovett, *Boston Medical and Surgical Journal*, 1908; 159: 131–138. Cited in Scobey, ibid reference 434.
445. Collins J, and Marchland HS. "Disease of primary motor neurones causing clinical picture of acute anterior poliomyelitis: result of poisoning by cyanide of potassium; clinical and experimental contribution to toxic effects of cyanide of potassium." *Journal of Nervous and Mental Disease*, 1908; 35: 417–426. Cited in Scobey, ibid reference 434.
446. Edsall DE. *Osler's System of Medicine*, Volume 1, 1907; p. 144. Cited in Scobey, ibid

reference 434.
447. Lambert SM. "A yaws campaign and an epidemic of poliomyelitis in Western Samoa." *Journal of Tropical Medicine and Hygiene*, 1936; 39: 41–46. Cited in Scobey, ibid reference 434.
448. Fiorini E. "Physics of rare events: insights on Napoleon death." *Nuclear Physics B– Proceedings Supplements*, 2009; 188: 365–370.
449. Scobey RR. "Is Human Poliomyelitis Caused by an Exogenous Virus." *Archives of Pediatrics*, 1954; 71 (4): 111–123. Commentary by Jim West.
[Online, accessed 7th September, 2009]. URL:http://www.harpub.co.cc/scobexog.htm
450. Emerson HC. "An epidemic of infantile paralysis in Western Massachusetts in 1908." *Boston Medical and Surgical Journal*, 1909; 151: 115–119. Commentary by Jim West.
[Online, accessed 7th July, 2009]. URL:http://www.harpub.co.cc/mass1908_2articles.htm
451. West J. *Images of Poliomyelitis: Polio in the United States*, Graph Timeline, US 1870–1998.
[Online, accessed 7th September, 2009]. URL:http://www.harpub.co.cc/pol_all.htm
452. West J. *Images of Poliomyelitis: Pesticide Introduction and Poliomyelitis*.
[Online, accessed 7th September, 2009]. URL:http://www.harpub.co.cc/pestintr.htm
453. Scobey RR. "Is human poliomyelitis caused by an exogenous virus?" *Archives of Pediatrics*, 1954; 71 (4): 111–123. Commentary by Jim West.
[Online, accessed 7th September, 2009]. URL:http://www.harpub.co.cc/scobexog.htm
454. Caverly (1894), Dana (1894), Free (1908). Cited in Lovett RW, "The occurrence of infantile paralysis in Massachusetts in 1908." Reported for the Massachusetts State Board of Health." *Boston Medical and Surgical Journal*, 1908; 159: 131–138.
[Online, accessed 7th July, 2009]. URL:http://www.harpub.co.cc/mass1908_2articles.htm
455. West J. "Pesticides and Polio."*Images of Poliomyelitis: A Critique of Scientific Literature*.
[Online, accessed 7th September, 2009]. URL:http://www.harpub.co.cc/overview.htm
456. Biskind MS. "Public health aspects of the new insecticides." *American Journal of Digestive Disease*, 1953; 20 (11): 331–341.
457. Biskind MS, and Bieber I. "DDT poisoning: a new syndrome with neuropsychiatric manifestations." *American Journal of Psychotherapy*, 1949; 3 (2): 261–270.
458. Biskind MS. "Statement on clinical intoxication from DDT and other new insecticides." Presented before a Select Committee to Investigate the Use of Chemicals in Food Products, US House of Representatives, December 12, 1950. *Journal of Insurance Medicine*, May, 1951.
459. Post Polio Health International. *Incidence Rates of Poliomyelitis in US*.
[Online, accessed 7th September, 2009]. URL:http://www.post-polio.org/ir-usa.html
460. Sabin AB. "The epidemiology of poliomyelitis: problems at home and among the armed forces abroad." *Journal of the American Medical Association*, 1947; 134 (9): 749–756.
461. Paul JR. "Poliomyelitis attack rates in American troops, 1940–1948." *The American Journal of Hygiene*, 1949; 50 (1): 57–62.
462. Paul JR. "Neurotropic Virus Diseases: Poliomyelitis." In: Lieutenant General LD Heaton, Colonel JB Coates Jr., and WP Havens Jr. (editors), *Internal Medicine in World War II*, Volume II, Infectious Diseases; Office of the Surgeon General, Department of the Army, Washington, DC, USA, 1963; pp. 91–99.
463. Paul JR, Havens WP Jr, and Van Rooyen CE. "Poliomyelitis in British and American troops in the Middle East; isolation of the virus from human faeces." *British Medical Journal*, 1944; 1 (4355): 841–843.
464. Caughey JE, and Porteous WM. "An epidemic of poliomyelitis occurring among troops in the Middle East." *Medical Journal of Australia*, 1946; 1: 5–10.

465. Hillman CC. "Poliomyelitis in the Philippine Islands." *Military Surgeon*, 1936; 79: 48–58.
466. Martin JK. "Local paralysis in children after injections." *Archives of Diseases of Childhood*, 1950; 25: 1–14.
467. McCloskey BP. "The relation of prophylactic inoculations to the onset of poliomyelitis." *The Lancet*, 1950; 255 (6606): 659–663.
468. Geffen DH. "The incidence of paralysis occurring in London children within four weeks after immunization." *Medical Officer*, 1950; 83: 137–140.
469. Bradford Hill A, Knowelden J. "Inoculation and poliomyelitis: a statistical investigation in England and Wales." *British Medical Journal*, 1950; 2 (4669): 1–6.
470. Editorial: "Inoculation and poliomyelitis." *The British Medical Journal*, 1950; 2 (4669): 28–29.
471. Toomey JA. "Second attacks of poliomyelitis." *American Journal of Disease in Children*, 1938; 56 95): 969–974.
472. Bridge EM, Clarke GH, and Abbe D. "Clinical immunity in poliomyelitis." *American Journal of Disease in Children*, 1946; 72 (5): 501–509.
473. Fox MJ, Madden WJ, and Kohn SE. "Recurrent poliomyelitis." *American Journal of Disease in Children*, 1948; 75 (3): 395–400.
474. Toomey JA. "Intranasal or gastrointestinal portal of entry in poliomyelitis." *Science*, 1935; 82 (2122): 200–201.
475. Klenner FR. "The treatment of poliomyelitis and other virus diseases with vitamin C." *Southern Medicine and Surgery*, 1949; 111 (7): 209–214.
476. Sandler BP. *Diet Prevents Polio*, The Lee Foundation for Nutritional Research, Milwaukee, Wisconsin, USA, 1951.
[Online, accessed 7th September, 2009]. URL:http://www.whale.to/v/sandler.html
477. Sandler, ibid reference 476, p. 43 and p. 146.
478. *Physicians' Desk Reference* (PDR), 55th edition. Medical Economics, Montvale, New Jersey, USA, 2001, p. 778.
479. West J. *Images of Poliomyelitis*. "Franklin D. Roosevelt at Campobello."
[Online, accessed 7th September, 2009]. URL:http://www.harpub.co.cc/fdr.htm)
480. Interview with J Sonnabend. "AIDS Inc", *Conspiracy Nation*, 1988; 7: (33): Part 4.
[Online, accessed 7th September, 2009].
URL:http://www.textfiles.com/conspiracy/CN/cn07-33.txt
481. Roberts J. *Fear of the Invisible: An Investigative Journey into a Reckless and Contaminated Medical Industry*, Impact Investigative Media Productions, Bristol, UK, 2008, p. 53.
482. Dalldorf G, and Sickles GM. "An unidentified, filterable agent isolated from the feces of children with paralysis." *Science*, 1948; 108 (2794): 61–62.
483. Enders JF, Weller TH, and Robbins FC. "Cultivation of the Lansing strain of poliomyelitis in cultures of various human embryonic tissues." *Science*, 1949; 109: 85–87.
484. Beddow Bayly M. *The Story of the Salk Anti-Poliomyelitis Vaccine*, "Statistical errors," 1956.
[Online, accessed 7th September, 2009]. URL:http://www.whale.to/vaccine/bayly.html
485. Offit PA. *The Cutter Incident, 50 Years Later: How America's First Polio Vaccine Led to the Growing Vaccine Crisis*, Yale University Press, New Haven, Connecticut, USA, 2005, pp. 42–44.
486. Offit, ibid reference 485, pp. 62–63.
487. Engel L. "The Salk vaccine: what caused the mess?" *Harpers Magazine*, August 1955, pp. 27–33.
488. Offit, ibid reference 485, pp. 61–62.
489. Offit PA. "The Cutter incident, 50 years later." *The New England Journal of Medicine*, 2005;

352 (14): 1411–1412.
490. Krasner G, and Mesh B. "The Salk Vaccine and the 'Disappearance' of Paralytic Polio: Is Paralysis a Viral Disease?" In: *Polio Awareness Day: Medical Myths Die Hard*, Part 1, 22nd September, 2006.
[Online, accessed 7th September, 2009]. URL:http://www.whale.to/a/krasner1.html
491. *New York Times*, May 11, 1956 Cited by Schippell TM. "The Salk monkey kidney juice." In: McBean, ibid reference 36, Chapter 10, "The hidden dangers in polio vaccine."
492. Shakespeare W. *Romeo and Juliet*, Act 2, Scene 2, Lines 46 and 47, 1594.
493. Scheibner V. *Hearings on Hepatitis B Vaccine*, "Letter to Miss Pinkerton," 16 June, 1999.
[Online, accessed 7th September, 2009].
URL:http://www.whale.to/vaccines/scheibner8.html)
493. James W. *Immunization, the Reality Behind the Myth*, 2nd edition, Bergin and Garvey (imprint of Greenwood Publishing Group), Westport, Connecticut, USA, 1995, p. 36.
495. Menkes JH. *Textbook of Child Neurology*, 5th edition, Williams and Wilkins, Baltimore, Maryland, USA, 1995, p. 420.
496. Goldman AS, Schmalstieg EJ, Freeman DH Jr, Goldman DA, and Schmalstieg FC Jr. "What was the cause of Franklin Delano Roosevelt's paralytic illness?" *Journal of Medical Biography*, 2003; 11 (4): 232–240.
497. Lyle WH. "An outbreak of a disease believed to have been caused by ECHO 9 virus." *Annals of Internal Medicine*, 1959; 51: 248–269.
498. Ramsay AM, Aberd MD, and O'Sullivan E. "Encephalomyelitis simulating poliomyelitis." *The Lancet*, 1956; 267 (6926): 761–764.
499. James W, ibid reference 493, p. 36. Citing the Los Angeles County Health Index, *Morbidity and Mortality*, "Reportable Diseases", 1967.
500. Rodale JI (editor-in-chief). *The Encyclopedia of Common Diseases*, Rodale Press, Emmaus, Pennsylvania, USA, 1962. Citing: *Illinois Medical Journal*, 1960; August and September editions. Reprinted in: *Child and Family*, 1980; 19: 195–213, 259–280.
501. Ratner H. *Nature, the Physician, and the Family: Selected Writings of, Herbert Ratner, MD*, MT Baggot (editor), AuthorHouse, Bloomington, Indiana, USA, 1962, pp. 259–264.
502. Sweet BH, and Hilleman MR. "The vacuolating virus, SV40." Proceedings of the Society for Experimental Biology and Medicine, 1960; 105: 420–427.
503. Eddy BE. "Tumors produced in hamsters by SV40." *Federal Proceedings*, 1962; 21: 930–935.
504. Immunization Safety Review Committee, Institute of Medicine of the National Academies. *Immunization Safety Review: SV 40 Contamination of Polio Vaccine and Cancer*, Stratton K, Alamario DA, and McCormick MC (editors), The National Academies Press, Washington, DC, USA; "Executive Summary", p. 5.
505. Kirschstein RL, and Gerber P. "Ependymomas produced after intracerebral inoculation of S40 into new-born hamsters." *Nature*, 1962; 195: 299–300.
506. Schein HM, and Enders JF. "Transformation induced by simian virus 40 in human renal cell cultures, I. Morphology and growth characteristics." *Proceedings of the National Academies of Sciences*, USA, 1962; 48 (7): 1164–1172.
507. Koprowski H, Ponten J, Jensen F, Ravdin RG, Moorhead P, and Saksela E. "Transformation of cultures of human tissue infected with simian virus 40." *Acta-Unio Internationalis Contra Cancorum*, 1963; 19: 362–367.
508. Jensen F, Koprowski H, Pagano JS, Ponten J, and Ravdin RG. "Autologous and homologous implantation of human cells transformed in vitro by simian virus 40." *Journal of the National Cancer Institute*, 1964; 32 (4): 917–937.
509. Horwini ME. "Simian virus 40 (SV40): a cancer causing monkey virus from FDA-

approved vaccines." *Albany Law Journal of Science and Technology*, 2003; 13 (3).
510. Bookchin D, and Schumacher J. *The Virus and the Vaccine: The True Story of a Cancer-Producing Monkey Virus, Contaminated Polio Vaccine, and the Millions of Americans Exposed*, St Martin's Press, New York, NY, USA, 2004.
511. Carlsen W. "Rogue virus in the vaccine: early polio vaccine harbored virus now feared to cause cancer in humans." *San Francisco Chronicle*, July, 2001.
512. "Questions and answers." *Journal of the American Medical Association*, 1961; 175 (8): 735–740.
513. American Academy of Pediatrics. *Report of Committee on Infectious Diseases*, American Academy of Pediatrics, Evanston, Illinois, USA, 1966, 47.
514. Fraumeni JF Jr, Ederer F, and Miller RW. "An evaluation of the carcinogenicity of the simian virus 40 in man." *Journal of the American Medical Association*, 1963; 185 (9): 713–718.
515. Fraumeni JF Jr. Stark CR, Gold E, an Lepow ML. "Simian virus 40 in polio vaccine follow-up of newborn recipients." *Science*, 1970; 167 (914): 59–63.
516. Letter from John T. Conner of Merck & Co. to Dr Leroy Burney, Surgeon General of the United States, dated 12/16/60; Plaintiff's Exhibit No. 54. In: *Sabin Polio Litigation, MDL 780, U.S.D.C. MD, Baltimore, Maryland*. Cited in Kops SP. "Oral polio vaccine and human cancer: a reassessment of SV40 as a contaminant based upon legal documents." *Anticancer Research*, 2000; 20 (6C): 4745–4749.
517. Meyer HM, Hopps HE, Rogers NG, Brooks BE, Berneheim BC, Jones WP, Nisalak A, and Douglas RD. "Studies on simian virus 40." *Journal of Immunology*, 1962; 88: 796–806.
518. Abraham R, Minor P, Dunn G, Modlin JF, and Ogra PL. "Shedding of virulent poliovirus revertants during immunization with oral poliovirus vaccine after prior immunization with inactivated polio vaccine." *The Journal of Infectious Diseases*, 1993; 168 (5): 1105–1109.
519. Lederle's *Cytomegalovirus Contingency Plan*, 4 August, 1972. Cited by Martin JW, Center for Complex Infectious Diseases, Rosemead, California, USA, *Detection of Stealth Viruses in Human Tissues*. Presented at a meeting entitled "Consultation on detection of simian megaloviruses in human tissues," National Institute of Allergy and Infectious Diseases, Rockville, Maryland, USA, July 1, 1996.
[Online, accessed 7th September, 2009]. URL:http://www.ccig.org/
520. Centers for Disease Control and Prevention. "Current trends paralytic poliomyelitis: United States, 1982 and 1983." *Morbidity and Mortality Weekly Report*, Nov 16, 1984; 33(45): 635.
521. Boffey PM. "Polio: Salk challenges safety of Sabin's live-virus vaccine." *Science*, 1977; 196 (4285): 35–36.
522. Sutter RW, Patriarca PA, Cochi SL, Pattansch MA, Kew OM, Hall DB, Brogan S, Malankar PG, Al-Ghassany AAK, Suleiman AJM, El-Bualy MS, Bass AG, and Alexander JP. "Outbreak of paralytic poliomyelitis in Oman: evidence for widespread transmission among fully vaccinated children." *The Lancet*, 1991; 338 (8769): 715–720.
523. Strebel PM, Aubert-Combiescu A, Ion-Nedelcu N, Biberi-Moroeanu S, Combiescu M, Sutter RW, Kew OM, Pallansch MA, Patriarca PA, and Cochi SL. "Paralytic poliomyelitis in Romania, 1984–1992." *American Journal of Epidemiology*, 1994; 140 (12): 1111–1124.
524. Strebel PM, Ion-Nedelcu N, Baughman AL, Sutter RW, and Cochi SL. "Intramuscular injections within 30 days of immunization with oral poliomyelitis vaccine: a risk factor for vaccine-associated paralytic poliomyelitis." *The New England Journal of Medicine*, 1995, 332 (8): 500–506.
525. Whale Vaccination Information Website. *Citations of Vaccine-associated Polio*.
[Online, accessed 7th September, 2009]. URL:http://www.whale.to/vaccine/polio6.html

526. Strebel PM, Sutter RW, Cochi SL, Biellik RJ, Brink EW, Kew OM, Pallansch MA, Orenstein WA, and Hinman AR. "Epidemiology of poliomyelitis in the United States one decade after the last reported case of indigenous wild virus-associated disease." *Clinical Infectious Disease*, 1992; 14 (2): 568–579.
527. Los Angeles County Health Index: *Morbidity and Mortality, Reportable Diseases, 1967*. Cited in: Kent C. "Drugs, bugs, and shots in the dark." *Health Freedom News*, Monrovia, California, January 1983, p. 26. Quoted by: James W, *Immunization, The Reality Behind the Myth*, Bergen and Garvey Publishers Inc, South Hadley, Massachusetts, USA, 1988, p. 28.
528. Krasner G. *Polio Awareness Day: Medical Myths Die Hard*, September 19, 2006.
    [Online, accessed 7th September, 2009].
    URL:http://www.whale.to/vaccine/Polio%20Awareness%20Day%20%20Medical%20Myths%20Die%20Hard.pdf
529. Centers for Disease Control and Prevention. "Outbreak of aseptic meningitis: Whiteside County, Illinois, 1995." *Morbidity and Mortality Weekly Report*, March 14, 1997; 46 (10): 221–224.
530. Dowsett EG, Ramsay AM, McCartney RA, and Bell EJ. "Myalgic encephalomyelitis: a powerful enteroviral infection?" *Postgraduate Medical Journal*, 1990; 66 (777): 526–530.
531. Dowsett EG. *The Late Effects of ME: Can They Be Distinguished from the Post-Polio Syndrome?* Presentation to the All Party Group of MPs on ME/PPS on 31st January, 2001. Published online by the Lincolnshire Post-Polio Library, February, 2001.
    [Online, accessed 7th September, 2009].
    URL:http://www.ott.zynet.co.uk/polio/lincolnshire/library/dowsett/lateeffectsme.html
532. Bruno RL, Frick NM, Creange S, Zimmerman JR, and Lewis T. "Polioencephalitis and the brain fatigue generator model of post-viral fatigue syndromes." *Journal of Chronic Fatigue Syndrome*, 1996; 2 (2/3): 5–27.
533. Bruno RL, Creange SJ, Frick NM. "Parallels between post-polio fatigue and chronic fatigue syndrome: a common pathophysiology?" *The American Journal of Medicine*, 1998; 105 (3A): 66S–73S.
534. Hyde B (editor). *M.E. Epidemics: The Clinical and Scientific Basis of Myalgic Encephalomyelitis/Chronic Fatigue Syndrome*, Nightingale Research Foundation, Ottawa, Ontario, Canada, 1992.
535. Bruno RL. *Dr Bruno's Response to People Who Write About "Poliovirus Causing CFS*, June 12, 2002.
    [Online, accessed 7th September, 2009].
    URL:http://www.ippso-world.org/ppsinfo/articles/bruno/response.html
536. Douglas WC. "Chronic fatigue syndrome: the hidden polio epidemic." *Second Opinion Newsletter*, 1996; 6 (8): 1–6.
537. Martin WJ. "Detection of viral related sequences in CFS patients using the polymerase chain reaction." In: Byron M Hyde (editor),*The Clinical and Scientific Basis of Myalgic Encephalomyelitis/Chronic Fatigue Syndrome*, Nightingale Research Foundation Press, Ottawa, Ontario, Canada, 1992, pp. 278–283.
538. Martin WJ. "Viral infection in CFS patients." In: Byron M Hyde (editor)*The Clinical and Scientific Basis of Myalgic Encephalomyelitis/Chronic Fatigue Syndrome*, , Nightingale Research Foundation Press, Ottawa, Ontario, Canada, 1992, pp. 325–327.
539. Martin WJ. Zeng LC, Ahmed K, and Roy M. "Cytomegalovirus-related sequences in an atypical cytopathic virus repeatedly isolated from a patient with the chronic fatigue syndrome." *American Journal of Pathology*, 1994; 145: 441–452.

540. Martin WJ, Ahmed KN, Zeng LC, Olsen J-S, Seward JG, and Seehrai JS. "African green monkey origin of atypical cytopathic 'stealth virus' isolated from a patient with chronic fatigue syndrome." *Clinical and Diagnostic Virology*, 1995; 4 (1): 93–103.
541. Martin WJ. "Stealth adaptation of an African green monkey simian cytomegalovirus." *Experimental and Molecular Pathology*, 1999; 66 (1): 3–7.
542. Martin WJ, and Glass RT. "Acute encephalopathy induced in cats with a stealth virus isolated from a patient with chronic fatigue syndrome." *Pathobiology*, 1995; 63 (3): 115–118.
543. Martin WJ, and Anderson D. "Stealth virus epidemic in the Mohave Valley: initial report of viral isolation." *Pathobiology*, 1997; 65 (1): 51–56.
544. Martin WJ, and Anderson D. "Stealth virus epidemic in the Mohave Valley: severe vacuolating encephalopathy in a child presenting with a behavioral disorder." *Experimental and Molecular Pathology*, 1999; 66 (1): 19–30.
545. Dang-Tan T, Mahmud SM, Puntoni R, and Franco EL. "Polio vaccines, simian virus 40, and human cancer: the epidemiologic evidence for a causal association." *Oncogene*, 2004; 23: 6535–6540.
546. Innis MD. "Oncogenesis and poliomyelitis vaccine." *Nature*, 1968; 219 (5157): 972–973.
547. Farwell JR, Dohrmann GJ, Marrett LD, and Meigs JW. "Effect of SV40 virus-contaminated polio vaccine on the incidence and type of CNS neoplasms in children: a population-based study." *Transactions of the American Neurological Association*, 1979; 104: 261–264.
548. Heinonen OP, Shapiro S, Monson RR, Hartz SC, Rosenberg L, and Slone D. "Immunization during pregnancy against poliomyelitis and influenza in relation to malignancy." *International Journal of Epidemiology*, 1973; 2 (3): 229–235.
549. Bergsagel DJ, Finegold MJ, Butel JS, Kupsky WJ, and Garcea RL. "DNA sequences similar to those of simian virus 40 in ependymomas and choroid plexus tumors of childhood." *The New England Journal of Medicine*, 1992; 326 (15): 988–993.
550. Lednicky JA, Garcea RL, Bergsagel DJ, and Butel JS. "Natural simian virus 40 strains are present in human choroid plexus and ependymoma tumors." *Virology*, 1995; 212 (2): 710–717.
551. Cicala C, Pompetti F, and Carbone M. "SV40 induces mesotheliomas in hamsters" *American Journal of Pathology*, 1993; 142 (5): 1524–1533.
552. Carbone M, Pass HI, Rizzo P, Marinetti M, Di Muzio M, Mew DJ, Levine AS, and Procopio A. "Simian virus 4-like DNA sequences in human pleural mesothelioma." *Oncogene*, 1994; 9 (6): 1781–1790.
553. De Rienzo A, Tor M, Sterman DH, Aksoy F, Albelda SM, and Testa JR. "Detection of SV40 DNA sequences in malignant mesothelioma specimens from the United States, but not from Turkey." *Journal of Cellular Biochemistry*, 2002; 84 (3): 455–459.
554. Hirvonen A, Mattson K, Karjalainen A, Ollkainen T, Tammilehto L, Hovi T, Vainio H, Pass HI, Di Resta I, Carbone M, and Linnainmaa K. "Simian virus 40 (SV40)-like DNA sequences not detectable in Finnish mesothelioma patients not exposed to SV40-contaminated polio vaccines." *Molecular Carcinogenesis*, 1999; 26 (2): 93–99.
555. Carbone M, Kratzke RA, and Testa JR. "The pathogenesis of mesothelioma." *Seminars in Oncology*, 2002; 29 (1): 2–17.
556. Bright RK, Kimchi ET, Shearer MH, Kennedy RC, and Pass HL. "SV40 Tag-specific cytotoxic T lymphocytes generated from the peripheral blood of malignant pleural mesothelioma patients." *Cancer Immunology, Immunotherapy*, 2002; 50 (12): 682–690.
557. Foddis R, De Rienzo A, Broccoli D, Bocchetta M, Stekala E, Rizzo P, Tosolini A, Grobelny JV, Jhanwar SC, Pass HI, Testa JR, and Carbone M. "SV 40 infection induces telomerase activity in human mesothelial cells." *Oncogene*, 2002; 21 (9): 1434–1442.

558. Carbone M, Kratzke RA, and Testa JR. "The pathogenesis of mesothelioma." *Seminars in Oncology*, 2002; 29 (1): 2–17.

559. Gazdar AF, and Carbone M. "Molecular pathogenesis of malignant mesothelioma and its relationship to simian virus 40." *Clinical Lung Cancer*, 2003; 5 (3): 177–181.

560. Carbone M, Rizzo P, Procopio A, Giuliano M, Pass HI, Gebhardt MC, Mangham C, Hansen M, Malkin DF, Bushart B, Pompetti F, Picci P, Levine AS, Bersagel JD, and Garcea RL. "SV40 sequences in human bone tumors." *Oncogene*, 1996; 13 (3): 527–535.

561. Testa JR, Carbone M, Hirvonen A, Khalili K, Krynska B, Linnainmaa K, Pooley FD, Rizzo P, Rusch V, and Xiao GH. "A multi-institutional study confirms the presence and expression of simian virus 40 in human malignant mesotheliomas." *Cancer Research*, 1998; 58 (2): 4505–4506.

562. Vilchez RA, Lednicky JA, Halvorson SJ, White ZS, Kozinetz CA, and Butel JS. "Detection of polyomavirus simian virus 40 tumor antigen DNA in AIDS-related systemic non-Hodgkin lymphoma." *Journal of Acquired Immune Deficiency Syndrome*, 2002; 29 (2): 109–116.

563. Vilchez RA, and Butel JS. "SV40 in bone cancers and non-Hodgkin's lymphoma." *Oncogene*, 2003; 22 (33): 5164–5172.

564. Martini F, Lazzarin L, Iaccheri L, Vignocchi B, Finocchiaro G, Magnani I, Serra M, Scotlandi K, Barbanti-Brodano G, and Tognon M. "Different simian virus 40 genome regions and sequences homologous with SV40 large T antigen in DNA of human brain and bone tumours and of leukocytes from blood donors." *Cancer*, 2002; 94 (4): 1037–1048.

565. Vilchez RA, and Butel JS. "Simian virus 40 and its association with human lymphomas." *Current Oncology Reports*, 2003; 5 (5): 372–379.

566. Butel JS, Arrington AS, Wong C, Lednicky JA, and Finegold MJ. "Molecular evidence of simian virus 40 infections in children." *Journal of Infectious Diseases*, 1999; 180 (3): 884–887.

567. Martini F, De Mattei M, Iaccheri L, Lazzarin L, Barbanti-Brodano G, Tognon M, and Gerosa M. "Human brain tumors and simian virus 40." *Journal of the National Cancer Institute*, 1995; 87 (17): 1331.

568. Martini F, Lazzarin L, Iaccheri L, Corallini A, Gerosa M, Trabanelli C, Calza N, Barbanti-Brodano G, and Tognon M. "Simian virus 40 footprints in normal human tissues, brain and bone tumors of different histotypes." *Developments in Biological Standardization*, 1998; 94: 55–66.

569. Huang H, Reis R, Yonekawa Y, Lopes JM, Kleihues P, and Ohgaki H. "Identification in human brain tumors of DNA sequences specific for SV40 large T antigen. *Brain Pathology*, 1999; 9 (1): 33–42.

570. Zhen HN, Zhang X, Bu XY, Zhang ZW, Huang WJ, Zhang P, Liang JW, and Wang XL. "Expression of the simian virus 40 large tumor antigen (Tag) and formation of Tag-p53 and Tag-pRb complexes in human brain tumors." *Cancer*, 1999; 86 (10): 2124–2132.

571. Martini F, Iaccheri L, Lazzarin L, Carinci P, Corallini A, Gerosa M, Iuzzolino P, Barbanti-Brodano G, and Tognon M. "SV40 early region and large T antigen in human brain tumors, peripheral blood cells, and sperm fluids from healthy individuals." *Cancer Research*, 1996; 56: 4820–4825.

572. Martini F, Iaccheri L, Lazzarin L, Carinci P, Corallini A, Gerosa M, Iuzzolino P, Barbanti-Brodano G, and Tognon M. "SV40 early region and large T antigen in human brain tumors, peripheral blood cells, and sperm fluids from healthy individuals." *Cancer Research*, 1997; 57 (15): 3319–3320.

573. Barbanti-Brodano G, Sabbioni S, Martini F, Negrini M, Corallini A, and Tognon M. "Simian virus 40 infection in humans and association with human diseases: results and

hypotheses." *Virology*, 2004; 318 (1): 1–9.
574. Zhen H, Zhang X, Zhang Z, Fei Z, He X, Liang J, Huang W, Liu X, and Zhang P. "Simian virus 40 large tumor antigen forms specific complexes with p53 and pRb in human brain tumors." *Chinese Medical Journal* [In English], 2001; 114 (4): 382–386.
575. Horwin M. *Simian Virus 40 (SV40) from FDA-Approved Polio Vaccine*, SV40 Foundation. [Online, accessed 7th September, 2009]. URL:http://www.sv40foundation.org
576. Butel JS, Jafar S, Wond C, Arrington AS, Opekun AR, Finegold MJ and Adam E. "Evidence of SV40 infections in hospitalized children." *Human Pathology*, 1999; 30 (12): 1496–1502.
577. Butel JS, and Lednicky JA. "Response re: Cell and molecular biology of simian virus 40: implications for human infections and disease." *Journal of the National Cancer Institute*, 1999; 91 (13): 1166–1167.
578. Rosa FW, Sever JL, and Madden DL. "Absence of antibody response to simian virus 40 after inoculation with killed poliovirus vaccine of mothers of offspring with neurologic tumors." *The New England Journal of Medicine*, 1988; 318 (22): 1469.
579. Rosa FW, Sever JL, and Madden DL.. "Response to: Neurologic tumors in offspring after inoculation of mothers with killed poliomyelitis vaccine." *The New England Journal of Medicine*, 1988; 319: 1226.
580. Brock B. *Paper Presented at the Workshop on Simian Virus 40 (SV40): A Possible Human Papillomavirus Workshop*, January 1997. At: Kops SP, SV40Cancer.com.
[Online, accessed 7th September, 2009]. URL:http://www.sv40cancer.com/paperled.asp
581. Kops SP. "Oral polio vaccine and human cancer: a reassessment of SV40 as a contaminant based upon legal documents." *Anticancer Research*, 2000; 20 (6C): 4745–4749. Also at: Kops SP, SV40Cancer.com.
[Online, accessed 7th September, 2009]. URL:http://www.sv40cancer.com/pap1.asp
582. Kops SP. *The Paper Trail: Correspondence with FDA, 1–6*. At: Kops SP, SV40Cancer.com [Online, accessed 7th September, 2009]. URL:http://www.sv40cancer.com/cor1.asp
583. Kops SP. *Oral Presentation to the Subcommittee on Human Rights and Wellness of the Committee on Government Reform: "The SV40 Virus: Has Tainted Polio Vaccine Caused an Increase in Cancer?"* September 10, 2003.
[Online, accessed 7th September, 2009]. URL:http://www.sv40cancer.com/oralpres.asp
584. Board on Health Promotion and Disease Prevention, Institute of Medicine. *Immunization Safety Review: SV40 Contamination of Polio Vaccine and Cancer*, The National Academies Press, Washington, DC, USA, 2002.
585. Cutrone R, Lednicky J, Dunn G, Rizzo P, Bocchetta M, Chumakov K, Minor P, and Carbone M. "Some oral poliovirus vaccines were contaminated with infectious SV40 after 1961." *Cancer Research*, 2005; 65: 10273–10279.
586. Melnick JL, and Stinebaugh S. "Excretion of vacuolating SV40 (papovavirus group) after ingestion as a contaminant of oral polio vaccine." *Proceedings of the Society for Experimental and Biological Medicine*, 1962; 109: 965–968.
587. Rizzo P, Di Resta I, Powers A, Ratner H, and Carbone M. "Unique strains of SV40 in commercial poliovaccines from 1955 not readily identifiable with current testing for SV40 infection." *Cancer Research*, 1999; 59: 6103–6108.
588. National Cancer Institute, US National Institutes of Health. *Studies Find No Evidence that SV40 is Related to Human Cancer*, 23 August, 2004.
[Online, accessed 7th September, 2009].
URL:http://www.cancer.gov/newscenter/pressreleases/SV40.
589. Wakefield AJ, Blaxhill M, Haley B, Ryland A, Hollenbeck D, Johnson J, Moody J, and

Stott C. "Response to Dr. Ari Brown and the Immunization Action Coalition." *Medical Veritas*, 2009; 6: 1907–1924.

590. US Food and Drug Administration, Vaccine Adverse Event Reporting System (VAERS), *News and Events: Statement of Susan S Ellenberg before the Subcommittee on Criminal Justice, Drug Policy and Human Resources House Committee on Government Reform*, May 18, 1999.
[Online, accessed 7th September, 2009].
URL:http://www.fda.gov/NewsEvents/Testimony/ucm115058

591. Rosenthani S, and Chen R. "The reporting sensitivities of two passive surveillance systems for vaccine adverse events." *American Journal of Public Health*, 1995; 85: 1706–1709.

592. Braun MM. *Vaccine Adverse Event Reporting System (VAERS): Usefulness and Limitations*, John Hopkins Bloomberg School of Public Health, Baltimore, Maryland, USA, 2006.
[Online, accessed 7th September, 2009].
URL;http://www.vaccinesafety.edu/VAERS/htm

593. Whale.to Website: *Medical Citations (Vaccination)*.
[Online, accessed 7th September, 2009].
URL:http://www.whale.to/vaccine/citations.html

594. Diodati C, Horowitz L, Scheibner V, and West E. "Vaccination: Part II–The Risks They Pose to Your Health." *Consumer Health* (Consumer Health Organization of Canada, Toronto, Ontario, Canada), 1999; volume 22, issue 5.
[Online, accessed 7th September, 2009].
URL:http://www.consumerhealth.org/articles/display.cfm?ID=19990705003020

595. King PG, And Goldman GS. "Key realities about autism, vaccines, vaccine-injury compensation, Thimerosal, and autism-related research." *Medical Veritas*, 2008; 5: 1610–1644.

596. Poling J, and Poling T. "Vaccines, autism and our daughter Hannah." *New York Times*, April 5, 2008.

597. Medical Advisory Committee of the Immune Deficiency Foundation. *The Clinical Presentation of the Primary Immunodeficiency Diseases : A Primer for Physicians*, Towson, Maryland, USA, 1992.

598. Van Hoff J, Schymura MJ, and Curnen MG. "Trends in the incidence of childhood and adolescent cancer in Connecticut, 1935–1979." *Medical and Pediatric Oncology*, 1988; 16 (2): 78–87.

599. Gurney JG, Davis S, Severson RK, Fang JY, Ross JA, and Robison LL. "Trends in cancer incidence among children in the U.S." *Cancer*, 1996; 78 (3): 532–541.

600. Bleyer WA. "What can be learned about childhood cancer from *Cancer Statistics Review*, 1973–1988." *Cancer*, 1993; 71 (10): 3229–3236.

601. Gurney JG, Davis S, Severson RK, Fang JY, Ross JA, and Robison LL. "Trends in cancer incidence among children in the U.S." *Cancer*, 1996; 78 (3): 532–541.

602. Gurney JG, Davis S, Severson RK, and Robison LL. "The influence of subsequent neoplasms on incidence trends in childhood cancer." *Cancer Epidemiology, Biomarkers and Prevention*, 1994; 3 (4): 349–351.

603. Bunin GR, Feuer EJ, Witman PA, and Meadows AT. "Increasing incidence of childhood cancer: report of 20 years experience from the greater Delaware Valley Pediatric Tumor Registry." *Paediatric and Perinatal Epidemiology*, 1996; 10 (3): 319–338.

604. Swenson AR, and Bushhouse SA. "Childhood cancer incidence and trends in Minnesota, 1988–1994." *Minnesota Medicine*, 1998; 81 (12): 27–32.

605. Linet MS, Ries LA, Smith MA, Tarone RE, and Devesa SS. "Cancer surveillance series: recent trends in childhood cancer incidence and mortality in the United States." *Journal of

the National Cancer Institute, 1999; 91 (12): 1051–1058.
606. Mangano JJ. "A rise in the incidence of childhood cancer in the United States." *International Journal of Health Services*, 1999; 29 (2): 393–408.
607. Moll UM, LaQuaglia M, Benard J, and Riou G. "Wild-type p53 undergoes cytoplasmic sequestration in undifferentiated neuroblastomas but not in differentiated tumors." *Proceedings of the National Academy of Sciences, USA*, 1995; 92 (10): 4407–4411.
608. Teitz T, Chang JC, Kitamura M, Yen TSB, and Kan YW. "Rhabdomyosarcoma arising in transgenic mice harboring the beta-globin locus control region fused with simian virus 40 large T antigen gene. *Proceedings of the National Academy of Sciences, USA*, 1993; 90 (7): 2910–2914.
609. DeCaprio JA, Ludlow JW, Figge J, Shew JY, Huang CM, Lee WH, Marsilio JY, Paucho E, and Livingston DM. "SV40 large tumor antigen forms a specific complex with the product of the retinoblastoma susceptibility gene." *Cell*, 1988; 54 (2): 275–283.
610. McWhirter WR, Dobson C, and Ring I. "Childhood cancer incidence in Australia, 1982–1991." *International Journal of Cancer*, 1998; 65 (1): 34–38.
611. Lotter V. "Epidemiology of autistic conditions in young children." *Social Psychiatry and Psychiatric Epidemiology*, 1967; 1 (4): 163–173.
612. Brask BH. "A prevalence investigation of childhood psychoses." Paper presented at the 16th Scandinavian Congress of Psychiatry, 1970. In: *Nordic Symposium on the Care of Psychotic Children*, Trykningssentral, Oslo, Norway, *Barnepsykiatrist Forening*, 1972: 145-153.
613. Fombonne E. "Epidemiology of autistic disorder and other pervasive developmental disorders." *Journal of Clinical Psychiatry*, 2005; 66 (Supplement 10): 3–8.
614. Fombonne E. "Epidemiological surveys of autism and other pervasive developmental disorders: an update." *Journal of Autism and Developmental Disorders*, 2003; 33 (4): 365–382.
615. Centers for Disease Control and Prevention. "Prevalence of autism spectrum disorders: Autism and Developmental Disabilities Monitoring Network, six sites, United States, 2000." *Morbidity and Mortality Weekly Report*, 2007; 56 (SS01): 1–11.
616. MacDermott S, Williams K, Ridley G, Glasson E, and Wray J. *The Prevalence of Autism in Australia: Can it be Established from Existing Data?* A report prepared for Australian Advisory Board on Autism Spectrum Disorders, Forestville, NSW, Australia, 2006.
617. Yasbak EF, Lang-Radosh KL. "Adverse outcomes associated with postpartum rubella or MMR vaccine." *Medical Sentinel*, 2001; 6 (3): 95–99.
618. Offit PA. "Inoculated against facts." *New York Times*, March 31, 2008.
619. Offit PA. "Vaccines and autism revisited—the Hannah Poling case." *The New England Journal of Medicine*, 2008; 358: 2089–2091.
620. Poling J. "Vaccines and autism revisited." Letters, *The New England Journal of Medicine*, 2008; 359: 655–656.
621. American Academy of Pediatricians. *A.L.A.R.M. Autism (Fact Sheet)*, January 2004. [Online, accessed 7th September, 2009]. URL:http://www.aap.org/healthtopics/autism.cfm
622. McDonald KL, Huq SI, Lix LM, Becker AB, and Kozyrskyj AL. "Delay in diphtheria, pertussis, tetanus vaccine is associated with a reduced risk of childhood asthma." *The Journal of Allergy and Clinical Immunology*, 2008; 121 (3): 626–631.
623. Classen DC, and Classen JB. "The timing of pediatric immunization and the risk of insulin-dependent diabetes." *Infectious Diseases in Clinical Practice*, 1997; 6 (7): 449–454.
624. Classen DC, and Classen JB. "Immunizations in the first month of life may explain the decline in incidence of IDDM in the Netherlands." *Autoimmunity*, 1999; 31: 43–45.

625. Classen JB, and Classen DC. "Public should be told that vaccines may have long term adverse effects." Letters, *British Medical Journal*, 1999; 318 (7177): 193.
626. Classen JB, and Classen DC. "Association between type 1 diabetes and Hib vaccine." Letters, *British Medical Journal*, 1999; 319 (7217): 1133.
627. Classen JB. "Diabetes epidemic follows hepatitis B immunization program." *New Zealand Medical Journal*, 1996; 109 (1022): 195.
628. Dokheel TM. "An epidemic of childhood diabetes in the United States? Evidence from Allegheny County, Pennsylvania." *Diabetes Care*, 1993; 16 (12): 1606–1611.
629. Gardner S, Bingley PJ, Sawtell PA, Weeks S, and Gale EA. "Incidence of insulin dependent diabetes is rising sharply in children under 5." *British Medical Journal*, 1997; 315 (7110): 713–716.
630. Kalokerinos A. *Medical Pioneer of the 20th Century: Dr. Archie Kalokerinos: An Autobiography*. Biological Therapies Publishing, Melbourne, Victoria, Australia, 2000.
631. Kalokerinos A. *Every Second Child*, Nelson, Melbourne, Victoria, Australia, 1974.
632. Kalokerinos A. Interview with Dr Kris Gaublomme, Genk, Belgium: *International Vaccine Newsletter*, June 1955.
[Online, accessed 7th September, 2009]. URL:http://www.whale.to/v/kalokerinos.html
633. Hume R, and Weyers E. "Changes in the leucocyte ascorbic acid concentration during the common cold." *Scottish Medical Journal*, 1973; 18: 3.
634. Kalokerinos A, and Dettman G. "Sudden death in infancy syndrome in Western Australia." *Medical Journal of Australia*, 1976; 2 (1): 31–32.
635. Dettman G. "Factor 'X', subclinical scurvy and S.I.D.S. Historical. Part 1." *The Australasian Nurses Journal*, 1978; 7 (7): 2–5.
636. Kalokerinos A, and Dettman G. "Aboriginal health: the gentle art of deception." *The Australasian Nurses Journal*, 1980; 10 (1): 14–15.
637. Kalokerinos A, and Dettman G. "Rubella immunisation: a tangle of absurdities and some comments." *The Australasian Nurses Journal*, 1981; 10 (11): 3–6.
638. Kalokerinos A. *The Vaccination Dilemma*, (video), 1992. Cited by HV Martin/Free-America, "Was the AIDS virus tested on expendable people?" *North American Investigative Journal*, 1995.
[Online, accessed 7th September, 2009].
URL:http://dmc.members.sonic.net/sentinel/naij4.html
639. Hadwen WR. "The fraud of vaccination." *The Truth*, January 3, 1923.
640. Hadwen WR. *Dare Doctors Think?* Verbatim Report: Great Meeting Held in Queen's Hall, London, Friday February 6, 1925. Published by The British Union for the Abolition of Vivisection, London, 1925.
641. Rook GA, and Stanford JL. "Given us this day our daily germs." *Immunology Today*, 1998; 19 (3): 113–116.
642. Reidler J, Braun-Fahrlander C, Eder W, Schreuer M, Waser M, Maisch S, Carr D, Schieri R, Nowak D, von Mutius E. (The ALEX Study Team, Salzburg, Austria). "Exposure to farming in early life and development of asthma and allergy: a cross-sectional survey." *The Lancet*, 2001; 358 (9288): 1129–1133.
643. Braun-Fahrlander C, Gassner M, Grize L, Neu U, Sennhauser FH, Varonier HS, Vuille JC, and Wuthrich B. (SCARPOL: Swiss Study on Childhood Allergy and Respiratory Symptoms with Respect to Air Pollution). "Prevalence of hay fever and allergic sensitization in farmers' children and their peers living in the same rural community." *Clinical and Experimental Allergy*, 1999; 29 (1): 28–34.
644. Strachan DP. "Family size, infection and atopy: the first decade of the 'hygiene

hypothesis'." *Thorax*, 2000; 55 (Supplement 1): S2–S10.
645. Kramer U, Heinrich J, Wist M, and Wichmann HE. "Age of entry to day nursery and allergy in later childhood." *The Lancet*, 1999; 353 (9151): 450–454.
646. Cramer DW, Welch WR, Cassells S, and Scully RE. "Mumps, menarche, menopause, and ovarian cancer." *American Journal of Obstetrics and Gynecology*, 1983; 147 (1): 1–6.
647. West RO. "Epidemiologic study of malignancies of the ovaries." *Cancer*, 1966; 19 (7): 1001–1007.
648. Menczer J, Modan M, Ranon L, and Golan A. "Possible role of mumps virus in the etiology of ovarian cancer." *Cancer*, 1979; 43 (4): 1375–1379.
649. Yazdanbakhsh M, Kremsner PG, and van Ree R. "Allergy, parasites, and the hygiene hypothesis." *Science*, 2002; 298 (5567): 490–494.
650. Ronne T. "Measles virus infection without rash in childhood is related to disease in later life." *The Lancet*, 1985; 1 (8419): 1–5.
651. Kucukosmanoglu E, Cetinkaya F, Akcay F, Pekun F. "Frequency of allergic diseases following measles." [In Spanish]. *Allergologia et Immunopathologia*, 2006; 34 (4): 146–149.
652. Shaheen SO, Aaby P, Hall AJ, Barker DJ, Heyes CB, Shiell AW, and Goudiaby A. "Measles and atopy in Guinea-Bissau." *The Lancet*, 1996; 347 (9018): 1792–1796.
653. Aim JS, Swartz J, Lilja G, Scheynius A, Pershagen G. "Atopy in children of families with an anthroposophical lifestyle." *The Lancet*, 1999; 353 (9163): 1485–1488.
654. Flotsrup H, Swartz J, Bergstrom A, Aim JS, Scheynius A, van Hage M, Waser M, Braun-Fahrlander C, Schram-Bijkerk D, Huber M, Zutavern A, von Mutius E, Ublagger E, Riedler J, Michaels KB, Pershagen B; (the Parsifal Study Group). "Allergic disease and sensitization in Steiner school children." *Journal of Allergy and Clinical Immunology*, 2006; 117 (1): 59–66.
655. Rosenlund H, Bergstrom A, Aim JS, Swartz J, Scheynius A, van Hage M, Johansen K, Brunekreef B, von Mutius E, Ege MJ, Riedler J, Braun-Fahriander C, Waser M, Pershagen B; (Parsifal Study Group). "Allergic disease and atopic sensitization in children in relation to measles vaccination and measles infection." *Pediatrics*, 2009; 123 (3): 771–778.
656. Rooth IB, and Bjorkman A. "Suppression of Plasmodium falciparum infections during concomitant measles or influenza but not during pertussis." *American Tropical Medicine and Hygiene*, 1992; 47 (5): 675–681.
657. Lepore L, Agosti E, Pennesi M, Barbi E, De Manzini A. "Long-term remission induced by measles infection and followed by immunosuppressive therapy in a case of refractory juvenile rheumatoid arthritis." *La Pediatria e Medical Chirurgia*, [In Italian] 1988; 10 (2): 191–193.
658. Simpanen E, van Essen R, and Isomaki H. "Remission of juvenile rheumatoid arthritis (Still's disease) after measles." *The Lancet*, 1977; 2 (8045): 987–988.
659. Yoshioka K, Miyata H, and Maki S. "Transient remission of juvenile rheumatoid arthritis after measles." *Acta Pediatrica Scandinavica*, 1981; 70 (3): 419–420.
660. Urbach J, Schirr D, and Abramov A. "Prolonged remission of juvenile rheumatoid arthritis (Still's disease) following measles." *Acta Paediatrica Scandinavica*, 1983; 72 (6): 917–918.
661. Bonjean M, and Prime A. "Suspensive effect of measles in psoriasic erythroderma of 12 years' duration." [In French], *Lyon Medical*, 1969; 222 (40): 839.
662. Fomkin KF. "Cure of psoriasis after co-existing measles." [In Russian],*Vestnik Dermatologi i Venerologii*, 1961; 35: 66-68.
663. Lintas N. "Case of psoriasis cured after recurrent measles." [In Italian], *Minerva Dermatologica*, 1959; 24 (4): 296–297.

664. Thiers H, Normand J, Fayolle J. "Suspensive effect of measles on chronic psoriasis in children: 2 cases." [In French], *Lyon Medical*, 1969; 222 (40): 839–840.
665. Sasco AJ, and Paffenbarger RS Jr. "Measles infection and Parkinson's disease." *American Journal of Epidemiology*, 1985; 122 (6): 1017–1031.
666. Yamamoto H, Yamano T, Niijima S, Kohyama J, and Yamanouchi H.n"Spontaneous improvement of intractable epileptic seizures following acute viral infections." *Brain and Development*, 2004; 26 (6): 377–379.
667. Cookson WO, and Moffatt MF. "Asthma: an epidemic in the absence of infection?" *Science*, 1997; 275 (5296): 41–42.
668. Matricardi PM, Rosmini F, Ferrigno L, Nisini R, Rapicetta M, Chionne P, Stroffolini T, Pasquini P, and D'Amelio R. "Cross sectional retrospective study of prevalence of atopy among Italian military students with antibodies against hepatitis A virus." *British Medical Journal*, 1997; 314 (7086): 999.
669. Yazdanbakhsh M, Kremsner PG, and van Ree R. "Allergy, parasites, and the hygiene hypothesis." *Science*, 2002; 298 (5567): 490–494.
670. Fortun P. "Scientists team up with an unlikely ally—hookworms." *News and Reviews*, University of Nottingham, UK, August 4, 2006.
[Online accessed 7th September, 2009].
URL:http://research.nottingham.ac.uk/Newsreviews/newsDisplay.aspx?id=270
671. Yamamoto H, Yamano T, Niijima S, Kohyama J, and Yamanouchi H. "Spontaneous improvement of intractable epileptic seizures following acute viral infections." *Brain and Development*, 2004; 26 (6): 377–379.
672. Shafren DR, Au GG, Nguyen T, Newcombe NG, Haley ES, Beagley L, Johansson ES, Hersey P, and Barry RD. "Systemic therapy of malignant human melanoma tumors by a common cold-producing enterovirus, Coxsackievirus A21." *Clinical Cancer Research*, 2004; 10 (Part 1): 53–60.
673. Au GG, Lindberg AM, Barry RD, and Shafren DR. "Oncolysis of vascular malignant human melanoma tumors by Coxsackievirus A21." *International Journal of Oncology*, 2005; 26 (6): 1471–1476.
674. Au GG, Lincz LF, Enno A, Shafren DR. "Oncolytic Coxsackievirus A21 as a novel therapy for multiple myeloma." *British Journal of Haematology*, 2007; 137 (2): 133–141.
675. Berry LJ, Au GG, Barry RD, and Shafren DR. "Potent oncolytic activity of human enteroviruses against human prostate cancer." *Prostate*, 2008; 68 (6): 577–587.
676. Skelding KA, Barry RD, and Shafren DR. "Systemic targeting of metastatic human breast tumor xenografts by Coxsackievirus A21." *Breast Cancer Research and Treatment*, 2009; 113 (1): 21–30.
677. Shafren DR, Sylvester D, Johansson ES, Campbell IG, and Barry RD. "Oncolysis of human ovarian cancers by echovirus type 1." *International Journal of Cancer*, 2005; 115 (2): 320–328.
678. Clarke P, Meintzer SM, Gibson S, Widmann C, Garrington TP, Johnson GL, and Tyler KL. "Reovirus-induced apoptosis is mediated by TRAIL." *Journal of Virology*, 2000; 74 (17): 8135–8139.
679. Hirasawa K, Nishikawa SG, Norman KL, Coffey MC, Thompson BG, Voon CS, Waisman DM, and Lee PWK. "Systemic reovirus therapy of metastatic cancer in immune-competent mice." *Cancer Research*, 2003; 63 (2): 348–353.
680. Thirukkumaran CM, and Morris DG. "Oncolytic viral therapy using reovirus." *Methods in Molecular Biology*, 2009; 542: 607–634.
681. Thirukkumaran CM, Nodwell MJ, Hirasawa K, Shi Z-Q, Diaz R, Luider J, Johnston RN, Forsyth PA, Magliocco AM, Lee P, Nishikawa S, Donnelly B, Coffey M, Trpkov K,

Fonseca K, Spurreff J, and Morris DG. "Oncolytic viral therapy for prostate cancer: efficacy of reovirus as a biological therapeutic." *Cancer Research*, 2010; 70 (6): 2435–2444.

682. MacKie RM, Stewart B, Brown SM. "Intralesional injection of herpes simplex virus 1716 in metastatic melanoma." *The Lancet*, 2001; 357 (9255): 525–526.

683. Varghese S, and Rabkin S. "Oncolytic herpes simplex virus vectors for cancer virotherapy." *Cancer Gene Therapy*, 2002; 9 (12): 967–978.

684. Steiner PE, and Loosli CG. "The effect of human influenza virus (Type A) on the incidence of lung tumors in mice." *Cancer Research*, 1950; 10: 385–392.

685. Zamai L, Ahmad M, Bennett IM, Azzoni L, Alnemri ES, and Perussia B. "Natural killer (NK) cell-mediated cytotoxicity: differential use of TRAIL and Fas ligand by immature and mature primary human NK cells." *Journal of Experimental Medicine*, 1998; 188 (12): 2375–2380.

686. Griffith TS, Wiley SR, Kubin MZ, Sedger LM, Maliszewski CR, and Fanger NA. "Monocyte-mediated tumoricidal activity via tumor necrosis factor- related cytokine, TRAIL. *Journal of Experimental Medicine*, 1999; 189 (8): 1343–1354.

687. Kayagaki N, Yamaguchi N, Nakayama M, Eto H, Okumura K, and Yagita H. "Type I interferons (IFNs) regulate tumor necrosis factor-related apoptosis-inducing ligand (TRAIL) expression on human T cells: a novel mechanism for the antitumor effects of type I IFNs." *Journal of Experimental Medicine*, 1999; 189 (9): 1451–1460.

688. Kayagaki N, Yamaguchi N, Nakayama M, Takeda K, Akiba H, Tsutsui H, Okamura H, Nakanishi K, Okumura K, and Yagita H. "Expression and function of TNF-related apoptosis-inducing ligand on murine activated NK cells." *Journal of Immunology*, 1999; 163 (4): 1906–1913.

689. Takeda K, Hayakawa Y, Smyth MJ, Kayagaki N, Yamaguchi N, Kakuta S, Iwakura Y, Yagita H, and Okumura K. "Involvement of tumor necrosis factor-related apoptosis-inducing ligand in surveillance of tumor metastasis by liver natural killer cells." *Nature Medicine*, 2001; 7 (1): 94–100.

690. Ishikawa E, Nakazawa M, Yoshinari M, and Minami M. "Role of tumor necrosis factor-related apoptosis-inducing ligand in immune response to influenza virus infection in mice." Journal of Virology, 2005; 79 (12): 7658–7663.

691. Brincks EL, Kucaba TA, Legge KL, and Griffith TS. "Influenza-induced expression of functional tumor necrosis factor-related apoptosis-inducing ligand (TRAIL) on human peripheral blood mononuclear cells." *Human Immunology*, 2008; 69 (10): 634–646.

692. Kotelkin A, Prikhod'ko EA, Cohen JI, Collins PL, and Bukreyev A. "Respiratory syncytial virus infection sensitizes cells to apoptosis mediated by tumor necrosis factor-related apoptosis-inducing ligand." *Journal of Virology*, 2003; 77 (17): 9156–9172.

693. Sedger LM, Shows DM, Blanton RA, Peschon JJ, Goodwin RG, Cosman D, and Wiley SR. "IFN-gamma mediates a novel antiviral activity through dynamic modulation of TRAIL and TRAIL receptor expression." *Journal of Immunology*, 1999; 163 (2): 920–926.

694. Wright P. "Smallpox vaccine triggered AIDs Virus: the World Health Organisation masterminded the 13-year vaccination campaign." *London Times*, May 11, 1987.

695. Gallo RC. *Virus Hunting: AIDS, Cancer, and the Human Retrovirus: A Story of Scientific Discovery*, New Republic/Basic Books, New York, NY, USA, 1991.

696. Wyllie A. "Two worlds, one hope." *The Scotsman*, December 1, 2007.

697. Green J, and Miller D. *AIDS: The Story of a Disease*, Grafton Books, London, UK, 1986, p. 66.

698. Noireau F. "HIV transmission from monkey to man." *The Lancet*, 1987; 1 (8548): 1498–1499.

699. Konotey-Ahulu FID. "Group specific component and HIV infection." *The Lancet*, 1987; 1 (8544): 1267–1269.
700. Mulder C. "Human virus not from monkeys." *Nature*, 1988; 333: 396.
701. Fukasawa M, Miura T, Hasegawa A, Morikawa S, Tsujimoto H, Miki K, Kitamura T, and Hayami M. "Sequence of simian immunodeficiency virus from African green monkey, a new member of HIV/SIV group." *Nature*, 1988; 333: 457–461.
702. Hymes KB, Cheung T, Greene JB, Prose NS, Marcus A, Ballard H, William DC, and Laubenstein LJ. "Kaposi's sarcoma in homosexual men: a report of eight cases." *The Lancet*, 1981; 2 (8247): 598–600.
703. Centers for Disease Control and Prevention. "Kaposi's sarcoma and pneumocystis pneumonia among homosexual men: New York City and California." *Morbidity and Mortality Weekly Report*, 1981; 30 (25): 305–308.
704. Centers for Disease Control and Prevention. "Pneumocystis pneumonia: Los Angeles." *Morbidity and Mortality Weekly Report*, 1981; 30 (21): 1–3.
705. Centers for Disease Control and Prevention. "Current trends update: acquired immunodeficiency syndrome in the San Francisco Cohort Study, 1978–1985." *Morbidity and Mortality Weekly Report*, 1985; 34 (38): 573–575.
706. Stevens CE, Taylor PE, Zang EA, Morrison JM, Harley EJ, Rodriguez de Cordoba S, Bacino C, Ting RC, Bodner AJ, Sarngadharan MG, Gallo RC, and Rubinstein P. "Human T-cell lymphotropic virus type III infection in a cohort of homosexual men in New York City." *Journal of the American Medical Association*, 1986; 255 (16): 2167–2172.
707. Centers for Disease Control and Prevention. "Current trends update on acquired immune deficiency syndrome (AIDS): United States." *Morbidity and Mortality Weekly Report*, 1982; 31 (37): 507–508, 513–514.
708. Koblin BA, van Benthem BHB, Buchbinder SP, Ren L, Vittinghoff E, Stevens CE, Coutinho RA, and van Griensven JP. "Long-term survival after infection with human immunodeficiency virus type 1 (HIV-1) among homosexual men in hepatitis B vaccine trial cohorts in Amsterdam, New York City, and San Francisco, 1978–1995." *American Journal of Epidemiology*, 1999; 150 (10): 1026–1030.
709. Harrison-Chirimuuta R, and Chirimuuta R. *AIDS and Africa: A Case of Racism vs Science?* [Online, accessed 7th September, 2009]. URL:http://www.virusmyth.com/aids/hiv/rcafrica.htm
710. "The AIDS 'plot' against blacks." *The New York Times*, May 12, 1992.
711. Jones JH. *Bad Blood: The Tuskagee Syphilis Experiment*, Free Press, New York, NY, USA, 1981.
712. Harris R, and Paxman J. *A Higher Form of Killing: The Secret History of Chemical and Biological Warfare*, Random House, London, UK, 1982. p. 265.
713. "Living with AIDS" *National Geographic*, 2005. [Online, accessed 7th September, 2009]. URL:http://ngm.nationalgeographic.com/ngm/0509/feature4/map.html
714. Scott DW, and Scott WLC. *AIDS: The Crime Beyond Belief*, Trafford Publishing, Bloomington, Indiana, USA, 2008.
715. Scott DW, and Scott WLC. *The Extremely Unfortunate Skull Valley Incident: Chronic Fatigue Syndrome, Acquired Immunodeficiency Syndrome, Gulf War Syndrome, and American Warfare*, The Chelmsford Publishers, Sudbury, Ontario, Canada, 1997.
716. Cantwell A Jr. *AIDS: The Mystery and the Solution*, Aries Rising, Los Angeles, California, USA, 1984.
717. Cantwell A Jr. *AIDS and the Doctors of Death*, Aries Rising, Los Angeles, California, USA,

1988.
718. Cantwell A Jr. *The Cancer Miracle: The Hidden Killer in Cancer, AIDS and Other Autoimmune Diseases*, Aries Rising, Los Angeles, California, USA, 1990.
719. Cantwell A Jr. *Queer Blood: The Secret AIDS Genocide Plot*, Aries Rising Press, Los Angeles, California, USA, 1993.
720. Martin HV. *Was the AIDS Virus Tested on Expendable People?* FreeAmerica, 1985.
[Online, accessed 7th September, 2009]. URL:http://www.whale.to/b/martin.html
721. Horowitz LG. *Emerging Viruses: AIDS and Ebola: Nature, Accident or Intentional?* Tetrahedron, Sandpoint, Idaho, USA, 1996.
722. Burnet FM. "Men or molecules? a tilt at molecular biology." *The Lancet*, 1966; 1 (7427): 37–39.
723. Vankin J. *Conspiracies, Cover-ups and Crimes: Political Manipulation and Mind Control in America*, Paragon House, New York, NY, USA,1996. Cited in Cantwell, ibid reference 719, p. 60.
724. US Congress Appropriations Committee Hearing. *Research, Development, Testing, and Evaluation of Synthetic Biological Agents, Appropriations for 1970, Hearings Before a Subcommittee on Appropriations, House of Representatives, Ninety-First Congress, First Session*. US Government Printing Service. Reposted on the Internet by PhilFam Committee, 22 June, 1998. Transcript of July 1, 1969 of Dr Donald MacArthur, Deputy Director of Defence, Research and Engineering. pp. 129–130.
[Online, accessed 7th September, 2009].
URL:http://panindigan.tripod.com/aidsdodhear.html
725. Allison AC, Beveridge WIB, Cockburn WC, East J, Goodman HC, Koprowski H, Lambert PH, van Loghemn JJ, Miescher PA, Mimms CA,,Notkins AI, and Torrigiani G. "Memoranda: Virus-associated immunopathology: animal models and implications for human disease." *Bulletin of the World Health Organisation*, 1972; 47 (2): 257–274.
726. Strecker RB. *The Strecker Memorandum*, a video from The Strecker Group, Eagle Rock, California, USA, 1983.
727. Grote J. "Bovine visna virus and the origin of HIV." Letter, *Journal of the Royal Society of Medicine*, 1988; 81 (10): 620.
728. Matsumoto G. *Vaccine A: The Covert Government Experiment That's Killing Our Soldiers and Why GIs Are Only the First Victims*, Basic Books, Cambridge, Massachusetts, USA, 2004.
729. UK Ministry of Defence. *Background to the Use of Medical Countermeasures to Protect British Forces during the Gulf War (Operation Grandby)*, Section 42, p.8. Cited in Matsumoto G, ibid reference 728, p. 84.
730. Matsumoto G, ibid reference 728, pp. 46–55.
731. Research Advisory Committee on Gulf War Veterans' Illnesses. *Gulf War Illness and the Health of Gulf War Veterans: Scientific Findings and Recommendations*, Washington, DC, USA, November 2008.
732. Fukuda K, Nisenbaum R, Stewart G, Thompson WW, Robin K, Washko RM, Noah DL, Barrett DH, Randall B, Herwaldt BL, Mawle AC, and Reeves WC. "Chronic multisymptom illness affecting Air Force veterans of the Gulf War." *Journal of the American Medical Association*, 1988; 280 (11): 981–988. Cited in Matsumoto G, ibid reference 728, p. 119 and p. 149.
733. CNN.com. *In Depth Specials: Gulf War Facts*.
[Online, accessed 7th September, 2009].
URL:http://webarchive.org/web.20070510125644/http://edition.cnn.com/SPECIALS/2001...

734. Kang H, Magee C, Mahan C, Lee K, Jackson L, and Matanoski G. "Pregnancy outcomes among U.S. Gulf War veterans: a population-based survey of 30,000 veterans." *Annals of Epidemiology*, 2001; 11 (7): 504–511.
735. Matsumoto G, ibid reference 728, pp. 146–155.
736. *The Newport Daily News*, Virginia, USA. "Effects of anthrax vaccine downplayed." Tuesday, December 20, 2005.
[Online, accessed 7th September, 2009].
URL:http://www.gulfwarvets.com/vaccine_downplayed.htm
737. Matsumoto G, ibid reference 728, pp. 155–165.
738. Asa PB, Wilson RB, Garry RF. "Antibodies to squalene in recipients of anthrax vaccine." *Experimental and Molecular Pathology*, 2002; 73: 19–27.
739. Phillips CJ, Matyas GR, Hansen CJ, Alving CR, Smith TC, and Ryan MAK. "Antibodies to squalene in US Navy Persian Gulf War veterans with chronic multisystem illness." *Vaccine*, 2009; 27 (29): 3921–3926.
740. Wade N. "Division of Biologics Standards: The boat that never rocked." *Science*, 1972; 175 (4027): 1225–1230.

PART TWO—BLINKERED SCIENCE AND THE VITAL FORCE

CHAPTER 6—How Do We Know?

Quote of Dr Martin Luther King Jr: from *Strength to Love*, 1963.

1. Aristotle. *Physics*, Book 2, Part 3, circa 350 BCE. Translated by RP Hardie and RK Grace, The Internet Classics Archive, Webatomics, DC Stevenson, classics@mit.edu.
[Online, accessed 18th July, 2009].
URL:http://classics.mit.edu/index.html
2. Aristotle. *The Metaphysics*, circa 350 BCE. Introduced and translated by H Lawson-Tancred, Penguin Classics, London, UK, 1998.
3. Plato. *The Republic*, circa 360 BCE. Translated by B Jowett, The Internet Classics Archive, Webatomics, DC Stevenson, classics@mit.edu.
[Online, accessed 18th July, 2009]. URL:http://classics.mit.edu/index.html
4. Blavatsky net—Theosophy. "Ancient Landmarks: Plato and Aristotle", *Theosophy*, September, 1939; 27 (11): 483–491.
[Online, accessed 18th July, 2009].
URL:http://www.wisdomworld.org/additional/ancientlandmarks/PlatoAndAristotle.html
5. Plato. *Phaedo*, circa 385 BCE. In: *Plato in Twelve Volumes*, volume 1, HN Fowler (translator), Harvard University Press, Cambridge, Massachusetts, USA, 1966.
6. Plato. *Symposium*, circa 385 BCE. Translated by B Jowett, The Internet Classics Archive, Webatomics, DC Stevenson, classics@mit.edu.
[Online, accessed 18th July, 2009]. URL:http://www.mit.edu/Plato/symposium/html
7. Plato. *Parmenides*, circa 370 BCE. Translated by B Jowett, The Internet Classics Archive, Webatomics, DC Stevenson, classics@mit.edu.
[Online, accessed 18th July, 2009].
URL:http://www.classics.mit.edu/Plato/parmenides.html
8. Plato. *Sophist*, circa 360 BCE. Translated by B Jowett, The Internet Classics Archive, Webatomics, DC Stevenson, classics@mit.edu.

[Online, accessed 18th July, 2009]. URL:http://classics.mit.edu/Plato/sophist.html
9. Plato. *Theaetetus*, circa 370 BCE. Translated by B Jowett, Project Gutenberg Literary Archive Foundation, Salt Lake City, Utah, USA.
[Online, accessed 18th July, 2009]. URL:http://gutenberg.org/dirs/1/7/2/1726/1726.txt
10. Plato. *Timaeus*, circa 360 BCE. Translated by B Jowett, Project Gutenberg Literary Archive Foundation, Salt Lake City, Utah, USA.
[Online, accessed 18th July, 2009]. URL:http://www.gutenberg.org/etext/1572
11. *The Matrix*. Written and directed by Andy Wachowski and Larry Wachowski. Executive producers: B Berman, A Mason, A Wachowski and L Wachowski. Productions companies: Groucho II Film Partnership, Silver Pictures, Village Road Show Pictures, and Warner Bros. Pictures, 1999.
12. Shakespeare W. *The Tempest*, Act IV, Scene 1, Line 155.
13. *The Bhagavad Gita: A Classic of Indian Spirituality*, introduced and translated by E Easwaran, Nilgiri Press, Blue Mountain Center of Meditation, Tomales, California, USA, 2007; chapters 7, 9, 10, and 11.
14. Lao Tzu. *Tao Te Ching*. translated by J Legge, Dover Publications Inc., Mineola, NY, USA, 1997.
15. Diels HA. *Die Fragmente der Vorskratiker* [Fragments of the Pre-Socratics], sixth edition, reviewed by W Kranz, Weidmann, Berlin, Germany, 1952; Fragments: 10, 60, 61, 62, 67, 88.
16. Stephenson M. *The Sage Age: Blending Science with Intuitive Wisdom*, Nightengale Press, Mequon, Wisconsin, USA, 2008; p. 126.
17. Sorokin PA. *Social and Cultural Dynamics*, 4 Volumes, American Book Company, New York, USA, 1937–41.
18. Capra F. *The Turning Point: Science, Society and the Rising Culture*, Fontana Paperbacks, Glasgow, Scotland, UK, 1982.
19. Rogers CR. *The Person of Tomorrow*, commencement address at Sonoma State College, Sonoma, California, USA, June 1969. Published in Sonoma State School Pamphlet; also published in *USIU Doctoral Society Journal*, 1970; 3 (1): 11–16.
20. Campbell J. *The Power of Myth, with Bill Moyers*. Betty Sue Flowers (editor) Doubleday, New York, NY, USA, 1988.
21. Harman W, and Rheingold H. *Higher Creativity: Liberating the Unconscious for Breakthrough Insights*, Jeremy P. Tarcher, Inc; distributed by St Martin's Press, New York, NY, USA, 1984.
22. Descartes R. *The Discourse on Method of Rightly Conducting the Reason, and Seeking for Truth in Sciences*, 1637. In: ES Haldane and GRT Ross (translators), *The Philosophical Works of Descartes*, Volume 1, Cambridge University Press, Cambridge, UK, 1981.
23. Descartes R. *Meditations on First Philosophy*, 1641. In: J Cottingham (editor and translator), *Meditations on First Philosophy, with Selections from the Objections and Replies*, Cambridge University Press, Cambridge, UK, 1996.
24. Suzuki D. and Levine J. *Cracking the Code*, Allen & Unwin, NSW, Australia, 1994, p 147.
25. Koffka K. *Principles of Gestalt Psychology*, Harcourt-Brace, New York, USA, 1935, p. 176.
26. Bacon F. *Novum Organum: Or True Directions Concerning the Interpretation of Nature*, 1620. B Montague (editor and translator), *The Works*, 3 volumes, Parry and MacMillan, Philadelphia, Pennsylvania, USA, 1854. Online: Hanover Historical Texts Project, 2001. [Online, accessed 20th July, 2009].
URL:http://history.hanover.edu/texts/Bacon/novorg.html
27. Kneale W. *Probability and Induction*, Part II, Clarendon Press, Oxford, UK, 1949.

28. *The Bible*: Genesis 1:26.
29. Rodis-Lewis G. "Limitations of the Mechanical Model in the Cartesian Conception of the Organism." In: *Descartes*, M Hooker (editor), Johns Hopkins University Press, Baltimore, Maryland, USA, 1978.
30. Randall JH. *The Making of the Modern Mind*, Columbia University Press, New York, NY, USA, 1976.
31. Einstein A, Podolsky B. and Rosen N. "Can quantum-mechanical description of physical reality be considered complete?" *Physical Review*, 1935; 47 (10): 777–780.
32. Schroedinger E. "Die gegenwaertige Situation in der Quantummechanik." *Naturwissenschaft*, 1935; 23: 807–812, 823–828, 844–849. ["The present situation in quantum mechanics: a translation of Schroedinger's cat paradox paper." Translated by JD Trimmer. *Proceedings of the American Philosophical Society*, 1980; 124 (5): 123–138.]
33. Bohr N. *Atomic Physics and Human Knowledge*, John Wiley & Sons, New York, NY, USA, 1958.
34. Heisenberg W. *Ordnung der Wirklichkeit* [Reality and Its Order], W Blum, H-P Duerr, and H Rechenberg (editors), Publisher: R Piper, Munich, Germany, 1984. English translation by MB Rumscheidt and N Lukens. Joechen Heisenberg, University of New Hamspshire, New Durham, New Hampshire, USA.
    [Online, accessed 20th July, 2009].
    URL:http://werner-heisenberg.unh.edu/t-OdW-english.htm#seg11
35. Capra F. *The Tao of Physics: An Exploration of the Parallels between Modern Physics and Eastern Mysticism*, Fontana Paperbacks, London, UK, 1983.
36. Heisenberg W. *Physics and Philosophy*, Allen & Unwin, London, UK, 1963.
37. Oppenheimer JR. *Science and the Common Understanding*, Oxford University Press, London, UK, 1954.
38. Jung CG, and Pauli W. *Atom and Archetype: The Pauli/Jung Letters, 1932–1958*. CA Meier (editor), D Roscoe (translator). Princeton University Press, Princeton, New Jersey, USA, 2001.
39. Gleich J. *Chaos: Making a New Science*, Penguin Books, New York, NY, USA, 1988.
40. Rosen R. *Theoretical Biology and Complexity*, Academic Press, New York, NY, USA, 1985.
41. Davies P. *The Cosmic Blueprint: New Discoveries in Nature's Creative Ability to Order the Universe*, Templeton Press, West Conshohocken, Pennsylvannia, USA, 2004.
42. Davies P, ibid reference 41, p. 100.
43. Burke J. *The Day the Universe Changed: A Personal View by James Burke*, BBC, London, UK, 1985.

CHAPTER 7—Two Ways to View Health and Disease

Quote of Upton Sinclair: from *The Jungle*, 1906.
1. Plaisted DA. *Estimates of the Number Killed by the Papacy in the Middle Ages and Later*, University of North Carolina, Chapel Hill, North Carolina, USA, 2006; Chapter 3: "The 50 million figure", p. 40; Chapter 4: "Alethia's estimate", pp. 50–52, 54, 55, 58.
   [Online, accessed 20th January, 2010].
   URL:http://www.cs.unc.edu/~plaisted/estimates.doc
2. Sobel D (editor). "Introduction." In: *Ways of Health: Holistic Approaches to Ancient and Contemporary Medicine*, Harcourt Brace Jovanovich, New York, NY, USA, 1979, pp. 15–16.
3. *The New Oxford Dictionary of English*, J Pearsall (editor), P Hanks (chief editor), Clarendon

Press, Oxford, UK, 1998.

CHAPTER 8—Vital Force, 1: Stuck in the Whole

1. Capra F. *The Tao of Physics: An Exploration of the Parallels between Modern Physics and Eastern Mysticism*, Fontana Paperbacks, London, UK, 1983.
2. Bohr N. *Atomic Physics and Human Knowledge*, John Wiley & Sons, New York, NY, USA, 1958.
3. Heisenberg W. *Physics and Philosophy*, Allen & Unwin, London, UK, 1963.
4. Oppenheimer JR. *Science and the Common Understanding*, Oxford University Press, London, UK, 1954.
5. Jung CG, and Pauli W. *Atom and Archetype: The Pauli/Jung Letters, 1932–1958*. CA Meier (editor), D Roscoe (translator). Princeton University Press, Princeton, New Jersey, USA, 2001.
6. Sheldrake R. *A New Science of Life: The Hypothesis of Formative Causation*. J.P. Tarcher, Inc. Los Angeles, California, USA, 1981.
7. Rosen R. *Theoretical Biology and Complexity*, Academic Press, New York, NY, USA, 1985.
8. Bateson G. *Steps to an Ecology of Mind: Collected Essays in Anthropology, Psychiatry, Evolution, and Epistemology*, University of Chicago Press, Chicago, Illinois, USA, 1972.
9. Bateson G. *Mind and Nature: A Necessary Unity*. Hampton Press, Cresskill, New Jersey, USA, 1979.
10. Hauck DW. *The Emerald Tablet: Alchemy of Personal Transformation*, Penguin Group, New York, NY, 1999. Cited in Sculley N. *Alchemical Healing: A Guide to Spiritual, Physical, and Transformational Medicine*, Bear and Company, Rochester, Vermont, USA, p. 321.
11. Chopra D. *Quantum Healing*, Bantum Books, New York, NY, USA, 1989, pp. 48–49.
12. Hippocrates. *De Alimento*, 400 BCE. In: *Hippocrates on Diet and Hygiene*, J Precope (editor and translator), Zeno, London, UK, 1952, p. 174. Cited in Jung CG, and Pauli W, ibid reference 19.
13. Koestler A. *The Roots of Coincidence*, Hutchinson, London, UK, 1972, p 137.
14. Watson L. *Lifetide: a Biology of the Unconscious*. Hodder and Stoughton, London, UK, 1979; 156–159.
15. Keyes K Jr. *The Hundredth Monkey*, Vision Books, Coos Bay, Oregon, USA, 1981.
16. Kawai M. "On the newly acquired behaviours of the natural troop of Japanese monkeys on Koshima Island." *Primates*, 1963; 4: 113–115. Cited in Watson L, ibid reference 14.
17. Kawai M. "Newly acquired behaviour of the neutral troop of Japanese monkeys on Koshima Island." *Primates*, 1965; 6: 1–30. Cited in Watson L, ibid reference 14.
18. Kawamura S. "The process of sub-culture propagation among Japanese monkeys." Cited in Southwick CH. *Primate Social Behavior*. Van Nostrand, Princeton, New Jersey, USA, 1963, p. 493.
19. Jung CG, and Pauli W. *The Interpretation of Nature and the Psyche*, 1. "Synchronicity: An Acausal Connecting Principle", Routledge and Kegan Paul, London, UK, 1955.
20. Capra F, ibid reference 1, pp. 178–207.
21. Capra F. *The Turning Point: Science, Society and the Rising Culture*, Fontana Paperbacks, London, UK, 1985, pp. 63–89.
22. Giorbran G. *Forever Everything: Learning to See Timelessness*, Barnes and Noble, Lyndhurst, New Jersey, USA, Chapter 18, 2006.

23. Heisenberg W. *Physics and Philosophy*, Harper & Row, New York, NY, USA, 1962. p. 139.
24. Born M, Einstein A, and Born H. *The Born-Einstein Letters: Correspondence between Albert Einstein and Max and Helwig Born from 1916 to 1955*. I Born (translator), Walker and Company, New York, NY, USA, 1971, pp. 90–91.
25. Jeans J. *The Mysterious Universe*, AMS Press, London, UK, 1933, p. 158.
26. Eddington A. *The Nature of the Physical World*. Cambridge University Press, Cambridge, UK, 1928, p. 276.

CHAPTER 9—Vital Force, 2: Spinning Energies

Quote of Albert Szent-Györgyi: from *Introduction to a Submolecular Biology*, 1960.

1. Liveson JA, and Ma DM. *Laboratory Reference for Clinical Neurophysiology*, Oxford University Press Inc, New York, NY, USA, 1992; pp. 387–388.
2. Koestler A. *The Roots of Coincidence*, Hutchinson, London, UK, 1972, p. 137.
3. Coryell DM. *Good Grief: Healing Through the Shadow of Loss*, Healing Arts Press, Rochester, Vermont, USA, 2004; "Letter to the reader", p. xvi.
4. "Chinese proverbs." ChooseChinese, Beijing Stanford Chinese Culture Co., Beijing, China. [Online, accessed 24th January, 2010]. URL:http://www.choosechinese.com/resource/html/18/1840.html
5. Koestler A, ibid reference 2, p. 59.
6. Burt C. "Psychology and Parapsychology". In: JR Smythies (editor)*Science and ESP*, London, UK, 1967, p 80.
7. Film clips of former US President George Bush, former British Prime Minister Tony Blair, and former Australian Prime Minister John Howard reveal their darting eyes in press conferences during and after the invasion of Iraq in 2003.

CHAPTER 10—Vital Force, 3: Signs of Intelligence

Quote of Sir Fred Hoyle: from 'Hoyle on evolution', *Nature*, volume 294, 12 November, 1981.

1. Van Hoven W. "Tannins and digestibility in Greater Kudu." *Canadian Journal of Animal Science*, 1984; 64 (Supplement): 177–178.
2. Backster C. "Evidence of a primary perception in plant life." *International Journal of Parapsychology*, 1968; 10 (4): 329–348.
3. Tomkins P, and Bird C. *The Secret Life of Plants*, Harper & Row Publishers Inc., New York, NY, USA, 1973.
4. Baxter C. *Primary Perception: Biocommunication with Plants, Living Foods and Human Cells*, White Rose Millennium Press, Anza, California, USA, 2003.
5. Commoner B. "Unraveling the DNA myth: the spurious foundation of genetic engineering." *Harper's Magazine*, Feb, 2001.
6. Commoner B, ibid reference 5, p. 43.
7. Ho M-W. Interview on Australia's ABC Radio National programme *Late Night Live* with presenter Philip Adams, 13 October, 2004.
8. Van Cappellen P, and Ingall IE. "Redox stability of the atmosphere and oceans by phosphorus-limited marine productivity." *Science*, 1996; 271 (5248): 493–496.

9. Society for Advancement of Education. "Sea plants regulate oxygen level: University of Texas at Austin researchers discover the role of phytoplankton in controlling atmospheric oxygen levels", *USA Today*, Vol 124, June 1, 1996.
10. *Star Wars, Episode IV: A New Hope*. Written and directed by George Lucas, produced by Gary Kurtz, George Lucas, and Rick McCallum, distributed by 20th Century Fox, 1977.
11. Commentary: Campbell J, and Moyers B. *The Power of Myth*, BS Flowers (editor). Doubleday, New York, NY, USA, 1988, pp. 144–145.
12. Baker R. *Sperm Wars: Infidelity, Sexual Conflict and Other Bedroom Battles*, Fourth Estate, London, UK, 1996.
13. Shrodinger E. *What is Life?* Cambridge University Press, Cambridge, UK, 1946, p. 77.
14. Koestler A. *The Ghost in the Machine*, Pan Books Ltd, Picador edition, London, UK, 1975, p. 127.
15. Waddington CH. *The Listener*, London, UK, 13th November, 1952. Quoted by Kostler A, ibid reference 14, p127.
16. Urey HC. "On the early chemical history of the Earth and the origin of life." *Proceedings of the National Academy of Sciences of the United States of America*, 1952; 38 (4): 351–363.
17. Miller SL. "A production of amino acids under possible primitive Earth conditions." *Science*, 1953; 117 (3046): 528–529.
18. Miller SL, and Urey HC. "Organic compound synthesis in the primitive Earth." *Science*, 1959; 130 (3370): 245–251.
19. Davison DB, and Burke JF. "Brute force estimation of the number of human genes using EST clustering as a measure." *IBM Journal of Research and Development*, 2001; 45 (3/4): 439.
20. Harrison PM, Kumar A, Lang N, Snyder M, and Gerstein M. "A question of size: the eukaryotic proteome and the problems in defining it." *Nucleic Acids Research*, 2002; 30 (5): 1083–1090.
21. Pray L. "Eukaryotic genome complexity." *Nature Education*, 2008; 1 (1).
22. Begley S. "Solving the next genome puzzle: identifying all our DNA was the easy part; now, bring on the proteome." *Newsweek*, February 19, 2001.
23. Neuweiler H, Doose S, and Sauer M. "A microscopic view of miniprotein folding: enhanced folding efficiency through formation of an intermediate." *Proceedings of the National Academy of Sciences of the United States of America*, 2006; 102 (46): 16650–16655.
24. Sela BA. "Titin: some aspects of the largest protein in the body." [In Hebrew]. *Harefuah*, 2002; 141 (7): 631–635, 665.
25. Coppedge JF Jr. *Evolution: Possible or Impossible?* Zondervan, Grand Rapids, Michigan, USA, 1973.
26. Davies P. *God and the New Physics*, Penguin, London, UK,1990, pp. 164–176.
27. Hutchings JA. "Evolutionary biology: the cod that got away." *Nature*, 2004; 428 (6986): 899–900.
28. Simpson S. "Survival of the smallest: returning the big ones to keep fisheries healthy." *Scientific American*, 2006; 294 (4): 17.
29. Cookson C. "Over-fishing produces a Darwinian revenge as only smaller cod survive." *Financial Times* (London), 28th August, 2007.
30. Penrose R. "Singularities and Time-Asymmetry." In: *General Relativity: An Einstein Centenary Survey*, SW Hawking and W Israel (editors), Cambridge University Press, Cambridge, UK, 1979. Cited in Davies P, ibid reference 26, p. 179.
31. Hoyle F. "Hoyle on evolution." *Nature*, 1981; 294 (5837): 105.
32. Bohm D. *Wholeness and the Implicate Order*, Ark Paperbacks, an imprint of Routledge &

Kegan Paul Ltd, London, UK, 1983.
33. Medawar P. "Remarks by the chairman, Mathematical Challenges to the Neo-Darwinian Interpretation of Evolution." *Wistar Institute Monograph No. 5*, P Moorhead and M Kaplan (editors), 1966.
34. Denton M. *Evolution: A Theory in Crisis*, Adler and Adler Publishers, Bethesda, Maryland, USA, 1985, pp. 327–328.
35. Bateson G. *Mind and Nature: A Necessary Unity*, Bantam Books, New York, NY, USA, 1985.
36. Sheldrake R. *A New Science of Life: The Hypothesis of Formative Causation*, J.P. Tarcher, Inc. Los Angeles, California, USA, 1981.
37. Bateson G, ibid reference 35, p. 230
38. Kauffman SA. *At Home in the Universe: The Search for Laws of Complexity*, Viking Press, New York, NY, USA, 1995.
39. Greene B. *The Elegant Universe: Superstrings, Hidden Dimensions, and Quest for the Ultimate Theory*, Jonathan Cape, London, UK, 1999, pp. 386–7.
40. Campbell J. *The Masks of God: Occidental Mythology*, Arkana, New York, NY, USA, 1991 (first published in 1964), p. 108
41. Aristotle. *Physics*, Book 2, Part 3, circa 350 BCE. Translated by RP Hardie and RK Grace, The Internet Classics Archive, Webatomics, DC Stevenson, classics@mit.edu. [Online, accessed 18th July, 2009]. URL:http://classics.mit.edu/index.html
42. Rosen R. "Some epistemological issues in physics and biology." In: BJ Hiley, and FD Peat (editors), *Quantum Implications: Essays In Honour of David Bohm*, Routledge and Kegan Paul, London, UK, 1987. Cited in Davies P. *The Cosmic Blueprint: New Discoveries in Nature's Creative Ability to Order the Universe*, Templeton Press, West Conshohocken, Pennsylvania, USA, 2004, p. 22, and p. 159.

CHAPTER 11—Health and Disease Revisited

Quote of Dr Arnold Mindell: from a lecture on the 'Dreambody', presented at the Process Work Institute, Portland, Oregon, USA, September 2001.
1. Sobel D (editor). "Introduction." In: *Ways of Health: Holistic Approaches to Ancient and Contemporary Medicine*, Harcourt Brace Jovanovich, New York, NY, USA, 1979, pp. 15–16.
2. Wetzer H. *The Typology of Adjectival Predication*, Mouton de Gruyter, a Division of Walter de Gruyter and Co, Berlin, Germany, 1996.
3. "Chinese proverbs." ChooseChinese, Beijing Stanford Chinese Culture Co., Beijing, China. [Online, accessed 24th January, 2010]. URL:http://www.choosechinese.com/resource/html/18/1840.html
4. Scheibner V. *Vaccination: 100 Years of Orthodox Research Shows That Vaccines Represent a Medical Assault on the Immune System*, Viera Scheibner, Blackheath, New South Wales, Australia, 1993; pp. 81–95.
5. Koch HK, and Dennison NJ. "Ambulatory medical care rendered in physicians' offices: United States, 1975." *Advance Data from Vital and Health Statistics*, No. 12, October 12, 1977, US Department of Health, Education, and Welfare, Washington, DC, USA.
6. Ezzati K. "Ambulatory medical care rendered in pediatricians' offices during 1975." *Advance Data from Vital and Health Statistics*, October 13, 1977, US Department of Health, Education, and Welfare, Washington, DC, USA.
7. Cherry DK, Woodwell DA, and Rechtsteiner EA. "National ambulatory medical care survey: 2005 summary." *Advance Data from Vital and Health Statistics*, No. 387, June 29,

2007, US Department of Health and Human Services, Centers for Disease Control and Prevention, and National Center for Health Statistics, Hyattsville, Maryland, USA.
8. Britt H, Miller GC, Charles J, Henderson J, Bayram C, Valenti L, Pan Y, Harrison C, Fahridin S, and O'Halloran J. "General practice activity in Australia, 1999–2000: changes over time data reference tables." *General Practice Series*, No. 26, Cat. no. GEP 26, Australian Institute of Health and Welfare, Canberra, ACT, Australia, 2009.

PART THREE—THE HUMAN CONTINUUM AND BEYOND

CHAPTER 12—The Human Continuum

Quote of Ronald David Laing: from *Did You Used to be RD Laing?* Video, Third Mind Productions, Vancouver, Canada, 1988.
1. Sagan C. *Cosmos*, MacDonald Futura Publishers, London, UK, 1981.
2. Liedloff J. *The Continuum Concept*, Futura Publications Ltd, London, UK, 1976.
3. Watson JB. *Psychological Care of Infant and Child*, WW Norton Company Inc, New York, NY, USA, 1928.
4. Aristotle. *De Anima (On the Soul)*, Book III, circa 350 BCE. Translated by JA Smith, The Internet Classics Archive, Webatomics, DC Stevenson, classics@mit.edu. [Online, accessed 7th February, 2010].
URL: http://classics.mit.edu/Aristotle/soul.3.iii.html
5. Rizvi SH. "Avicenna (Ibn Sina)." *Internet Encyclopedia of Philosophy*, J Fieser, and B Dowden (editors), 2006. [Online, accessed 7th February, 2010].
URL:http://www.iep.utm.edu/avicenna/#H2
6. Ibn Tufayl (Abu Bakr Muhammad). *Hayy Ibn Yaqzan* (The Living Son of the Vigilant), before 1185 AD. In: *Ibn Tufayl's Hayy Ibn Yaqzan, a Philosophical Tale*, L Gauthier (editor), Catholic Press, Beirut, Lebanon, 1936; re-published in L Goodman (translator), Twain Publishers, New York, NY, USA, 1972.
7. Bacon F. *Novum Organum: Or True Directions Concerning the Interpretation of Nature*, 1620. B Montague (editor and translator), *The Works*, 3 volumes, Parry and MacMillan, Philadelphia, Pennsylvania, USA, 1854. Online: Hanover Historical Texts Project, 2001. [Online, accessed 20th July, 2009].
URL:http://history.hanover.edu/texts/Bacon/novorg.html
8. Locke J. *An Essay Concerning Human Understanding*, R Woodhouse (editor), Penguin Books, New York, NY, USA, 1997, p. 307.
9. Plato. *Phaedo*, circa 385 BCE. In: *Plato in Twelve Volumes*, volume 1, HN Fowler (translator), Harvard University Press, Cambridge, Massachusetts, USA, 1966.
10. Plato. *Apology*, circa 390 BCE. Translated by B Jowett, The Internet Classics Archive, Webatomics, DC Stevenson, classics@mit.edu.
[Online, accessed 8th February, 2010]. URL:http://classics.mit.edu/Plato/apology.html
11. Plato. *The Republic*, Book 6, circa 360 BCE. Translated by B Jowett, The Internet Classics Archive, Webatomics, DC Stevenson, classics@mit.edu.
[Online, accessed 18th July, 2009]. URL:http://classics.mit.edu/index.html
12. Kirk GS. "Popper on science and the Presocratics." *Mind*, 1960; 69 (275): 318–339.
13. Scherer KR. *Plato's legacy: relationships between cognition, emotion, and motivation*. Summary of introductory parts of keynote addresses of the Societe Psychologique de Quebec, 1993, and the Assoziatione Italiana de la Psicologia delle Emozioni, Milano, Italy, 1994.

[Online, accessed 8th February, 2010].
URL:http://www.unige.ch/fapse/emotion/publications/pdf/plato.pdf

14. Descartes R. "Treatise on the Passions of the Soul", 1649. In: *The Philosophical Works of Descartes*, ES Halden, and GRT Ross (translators), Cambridge University Press, Cambridge, UK, 1967.
15. Descartes R. *The Discourse on Method of Rightly Conducting the Reason, and Seeking for Truth in Sciences*, 1637. In: ES Haldane and GRT Ross (translators), *The Philosophical Works of Descartes*, Volume 1, Cambridge University Press, Cambridge, UK, 1981.
16. Fantz RL. "The origin of form perception." *Scientific American*, 1961; 204: 66–72.
17. Fantz RL. "Pattern vision in newborn infants." *Science*, 1963; 14 (3564): 296–297.
18. Gardner HE. *Frames of Mind: The Theory of Multiple Intelligences*, Basic Books, New York, NY, USA, 1993.
19. Mithen S. *The Prehistory of the Mind: A Search for the Origins of Art, Religion and Science*, Thames and Hudson, London, UK, 1996.
20. Mithen S, ibid reference 19, p. 10.
21. Chomsky N. *Rules and Representations*, Basil Blackwell, Oxford, UK, 1980.
22. Mithen S, ibid reference 19, p. 54.
23. Tolman EC. "Cognitive maps in rats and men." *The Psychological Review*, 1948; 55 (4): 189–208.
24. Jung CG. "Archetypes and the Collective Unconscious", translated by RFC Hull. In: *Collected Works of CG Jung*, volume 9, part 1, Pantheon, New York, NY, USA, 1959, p. 43.
25. Goldsmith E. "Towards a unified science: trial and error?" *Ecologist*, 1972; 2 (7): 32.
26. Richter CP. "Biology of drives." *Journal of Comparative and Physiological Psychology*, 1947; 40 (3): 129–134.
27. Warren-Davis A. "The ancient roots of herbal medicine." Lecture given for the Herb Society at the Royal Horticultural Society Lecture Hall, London, UK, on 6th March, 1980. *New Herbal Practitioner*, December, 1980; 7 (1): 35–42.
28. Foucault M. *The Order of Things: An Archaeology of the Human Sciences*, Pantheon Books, New York, NY, USA, 1970.
29. Boehme J. *The Signature of All Things*, James Clarke and Co Ltd, Cambridge, UK, 1969.
30. Pearce JMS. "The doctrine of signatures." *European Neurology*, 2008; 60: 51–52.
31. Clauss M. "The potential interplay of posture, digestive anatomy, density of ingesta and gravity in mammalian herbivores: why sloths do not rest upside down." *Mammalian Review*, 2004; 34 (3): 241–245.
32. Diamond J. *Guns, Germs and Steel: A Short History of Everybody for the Last 13,000 years*, Vintage, London, UK, 1998.
33. Huffman MA, Gotoh S, Izutsu D, Koishimizu K, and Kalunde MS. "Further observations on the use of the medicinal plant *Vernonia amygdalina (Del)* by a wild chimpanzee, its possible effect on parasite load, and its phytochemistry." *African Study Monographs*, 1993; 14 (4): 227–240.
34. Stuart-Macadam P. *Sex and Gender in Paleopathological Perspectives*, AL Grauer, and PL Stuart-Macadam (editors), Cambridge University Press, Cambridge, UK, 1998.
35. MacLennan WJ. "History of arthritis and bone rarefaction evidence from paleopathology onwards", *Scottish Medical Journal*, 1999 Feb; 44 (1): 18–20.
36. Larsen CS. "Biological changes in human populations with agriculture." *Annual Review of Anthropology*, 1995; 24, pp. 185–213.
37. Larsen CS. *Post-Pleistocene Human Evolution: Bioarcheology of the Agricultural Transition*,

Paper presented to the 14th International Congress of Anthropological and Ethnological Sciences, Williamsburg, Virginia, USA, July 26–August 1, 1998.

38. Leroi-Gourhan A. "The flowers found with Shanidar IV, a Neanderthal burial in Iraq." *Science*, 1975; 190 (4214): 562–564.
39. Solecki RS. "Shanidar IV, a Neanderthal flower burial in northern Iraq." *Science*, 1975; 190 (4217): 880–881.
40. Riley CR. *Rising Life Expectancy: A Global History*, Cambridge University Press, Cambridge, UK, 2001: pp. 2 and 21.
41. Hawkes K. "Grandmothers and the evolution of human longevity." *American Journal of Human Biology*, 2003; 15 (3): 380–400.
42. Gurven M, and Kaplan H. "Longevity among hunter-gatherers: a cross cultural examination." *Population and Development Review*, 2007; 33 (2): 321–365.
43. Petrie CC. *Tom Petrie's Reminiscences of Early Queensland (Dating from 1937)*, first published by Watson & Ferguson, Brisbane, Queensland, 1904. Re-published by University of Queensland Press Paperbacks, St Lucia, Queensland, Australia, 1992.
44. McCloy P. "Becoming an elder." *Manzine*, Issue 1, 23 June, 2001.
[Online, accessed 14th January, 2010].
URL:http://www.manhood.com.au/manhood.nsf/8178b1c14b1e9b6b8525624f0062fe9f/0551d6316ec5001f4a256a740043263a!OpenDocument
45. Ship SJ, and Tarbell R. *Our Nations' Elders Speak: Ageing and Cultural Diversity, A Cross-Cultural Approach*, published by the National Indian and Inuit Community Health Representatives Organization (NIICHRO), Kahnawake, Quebec, Canada, 1997.
[Online accessed 14th January, 2010].
URL:http://www.niichro.com/Elders/Elders7.html
46. White JP, and Mulvaney DJ. "Creation and discovery." In: DJ Mulvaney and JP White (editors), *Australians to 1788*, Fairfax, Syme and Weldon, Sydney, NSW, Australia, 1987, p. 117.
47. M Walsh and C Yallop (editors). *Language and Culture in Aboriginal Australia*, Aboriginal Studies Press, Canberra, ACT, Australia, 1993.
48. Elkin AP. *Aboriginal Men of High Degree*, 1st edition: 1945; 2nd edition: University of Queensland Press, St Lucia, Queensland, Australia, 1977.
49. Reid J, and Trompf P(editors). *The Health of Aboriginal Australia*, Harcourt Brace Jovanovich Publishers, Sydney, NSW, Australia, 1991, pp. 1–3.
50. Cowlishaw G. "Infanticide in Aboriginal Australia." *Oceania*, 1978; 48 (4): 262–283.
51. Abbie AA. *The Original Australians*, AH and AW Reed, Sydney, NSW, Australia, 1970.
52. O'Dea K, Jewell PA, Whiten A, Altmann SA, Strickland SS, and Oftedal OT. "Traditional diet and food preferences of Australian Aboriginal Hunter-Gatherers." *Philosophical Transactions of the Royal Society of London: Biological Sciences*, 1991; 334 (1270): 233–241.
53. O'Dea K. "Marked improvement in carbohydrate and lipid metabolism in diabetic Australian Aborigines after temporary reversion to traditional lifestyle." *Diabetes*, 1984; 33 (6): 593–603.
54. O'Dea K. "Online opinion." *Nuclear Territory News*, 25 March, 2008.
[Online, accessed 10th February, 2010]. URL:http://ntne.ws/articles/article.php?id=2937
55. Personal correspondence with Professor Kerin O'Dea, 14 February, 2010.

CHAPTER 13—Beyond the Continuum

Quote of John Steinbeck: from *Travels with Charley*, 1962.

1. Leakey RE. *The Making of Mankind*, Michael Joseph Ltd, London, UK, 1981, pp. 184–217.
2. Solis RS, Haas J, and Creamer W. "Dating Caral, a preceramic site in the Supe Valley on the central coast of Peru." *Science*, 2001; 292 (5517): 723–726.
3. Haas J, Creamer W, and Ruiz A. "Dating the Late Archaic occupation of the Norte Chico region in Peru." *Nature*, (Letters), 2004; 432: 1020–1023.
4. Adams REW. *Prehistoric Mesoamerica*, University of Oklahoma Press, Norman, Oklahoma, USA, 1991.
5. Wheeler M. *The Indus Civilization*, Cambridge University Press, Cambridge, UK, 1953.
6. Chang K-C, and Xu P, S Allan (editor), The *Formation of Chinese Civilization: An Archaeological Perspective*, Yale University Press, Newhaven, Connecticut, USA, 2005.
7. Leakey RE, ibid reference 1, p. 200.
8. Cordain L, Miller JB, Eaton SB, Mann N, Holt SHA, and Speth JD. "Plant-animal subsistence ratios and macronutrient energy estimations in worldwide hunter-gatherer diets." *American Journal of Clinical Nutrition*, 2000; 71 (3): 682–692.
9. Itan Y, Powell A, Beaumont M, Burger J, and Thomas M. "Origins of lactase persistence in Europe." *Public Library of Science (PLoS): Computational Biology*, 5 (8): e1000491. doi: 10.1371/journal.pcbi.1000491
10. Swallow DM. "Genetics of lactase persistence and lactose intolerance." *Annual Review of Genetics*, 2003; 37: 197–219.
11. Mulcare CA, Weale ME, Jones AL, Connell B, Zeitlyn D, Tarekegn A, Swallow DM, Bradman N, and Thomas MG. "The T allele of a single-nucleotide polymorphism 13.9 kb upstream of the lactase gene (LCT) (C-13.9kbT) does not predict or cause the lactase-persistence phenotype in Africans." *American Journal of Human Genetics*, 2004; 74 (6): 1102–1110.
12. Ingram CJ, Elamin MF, Mulcare CA, Weale ME, Tarekegn A, Raga TO, Bekele E, Elamin FM, Thomas MG, Bradman N, and Swallow DM. "A novel polymorphism associated with lactose tolerance in Africa: multiple causes for lactase persistence?" *Human Genetics*, 2007; 120 (6): 779–788.
13. Tishkoff SA, Reed FA, Ranciaro A, Voight BF, Babbitt CC, Silverman JHS, Powell K, Mortensen HM, Hirbo JB, Osman M, Ibrahim M, Omar SA, Lema G, Nyambo TB, Ghori J, Bumpstead S, Pritchard JK, Wray GA, and Deloukas P. "Convergent adaptation of human lactase persistence in Africans and Europeans." *Nature Genetics*, 2007; 39 (1): 31–40.
14. Wadley G, and Martin A. "The origins of agriculture: a biological perspective and a new hypothesis." *Australian Biologist*, 1993; 6: 96–105.
15. Kano, T. Muavwa, M. "Feeding ecology of the pygmy chimpanzees (*Pan paniscus*) at Wamba." In: *The Pigmy Chimpanzee: Evolutionary Biology and Behavior*, R.L. Susman (editor), Plenum Press, New York, NY, USA, 1984, pp. 233–274.
16. Badrian N, and Malenky R. "Feeding ecology of *Pan paniscus* in the Lomko Forest, Zaire." In: *The Pigmy Chimpanzee: Evolutionary Biology and Behavior*, RL Susman (editor). Plenum Press, New York, NY, USA, 1984, pp. 275–299.
17. Goodall J. *The Chimpanzees of Gombe: Patterns of Behavior*, Bellknap Press of the Harvard University Press, Cambridge, Massachusetts, USA, 1986, p. 232.
18. Food and Agriculture Organization (FAO) of the United Nations (UN). *The State of the World's Plant Genetic Resources for Food and Agriculture*, Rome, Italy, 1997, p. 14.
19. Lucretius (Titus Lucretius Carus). *De Rerum Natura (Of the Nature of Things)*, 50 BCE. Book

One: "Substance is eternal"; Book Two: "Atomic Forms and Their Combinations"; Book Five: "The World is Not Eternal", "Origins of Vegetable and Animal Life", and "Beginnings of Civilization"; translated by WE Leonard, produced by L Kurnaz and D Widger, Project Gutenberg eBook, 2008.
[Online, accessed 10th February, 2010]. URL:http://www.gutenberg.org/files/785/785-h/785-h.htm

20. Lucien of Samosata, *Cronosolon*, 2nd century AD. In: *The Works of Lucien of Samosata*, translated by HW Fowler and FG Fowler, The Clarendon Press, Oxford, UK, 1905, volume IV; scanned, proofed and formatted by JB Hare at sacred-texts.com.
[Online, accessed 10th February, 2010].
URL:http://www.sacred-texts.com/cla/luc/fowl/index.htm

21. Bachofen JJ. *Das Mutterrecht. Eine Untersuchung uber die gynaikokratie der alten Welt nach ihrer religiosen und rechtlichen Natur (The Mother Right. An Examination of Female Rule in the Old World from their Religious and Legal Nature)*. Volume 1. Krais and Hoffman, Stuttgart, Germany, 1861; reprinted by B Schwabe, Basel, Germany, 1948.

22. Bachofen JJ. *Myth, Religion, and Mother Right: Selected Writings of JJ Bachofen*, translated by R Manheim, Princeton University Press, Princeton, New Jersey, USA, 1973.

23. Campbell J. *The Masks of God: Primitive Mythology*, volume I, first published 1959; Arkana (Penguin), New York, NY, USA, 1991.

24. Campbell J. *The Masks of God: Oriental Mythology*, volume II, first published 1962; Arkana (Penguin), New York, NY, USA, 1991.

25. Campbell J. *The Masks of God: Occidental Mythology*, volume III, first published 1964; Arkana (Penguin), New York, NY, USA, 1991.

26. Campbell J. *The Masks of God: Creative Mythology*, volume IV, first published 1968; Arkana (Penguin), New York, NY, USA, 1991.

27. Campbell J. *Historical Atlas of World Mythology*, Volume I: *The Way of the Animal Powers*, Part 1: *Mythologies of the Primitive Hunters and Gatherers*; Part 2: *Mythologies of the Great Hunt* , first published byAlfred van der Marck Editions, New York, NY, USA, 1983; reprinted by Harper and Row, New York, NY, USA, 1988.

28. Campbell J. *Historical Atlas of World Mythology*, Volume II: *The Way of the Seeded Earth*, Part 1: *The Sacrifice*; Part II: *Mythology of the Primitive Planters: The North Americas*; *Mythologies of the Primitive Planters: The Middle and Southern Americas*, edited by R Walter, Harper and Row, New York, NY, USA, 1989.

29. Stone M. *When God Was a Woman*, Barnes and Noble, New York, NY, USA, 1976.

30. Gimbutas M. *The Language of the Goddess: Unearthing the Hidden Symbols of Western Civilization*, Thames and Hudson, London, UK, 2001.

31. Guiley RE. *Harpers Encyclopedia of Mystical and Paranormal Experiences*, HarperCollins Publishers, New York, NY, USA, 1991, p. 239.

32. Gray HF. "Sewerage in ancient and medieval times." Presented at the Spring Meeting of the California Sewage Works Association, Avalon, Catalina Island, California, USA, May 20, 1940; *Sewage Works Journal*, 1940; 12 (5): 939–946.

33. Schladweiler J. *Tracking Down the Roots of Our Sanitary Sewers*, Arizona Water Association, Prescott, Arizona, USA, 2004.
[Online, accessed 10th February, 2010].
URL: http://www.sewerhistory.org/chronos/roots.htm

34. Creamer W, Ruiz A, and Hass J. "Archaeological investigation of Late Archaic sites (3000–1800 B.C) in the Pativilca Valley, Peru." *Fieldiana Anthropology*, 2007; 40: 1–78.

35. Shaikh KH, and Ashfaque SM. *Moenjodaro: a 5000-year-old-legacy*, United Nations

Educational, Scientific and Cultural Organization (UNESCO), Paris, France, 1981.

36. Dyer J. *Ancient Britain*, BT Batsford Ltd, London, UK, 1995, p. 80.
37. Ellerbe H. *The Dark Side of Christian History*, Morningstar and Lark, Orlando, Florida, USA, 1995, pp. 41–45.
38. Gray HF, ibid reference 32, p. 943.
39. Paige JC, and Harrison LS. *Out of the Vapors: A Social and Architectural History of Bathhouse Row*, Hot Springs National Park, Arkansas, USA, US Department of the Interior/National Park Service, 1988, p. 5.
40. Daileader P. *The Late Middle Ages*, (DVD) The Teaching Company, LLC, Chantilly, Virginia, USA, 2007.
41. De Costa C. "St Anthony's fire and living ligatures: a short history of ergometrine." *The Lancet*, 2002; 359 (9319): 1768–1770.
42. Lamason RL, Mohideen M-APK, Mest JR, Wong AC, Norton HL, Aros MC, Jurynec MJ, Moa X, Humphreville VR, Humbert JE, Sinha S, Moore JL, Jagadeeswaren P, Zhao W, Ning G, Makalowska I, McKeigue PM, O'Donnell D, Kittles R, Parra EJ, Mangini NJ, Grunwald DJ, Shriver MD, Canfield VA, and Cheng KC. "SLC24A5, a putative cation exchanger, affects pigmentation in zebrafish and humans." *Science*, 2005; 310 (5755): 1782–1786.
43. Schaffner SF, and Sabeti PC. "Evolutionary adaptation in the human lineage." *Nature Education*, 2008; 1 (1).
44. Mogelonsky M. "Milk doesn't always do a body good." *American Demographics*, January 1995. Cited in: The National Medical Association, ibid reference 45.
45. The National Medical Association (US). "Consensus Report of the National Medical Association (US): The Role of Dairy and Dairy Nutrients in the Diet of African Americans." WJ Wooten and W Price (editors), *Journal of the National Medical Association*, 2004; 96 (12, Supplement): 1–33.
46. Scheibner V. *Vaccination: 100 Years of Orthodox Research Shows That Vaccines Represent a Medical Assault on the Immune System*, Viera Scheibner, Blackheath, New South Wales, Australia, 1993; pp. 81–95.
47. Livi-Bacci M. *A Concise History of World Population*, 4th Edition, Blackwell Publishing Ltd, Oxford, UK, 2007. pp. 44–48.
48. Suzuki D, and Levine R. *Cracking the Code*, Allen & Unwin, Sydney, NSW, Australia, 1994.
49. Tsaras G, Owusu-Ansah A, Boateng FO, and Amoateng-Adjepong Y. "Complications associated with sickle cell trait: a brief narrative review." *American Journal of Medicine*, 2009; 122 (6): 507–512.
50. Kwiatkowski DP. "How malaria has affected the human genome and what human genetics can teach us about malaria." *American Journal of Human Genetics*, 2005; 77: 171–192.
51. Hill AVS, Allsopp CEM, Kwiatkowski D, Anstey NM, Twumasi P, Rowe PA, Bennett S, Brewster D, McMichael AJ, and Greenwood BM. "Common West African HLA antigens are associated with protection from severe malaria." *Nature*, 1991; 352: 595–600.
52. World Health Organization. Fact Sheet No. 4: *Malaria*. Updated in 2009. [Online, accessed 12th February, 2010]. URL: http://www.who.int/mediacentre/factsheets/fs094/en/
53. Stuart-Macadam P. *Sex and Gender in Paleopathological Perspectives*, AL Grauer, and PL Stuart-Macadam (editors), Cambridge University Press, Cambridge, UK, 1998.
54. MacLennan WJ. "History of arthritis and bone rarefaction evidence from paleopathology onwards", *Scottish Medical Journal*, 1999 Feb; 44 (1): 18–20.

55. Larsen CS. "Biological changes in human populations with agriculture." *Annual Review of Anthropology*, 1995; 24: 185–213.
56. Larsen CS. *Post-Pleistocene Human Evolution: Bioarcheology of the Agricultural Transition*, paper presented to the 14th International Congress of Anthropological and Ethnological Sciences, Williamsburg, Virginia, USA, July 26–August 1, 1998. In: PS Ungar, and MF Teaford (editors), *Human Diet: Its Origin and Evolution*, Bergin and Garvey, Westport, Connecticut, USA, 2002, pp. 19–35.
57. Gore A (presenter). *An Inconvenient Truth*, Director: Davis Guggenheim; Producer: Laurie David; Studios: Paramount Classics and United International Pictures. Released: 24 May, 2006.
58. Abramov O, an Mojzsis S. "Microbial habitability of the Haldean Earth during the late heavy bombardment." *Nature*, 2009; 459 (7245): 419–422.
59. Korsten L, Sivakumar D, Rolle R, Vermulen H, and Njie D. *Horticultural Chain Management for Eastern and Southern Africa: A Theoretical Manual*, published by Commonwealth Secretariat, London, UK, in conjunction with the Food and Agriculture Organization of the United Nations, Rome, Italy, 2008, p. 85.
60. Carson R. *Silent Spring*. Penguin Books Ltd, Ringwood, Victoria, Australia, 1962.
61. Collison DR, and Hall T. *Why Do I Feel So Awful?* Angus and Robertson Publishers, North Ryde, NSW, Australia, 1989, p. 252.
62. Crumpler D. *Chemical Crisis: One Woman's Story. Humanity's Future?* Scribe Publications, Newham, Australia, 1994, pp. 113–114.
63. Suzuki D. *Inventing the Future*. Allen and Unwin, Sydney, Australia, 1990, p. 135. Cited in Crumpler D, ibid reference 62, p. 194.
64. Rosenstock L, Keifer M, Daniell W, McConnell R, Claypoole K, and the Pesticide Health Effects Study Group (University of Washington). "Chronic central nervous system effects of acute organophosphate pesticide poisoning." *The Lancet*, 1991; 338 (7245): 223–227.
65. Collison DR and Hall T, ibid reference 61, p. 338.
66. New Zealand Food Safety Authority. *2003/2004 New Zealand Total Diet Survey: Analytic Results–Third Quarter*, Dr RW Vannoort, project leader. Institute of Environmental Science and Research Ltd, for New Zealand Food Safety Authority, Wellington, New Zealand, 8 July, 2004.
67. Kedgley S (MP for the Green Party of Aeotearoa/New Zealand). *Food for Thought*, 31 August, 2004. [Online, accessed 24th July, 2009]. URL:http://www.greens.org,nz/node/17713
68. World Health Organization. *Safe Use of Pesticides: Twentieth Report of the WHO Expert Committee on Insecticides*, Technical Report Series, No. 513, Geneva, Switzerland, 1973.
69. Jeyaratnam J. "Acute pesticide poisoning: a major global health problem." *World Health Statistics Quarterly*, 1990; 43 (3): 139–44. Cited in *30 Years after Silent Spring: The Poisoning Continues*, Greenpeace, Sydney, NSW, Australia, 1992.
70. Reeves M, Schwind K, and Silberblatt R. "The invisible epidemic: global acute pesticide poisoning." *The Magazine of Pesticide Action Network North America*, Spring, 2006. [Online, accessed 24th July, 2009]. URL:http://magazine.panna.org/spring2006/inDepthGlobalPoisoning.html
71. Pan American Health Organization. "Epidemiological situation of acute pesticide poisoning in Central America, 1992–2000." *Epidemiological Bulletin*, 2002; 23 (3): 5–9.
72. Schettler T, Solomon G, Kaplan J, Valenti M, Burns P, and Huddle A. *Generations at Risk: How Environmental Toxicants May Affect Reproductive Health in California*, A report by Physicians for Social Responsibility (Greater San Fransisco and Los Angeles Chapters)

and the California Public Interest Research Group Charitable Trust, San Francisco, California, USA, November, 1998.

73. Mohammad O, Walid AA, and Ghada K. "Chromosomal aberrations in human lymphocytes from two groups of workers occupationally exposed to pesticides in Syria." *Environmental Research*, 1995; 70 (1): 24–29. Cited in Schettler T, et al., ibid reference 72, p. 69.

74. Eil C, and Nisula, B.C. "The binding properties of pyrethroids to human skin fibroblast androgen receptors and to sex hormone binding globulin." *Journal of Steroid Biochemistry*, 1990; 35 (3–4): 409–414. Cited in Schettler T, et al., ibid reference 72, p. 75.

75. Colborn T, vom Saal FS, and Soto AM. "Developmental effects of endocrine-disrupting chemicals in wildlife and humans." *Environmental Health Perspectives*, 1993; 101 (5): 378–384.

76. Ahlbom J, Fredriksson A, and Eriksson P. "Neonatal exposure to a type-1 pyrethroid (bioallethrin) induces dose-response changes in brain muscarinic receptors and behavior in neonatal and adult mice." *Brain Research*, 1994; 645 (1–2): 318–324. Cited in Schettler T, et al., ibid reference 72, p. 75.

77. Martin MF. "Estimates of Vietnamese exposure to Agent Orange." In: *Vietnamese Victims of Agent Orange and U.S.-Vietnam Relations*, Congressional Research Service Report for Congress, Washington, DC, USA. May 28, 2009, pp. 12–13.

78. Takacs P, Martin PA, and Struger J. *Pesticides in Ontario: A Critical Assessment of Potential Toxicity of Agricultural Products to Wildlife, With Consideration for Endocrine Disruption*, Volume 2. "Triazine Herbicides, Glyphosate, and Metolachlor", Technical Report Series No. 369, Canadian Wildlife Service, Ontario Region, Burlington, Ontario, Canada, 2002, p. 6.

79. Hardell L, and Eriksson M. "A Case-control study of non-Hodgkin lymphoma and exposure to pesticides." *Cancer*, 1999; 85 (6): 1353–1360.

80. Bolognesi C, Bonatti S, Degan P, Gallerani E, Peluso M, Rabboni R, Roggieri P, and Abbondandolo A. "Genotoxic activity of glyphosate and its technical formulation." *Journal of Agricultural and Food Chemistry*, 1997; 45: 1957–1962. Cited in Takacs P, ibid reference 78, p. 71.

81. Yousef MI, Salem MH, Ibrahim HZ, Helmi S, Seehy MA, and Bertheussen K. "Toxic effects of carbofuran and glyphosate on semen characteristics in rabbits." *Journal of Environmental Science and Health*, Part B (Pesticides, Food Contaminants and Agricultural Wastes), 1995; 30 (4): 513–534. Cited in Takacs P, reference 78, p. 80.

82. Yousef MI, Bertheussen K, Ibrahim HZ, Helmi S, Seehy MA, and Salem MH. "A sensitive sperm-motility test for the assessment of cytotoxic effect of pesticides. *Journal of Environmental Science and Health*, Part B (Pesticides, Food Contaminants and Agricultural Wastes), 1996; 31 (1): 99–115. Cited in Takacs P, ibid reference 78, p. 80.

83. El-Gendy KS, Aly NM, and El-Sebae AH. "Effects of edifenphos and glyphosate on the immune response and protein biosynthesis of bolti fish (Tilapia nilotica)." *Journal of Environmental Science and Health*, Part B (Pesticides, Food Contaminants and Agricultural Wastes), 1998; 33 (2): 135–149. Cited in Takacs P, ibid reference 78, p. 80.

84. Wetzel LT, Luempert III LG, Breckenridge CB, Tisdel MO, Stevens JT, Thakur AK, Extrom PJ, and Eldridge JC. "Chronic effects of atrazine on estrus and mammary tumor formation in female Sprague-Dawley and Fischer 344 rats." *Journal of Toxicology and Environmental Health*, 1994; 43 (2): 169–182.

85. Kettles MA, Browning SR, Prince TS, and Horstman SW. "Triazine herbicide exposure and breast cancer incidence: an ecologic study of Kentucky counties." *Environmental*

Health Perspectives, 1997; 105 (11): 1222–1227.
86. Illinois Environmental Protection Agency. *Report on Endocrine Disrupting Chemicals*. Illinois EPA, Springfield, Illinois, USA, February, 1997.
87. Larson SJ, Capel PD, and Majewski MS. *Pesticides in Surface Waters: Distribution Trends and Governing Factors*, Ann Arbor Press Inc, Chelsea, Michigan, USA, 1997, p. 194. Cited in Illinois EPA report, ibid reference 86.
88. Keith LH. *Environmental Endocrine Disruptors: A Handbook of Property Data*, Wiley Interscience, New York, NY, USA, 1997. Cited in Illinois EPA report, ibid reference 86.
89. Rifkin J, and Howard T. "Entropy in Agriculture." NCAP News, vol 3, no. 2, 1982, pp 2–3 [reprinted from *Entropy: A New Worldview*, Viking Press, New York, NY, USA, 1980]. Cited in Crumpler D, ibid reference 62, p. 189.
90. Benbrook CM, Groth III E, Halloran JM, Hansen MK, and Marquardt S. *Pest Management at the Crossroads*, Consumers Union, Yonkers, NY, USA, 1996.
91. Heap I. *International Survey of Herbicide Resistant Weeds*, Herbicide Resistance Action Committee (HRAC), the North American Herbicide Resistance Action Committee (NAHRAC), and the Weed Science Society of America (WSSA), Corvallis, Oregon, USA. [Online, accessed 25th July, 2009]. URL:http://www.weedscience.org/In.asp
92. Barber M, and Whitehead JEM. "Bacteriophage types in penicillin-resistant staphylococcal infection." *British Medical Journal*, 1949; 2 (4627): 565–569.
93. Akiba TK, Koyama K, Ishiki Y, Kimura S, and Fukushima T. "On the mechanism of the development of multple-drug-resistan clones of Shigella." [In Japanese]. *Japanese Journal of Microbiology*, 1960; 4: 219–227.
94. Barber M. "Methicillin-resistant Staphylococci." *Journal of Clinical Pathology*, 1961; 14 (4): 385–393.
95. Mendez B, Tachibana C, and Levy SB. "Heterogeneity of tetracycline resistance determinants." *Plasmid*, 1980; 3 (2): 99–108.
96. Bentorcha F, De Cespedes G, and Horaud T. "Tetracycline resistance heterogeneity in Enterococcus faecium." *Antimicrobial Agents and Chemotherapy*, 1991; 35 (5): 808–812.
97. Stirland RM, and Shotts N. "Antibiotic resistant Streptococci in the mouths of children treated with penicillin." *The Lancet*, 1967; 289 (7487): 405–408.
98. Ronald AR, Eby J, and Sherris JC. "Susceptibility of Neisseria gonorrhoeae to penicillin and tetracycline." *Antimicrobial Agents and Chemotherapy*, 1968; 8: 431–434.
99. Witte E. "Medical consequences of antibiotics in agriculture." *Science*, 1998; 279 (5353): 996–997.
100. Langlois C, Cromwell GL, Stahly TS, Dawson KA, and Hays VW. "Antibiotic resistance of fecal coliforms after long-term withdrawal of therapeutic and subtherapeutic antibiotic use in a swine herd." *Applied and Environmental Microbiology*, 1983; 46 (6): 1433–1434.
101. Australian Joint Expert Advisory Committee on Antibiotic Resistance (JETACAR). *The Use of Antibiotics in Food-Producing Animals: Antibiotic-Resistant Bacteria in Animals and Human*, Report of JETACAR, Commonwealth Department of Health and Aging, and the Commonwealth Department of Agriculture, Fisheries and Forestry, Canberra, ACT, Australia, September, 1999.
102. Chapin A, Rule A, Gibson K, Buckley T, and Schwab K. "Airborne multidrug-resistant bacteria isolated from a concentrated swine feeding operation." *Environmental Health Perspectives*, 2005; 113 (2): 137–142.
103. Smith TL, Pearson ML, Wilcox KR, Cruz C, Lancaster MV, Robinson-Dunn B, Tenover FC, Zervos MJ, Band JD, White E, and Jarvis WR. "Emergence of vancomycin resistance in Staphylococcus aureus. Glycopeptide-intemediate Staphylococcus aureus Working

Group." *The New England Journal of Medicine*, 1999; 340 (7): 493–501.
104. Horodniceanu T, and Delbos F. "Group D streptococci in human infections: identification and sensitivity to antibiotics." [In French]. *Annales de Microbiologie*, 1980; 131B (2): 131–144.
105. Moran JS, and Zenilman JM. "Therapy for gonococcal infections: options in 1989." *Reviews of Infectious Diseases*, 1990; 12 (Supplement 6): 633–644.
106. Albricht WC, Monnet DL, and Harbarth S. "Antibiotic selection pressure and resistance in Streptococcus pneumoniae and Streptococcus pyogenes." *Emerging Infectious Diseases*, 2004; 10 (3): 514–517.
107. Maree CL, Daum RS, Boyle-Vavra S, Matayoshi K, and Miller LG. "Community-associated methicillin-resistant Staphylococcus aureus isolates causing healthcare-associated infections." *Emerging Infectious Diseases*, 2007; 13 (2): 236–242.
108. Arias CA, and Murray BE. "Antibiotic-resistant bugs in the 21st century: a clinical super-challenge." *The New England Journal of Medicine*, 360 (5): 439–443.
109. Pimentel D, and Grenier A. "Environmental and socio-economic costs of pesticide use." In: *Techniques for Reducing Pesticide Use*, D Pimental (editor), John Wiley and Sons, New York, pp. 51–78. Cited in Mitchell JA, "The attack of the killer fungus." In: *IPM Practitioner*, 2001; 23 (1): 5. Bio-Integral Resonance Center, W Quarles (editor), Berkeley, California, USA.
110. Pimentel D, Krummel J, Gallahan D, Hough J, Merrill A, Schreiner I, Vittum P, Koziol F, Back E, Yen D, and Fiance S. "Benefits and costs of pesticide use in US food production," *BioScience*, 1978; 28 (12): 778–784.
111. Rifkin J, and Howard T, ibid reference 89, pp. 138–139.
112. International Food Policy Research Institute and Rockefeller Foundation. *Facts and Figures: International Agriculture Research*, Rockefeller Foundation, New York, USA, 1990.
113. Shea K. "Protecting our children from environmental hazards in the face of limited data: a precautionary approach is needed." *The Journal of Pediatrics*, 2004; 145 (2): 146–148.
114. Murmann JP. "Chemical industries after 1850." In: J Mokyr (editor), *Oxford Encyclopedia of Economic History*, Oxford University Press, Oxford, UK, 2003, pp. 398–406.
115. Mitchell JD. "Nowhere to hide: the global spread of high-risk synthetic chemicals." *World Watch* (publication of the Worldwatch Institute, Washington, DC, USA) 1997; 10 (2): 26–36.
116. Landrigan PJ, Schechter CB, Lipton JM, Fahs MC, and Schwartz J. "Environmental pollutants and disease in American children: estimates of morbidity, mortality, and costs for lead poisoning, asthma, cancer, and developmental disabilities." *Environmental Health Perspectives*, 2002; 110 (7): 721–728.
117. CAS Chemical Registry System, a Division of the American Chemical Society. [Online, accessed 29th July, 2009]. URL:http://www.cas.org/expertise/cascontent/registry/regsys.html
118. US Centers for Disease Control and Prevention (CDC). *Third National Report on Human Exposure to Environmental Chemicals*, 2005, National Center for Environmental Health, Publication no. 05-0570, Atlanta, Georgia, USA, July 2005.
119. Pesticide Action Network North America (PANNA). *CDC Body Burden Study Finds Widespread Pesticide Exposure*, Pesticide Action Network Updates Services (PANUPS), San Francisco, California, USA, July 22, 2005.
[Online, accessed 29th July, 2009].
URL:http://www.panna.org/legacy/panups/panup_200550722.dv.html
120. CDC Report, ibid reference 118, "Introduction", p. 4.

121. Environmental Working Group (EWG). *BodyBurden: The Pollution inPeople. Executive summary: What We Found*, EWG, Washington DC, USA, January 20, 2003.
[Online, accessed 9th July, 2009].
URL:htttp://archive.ewg.org/reports/bodyburden1/es.php
122. WWF–World Wide Fund for Nature (UK). *Contamination: The Result of WWF's Biomonitoring Survey*, WWF-UK, Godalming, Surrey, UK. November 2003.
[Online, accessed 29th July, 2009].
URL:http://www.wwf.org.uk/filelibrary/pdf/biomonitoringresults.pdf
123. WWF–World Wide Fund for Nature (UK). *Contamination: The Next Generation. Results of the Family Chemical Contamination Survey*, WWF-UK, Godalming, Surrey, UK. October, 2004.
[Online, accessed 29th July, 2009].
URL:http://www.wwf.org.uk/filelibrary/pdf/family_biomonitoring.pdf
124. Harden F, Muller J, and Toms L. "Organochlorine pesticides (OCPs) and polybrominated diphenyl ethers (PBDEs) in the Australian population: Levels in human milk." January 2005, Environment Protection and Heritage Council, Canberra, ACT, Australia.
125. Harden F, Muller J, and Toms L. *Breastmilk Testing in Australia*, National Toxics Network, Bangalow, NSW, Australia, 2005.
[Online, accessed 24th July, 2009]. URL:http://www.oztoxics.org/ntn/breastmilk.html
126. EWG Group. *Body Burden–The Pollution in Newborns: A Benchmark Investigation of Industrial Chemicals, Pollutants and Pesticides in Umbilical Cord Blood*. Environmental Working Group, Washington, DC, USA, July 14, 2005.
127. Onstot J, Ayling J, and Stanley J. "Characterization of HRGC/MS unidentified peaks from the analysis of human adipose tissue." Volume 1: *Technical Approach*, US Environment Protection Agency, Washington, DC, USA, 1987.
128. Schafer KS. *Biomonitoring: A Tool Whose Time Has Come*, Pesticide Action Network North America (PANNA), San Francisco, California, USA, 2008.
[Online, accessed 12th February, 2010].
URL:http://www.panna.org/legacy/gpc/gpc_200404.14.1.02.dv.html
129. Poulos A. *The Silent Threat*, Published by Professor Alfred Poulos, PO Box 627, Magill, South Australia, Australia, 2005.
130. Personal correspondence with Professor Alfred Poulos, October 2005.
131. Moyers B. *Trade Secrets: A Moyer's Report*, Program transcript of Public Broadcasting Service, Sherry Jones (producer), Bill Moyers (presenter), Public Affairs Television, Arlington, Virginia, USA, March 26, 2001.
132. Personal correspondence with Professor Philip Landrigan, November, 2005.
133. Steering Committee on Identification of Toxic and Potentially Toxic Chemicals for Consideration by the National Toxicology Program, National Research Council. *Toxicity Testing: Strategies to Determine Needs and Priorities*, National Academy of Sciences, the National Academies Press, Washington DC, USA, 1984.
134. Environmental Defense Fund, Environmental Health Program. *Toxic Ignorance: The Continuing Absence of Basic Health Testing for Top-selling Chemicals in the United States*. Environmental Defense Fund Inc, New York, NY, USA, 1997.
135. Tattersal A. "Is EPA registration a guarantee of pesticide safety?" *Journal of Pesticide Reform* (publication of the Northwest Coalition for Alternatives to Pesticides, Eugene, Oregon, USA), 1986; 6 (1): 40–42.
136. Collison DR, and Hall T, ibid reference 61, p. 347.
137. Mott , and Snyder K. *Pesticide Alert: A Guide to Pesticides in Fruit and Vegetables*, Sierra

Club, San Francisco, USA, 1987, p. 8. Cited in Crumpler D, ibid reference 62, p. 123.
138. Poulos A, ibid reference 129, p. 13.
139. vom Saal FS, and Soto AM. "Developmental effects of endocrine-disrupting chemicals in wildlife and humans." *Environmental Health Perspectives*, 1993; 101 (5): 378–384.
140. Nagel SC, vom Saal FS, Thayer KA, Dhar MG, Boechler M, and Welshons WV. "Relative binding affinity-serum modified access (RBA-SMA) assay predicts the relative in vivo bioactivity of the xenoestrogens bisphenol A and octylphenol." *Environmental Health Perspectives*, 1997; 105 (1): 70–76.
141. Andersen HR, Andersson A-M, Arnold SF, Autrup H, Barfoed M, Beresford NA, Bjerregaard P, Christiansen LB, Gissel B, Hummel R, Jorgensen EB, Korsgaard B, Le Guevel R, Leffers H, McLachlan J, Moller A, Nielsen JB, Olea N, Oles-Karasko A, Pakdel F, Pedersen KL, Perez P, Skakkeboek NE, Sonnenschein C, Soto AM, Sumpter JP, Thorpe SM, and Grandjean P. "Comparison of short-term estrogenicity tests for identification of hormone-disrupting chemicals." *Environmental Health Perspectives*, 1999; 107 (supplement 1): 89–108.
142. Colborn T, Dumanoski D, and Myers JP. *Our Stolen Future*, Penguin Books, New York, NY, USA, 1997, parts 3 and 4.
143. Lambrecht B. "Chemicals may threaten reproduction, scientists say." *St Louis Post-Dispatch*, April 8, 1996, p. 17B.
144. Personal correspondence from Professor Peter Dingle, October, 2005.
145. Yokel RA, Allen DD, and Meyer JJ. "Studies of aluminum neurobehavioral toxicity in the intact mammal." *Journal of Cellular and Molecular Neurobiology*, 1994; 14 (6): 791–808.
146. Kawahara M. "Effects of aluminum on the nervous system and its possible link with neurodegenerative diseases." *Journal of Alzheimer's Disease*, 2005; 8 (2): 171–182.
147. Altmann P, Cunningham J, Dhaneshall U, Ballard M, Thompson J, and Marsh F. "Disturbance of cerebral function in people exposed to drinking water contaminated with aluminium sulphate: retrospective study of the Camelford water incident." *British Medical Journal*, 1999; 319   (7213): 807–811.
148. Poulos A, ibid reference 129, pp. 87–92.
149. Poulos A, ibid reference 129, pp. 50–52.
150. Taubert P. *Your Health and Food Additives*. 1989. Comsafe Consultancy, Murray Bridge, South Australia, Australia.
151. Statham B. *The Chemical Maze: Your Guide to Food Additives and Cosmetic Ingredients*. 2002. Published by POSSIBILITY.COM, P.O. Box 4125, Candelo, NSW, Australia.
152. Collison DR, and Hall T, ibid reference 61, p. 116.
153. Dingle P. "Chemicals, kids and cancer: why kids are particularly vulnerable to toxic home chemicals." Published in *byronchild/Kindred* Magazine (K. Wendorf [editor], Mullumbimby, NSW, Australia), September, 2006.

CHAPTER 14—Drowning in a Sea of Electropollution

Quote of George Orwell: from *My Few Wise Words of Wisdom*, Charles Walker, 2000.
1. Howe LM. *British Cell Phone Safety Alert and An Interview with Robert O. Becker, M.D.*, Earthfiles, 14 May, 2000.
   [Online, accessed 1st August, 2009]. URL:http:www.earthfiles.com
2. Becker RO, and Selden G. *The Body Electric: Electromagnetism and the Foundation of Life*; 1985. Quill, William Morrow, New York, NY, USA, pp. 259–307.

3. Becker RO, and Selden G, ibid reference 2, p. 273.
4. Becker RO, and Selden G, ibid reference 2, p. 259.
5. Hamer JR. *Biological Entrainment of the Human Brain by Low-frequency Radiation*, Northrop Space Laboratories, Hawthorne, California, USA, NSL Report no. 65, 1965: pp. 65–199.
6. Hamer JR. "Effects of low level, low frequency electric fields on human time judgement." *Proceedings of Fifth Biometeorological Congress, Montreux, Switzerland*, SW Tromp and WW Weihe (editors), Springer-Verlag, Amsterdam, The Netherlands, 1969.
7. Konig HL. "Behavioral changes in human subjects associated with ELF electric fields." In: *ELF and VLF Electromagnetic Field Effects*, MA Persinger (editor), Plenum Press, New York, NY, USA, 1974, pp. 81–99.
8. Schumann WO. "On the characteristic oscillations of a conducting sphere which is surrounded by an air layer and an ionospheric shell." [In German], *Zeitshrift fuer Naturforschung*, 1952; 7 (A): 149–154.
9. Konig HL. "ELF and VLF signal properties: physical characteristics." In: *ELF and VLF Electromagnetic Field Effects*, MA Persinger (editor), Plenum Press, New York, NY, USA, 1974, pp. 9–34.
10. Achkasova YN, Pyatkin KD, Bryzqunova NI, Sarachan TA, and Tyshkevich LV. "Very low frequency and small intensity electromagnetic and magnetic fields as an ecological factor." *Journal of Hygiene, Epidemiology, Microbiology and Immunology*, 1978; 22 (4): 415–420.
11. Becker RO, and Selden G, ibid reference 2, p. 24.
12. Zhadin MN. "Review of Russian literature on biological action of DC and low-frequency AC magnetic fields." *Bioelectromagnetics*, 2001; 22 (1): 27–45.
13. Sandstrom M, Wilen J, Oftedal G, and Hanssen Mild K "Mobile phone use and subjective symptoms. Comparison of symptoms experienced by users of analogue and digital mobile phones." *Occupational Medicine* (London), 2001; 51 (1): 25–35.
14. Hocking B. "Preliminary report: symptoms associated with mobile phone use." *Occupational Medicine* (London), 1998; 48 (6): 357–360.
15. Oftedal G, Wilen J, Sandstrom M, and Mild KH. "Symptoms experienced in connection with mobile phone use." *Occupational Medicine* (London), 2000; 50 (4): 237–245.
16. Santini R, Seigne M, Bonhomme-Faivre L, Bouffet S, Defrasne E, and Sage M. "Symptoms experienced by users of digital cellular phones: a study of a French engineering school." *Electromagnetic Biology and Medicine*, 2002; 21 (1): 81–88.
17. Hocking B. "Microwave sickness: a reappraisal." *Occupational Medicine* (London), 2001; 51 (1): 66–69.
18. Hocking B, and Westerman R. "Neurological effects of radiofrequency radiation," *Occupational Medicine* (London), 2003; 53 (2): 123–127.
19. Szyjkowska A, Bortkiewicz A, Szymczak W, and Makowiec-Dabrowska T. "Subjective symptoms related to mobile phone use: a pilot study." [In Polish]. *Polski Merkuriusz Lekarski* (Poland), 2005; 19 (112): 529–532.
20. Santini R, Santini P, Danze JM, Le Ruz P, and Seigne M. "Investigation on the health of people living near mobile telephone relay stations: I/Incidence according to distances and sex." [In French]. *Pathologie-Biologie* (Paris), 2002; 50 (6): 369–373.
21. Santini R, Santini P, Danze JM, Le Ruz P, and Seigne M. "Symptoms experienced by people in the vicinity of base stations: II/Incidences of age, duration of exposure, location of subjects in relation to the antennas and other electromagnetic factors." [In French]. *Pathologie-Biologie* (Paris), 2003; 51 (7): 412–415.
22. Hutter HP, Moshammer H, Wallner P, and Kundi M. "Subjective symptoms, sleeping

problems, and cognitive performance in subjects living near mobile phone base stations." *Occupational and Environmental Medicine*, 2006; 63 (5): 307–313.
23. Navarro EA, Segura J, Portoles M, and Gomez-Perretta C. "The microwave syndrome: a preliminary study in Spain." *Electromagnetic Biology and Medicine*, 2003; 22 (2&3): 161–169.
24. Oberfeld G, Navarro AE, Portoles M, Maestu C, and Gomez-Perretta C. *The Microwave Syndrome: Further Aspects of a Spanish Study*, Presented at an International Conference in Kos, Greece, in May 2004.
[Online, accessed 1st August 2009].
URL:http://www.apdr.info/electrocontaminacion/Documentos/Investigacion/ESTUDOS%20EPIDEMIOLOXIDOS%20E%20ANTENAS/The%20Microwave%20Syndrome%20%20Further%20Aspects%20of%20a%20Spanish%20 Study.pdf
25. Bortkiewicz A, Zmyslony M, Szyjkowska A, and Gadzicka E. "Subjective symptoms reported by people living in the vicinity of cellular phone base stations: review." [In Polish]. *Medycyna Pracy* (Poland), 2004; 55 (4): 345–351.
26. Abdel-Rassoul G, El-Fateh OA, Salem MA, Michael A, Farahat F, El-Batanouny M, and Salem E. "Neurobehavioral effects among inhabitants around mobile phone base stations." *Neurotoxicology*, 2007; 28 (2): 434–440.
27. Zwamborn APM, Vossen SHJA, van Leersum BJAM, Ouwens MA, and Makel WN. *Effects of Global Communication System Radio-frequency Fields on Wellbeing and Cognitive Functions of Human Subjects With and Without Subjective Complaints*, Sept. 2003. Netherlands Organisation for Applied Scientific Research (TNO), Report No. FEL-03-C148, The Hague, The Netherlands, pp. 1–89.
28. Sadchikova MN. "State of the nervous system under the influence of UHF." *The Biological Action of Ultrahigh Frequencies*, AA Letavet and ZV Gordon (editors), Academy of Medical Sciences, Moscow, USSR, 1962, pp. 25–29.
29. Sadchikova MN. "Clinical manifestation of reactions to microwave irradiation in various occupational groups." In: *Biologic Effects and Health Hazards of Microwave Radiation, Proceedings of an International Symposium*, sponsored by the WHO, Warsaw, 15–18 Oct., 1973. P Czerski (editor), Polish Medical Publications, Warsaw, Poland, pp. 261–267.
30. Wilson BW, Chess EK, and Anderson LE. "60-Hz electric-field effects on pineal melatonin rhythms: Time course for onset of recovery." *Bioelectromagnetics*, 1986; 7 (2): 239–242.
31. Wilson BW, Wright CW, Morris JE, Buschbom RL, Brown DP, Miller DL, Sommers-Flannigan R, and Anderson LE. "Evidence for an effect of ELF electromagnetic fields on human pineal gland function." *Journal of Pineal Research*, 1990; 9 (4): 259–269.
32. Pfluger DH, and Minder CE. "Effects of exposure to 16.7 Hz magnetic fields on urinary 6-hydroxymelatonin sulphate excretion of Swiss railway workers." *Journal of Pineal Research*, 1996; 21 (2): 91–100.
33. Lai H, and Singh NP. "Melatonin and N-tert-butyl-alpha-phenylnitrone block 60-Hz magnetic field-induced DNA single and double strand breaks in rat brain cells." *Journal of Pineal Research*, 1997; 22 (3): 152–162.
34. Lai H, and Singh NP. "Melatonin and a spin-trap compound block radiofrequency electromagnetic radiation-induced DNA strand breaks in rat brain cells." *Bioelectromagnetics*, 1997; 18 (6): 446–454.
35. Wood AW, Armstrong SM, Sait ML, Devine L, and Martin MJ. "Changes in human plasma melatonin profiles in response to 50 Hz magnetic field exposure." *Journal of Pineal Research*, 1998; 25 (2): 116–127.
36. Karasek M, Woldanska-Okonska M, Czernicki J, Zylinska K, and Swietoslawski J. "Chronic exposure to 2.9 mT, 40 Hz magnetic field reduces melatonin concentrations in

humans." *Journal of Pineal Research*, 1998; 25 (4): 240–244.
37. Rosen LA, Barber I, and Lyle DB. "A 0.5 G, 60 Hz magnetic field suppresses melatonin production in pinealocytes." *Bioelectromagnetics*, 1998; 19 (2): 123–127.
38. Arnetz BB, and Berg M. "Melatonin and adrenocorticotropic hormone levels in video display unit workers during work and pleasure." *Journal of Occupational and Environmental Medicine*, 1996; 38 (11): 1108–1110.
39. Stark KD, Krebs T, Altpeter E, Manz B, Griot C, and Abelin T. "Absence of chronic effect of exposure to short-wave radio broadcast signal on salivary melatonin concentrations in dairy cattle." *Journal of Pineal Research*, 1997; 22 (4): 171–176.
40. Burch JB, Reif JS, Noonan CW, Ichinose T, Bachand AM, Koleber TL, and Yost MG. "Melatonin metabolite excretion among cellular telephone users." *International Journal of Radiation Biology*, 2002; 78 (11): 1029–1036.
41. Burch JB, Reif JS, and Yost MG. "Geomagnetic disturbances are associated with reduced nocturnal excretion of a melatonin metabolite in humans." *Neuroscience Letters*, 1999; 266 (3): 209–212.
42. Altpeter ES, Krebs T, Pfluger DH, von Kanel J, Blattmann R, Emmenegger D, Cloetta B, Rogger U, Gerber H, Manz B, Coray R, Baumann R, Staerk K, Griot C, and Abelin T. *Study on Health Effects of the Shortwave Transmitter Station of Schwarzenburg, Berne, Switzerland*, BEW Publication Series, Study No. 55. The Federal Office of Energy, Berne, Switzerland, 1995.
43. Abelin T, Altpeter E, and Roosli M. "Sleep disturbances in the vicinity of the short-wave broadcast transmitter Schwarzenburg." *Somnologie*, 2005; 9 (4): 203–209.
44. Verkasalo PK, Kaprio J, Varjonen J, Romanov K, Heikkila K, and Koskenvuo M. "Magnetic fields of transmission lines and depression." *American Journal of Epidemiology*, 1997; 146 (12): 1037–1045.
45. Beale IL, Pearce NE, Conroy DM, Henning MA, and Murrell KA. "Psychological effects of chronic exposure to 50 Hz magnetic fields in humans living near extra-high-voltage transmission lines." *Bioelectromagnetics*, 1997; 18 (8): 584–594.
46. Zyss T, Dobrowolski JW, and Krawczyk K. "Neurotic disturbances, depression and anxiety disorders in the population living in the vicinity of overhead high-voltage transmission line 400 kV. Epidemiological pilot study." [In Polish]. *Medycyna Pracy* (Poland), 48 (5): 495–505.
47. Perry FS, Reichmanis,M, Marino AA, and Becker RO. "Environmental power-frequency magnetic fields and suicide." *Health Physics*, 1981; 41 (2): 267–277.
48. Van Wijngaarden E, Savitz DA, Kleckner RC, Cai J, and Loomis D. "Exposure to electromagnetic fields and suicide among electric utility workers: a nested case-control study." *The Western Journal of Medicine*, 2000; 173 (2): 94–100.
49. Sandyk R, Anastasiadis PG, Anninos PA, and Tsagas N. "The pineal gland and spontaneous abortions: implications for therapy with melatonin and magnetic field." *International Journal of Neuroscience*, 1992; 62 (3–4): 243–250.
50. O'Connor RP, and Persinger MA. "Geophysical variables and behavior: LXXXII. Strong association between sudden infant death syndrome and increments of global geomagnetic activity: possible support for the melatonin hypothesis." *Perceptual and Motor Skills*, 1997; 84 (2): 395–402.
51. Reiter RJ. "Melatonin suppression by static and extremely low frequency electromagnetic fields: relationship to the reported increased incidence of cancer." *Reviews on Environmental Health*, 1994; 10 (3–4): 171–186.
52. Goldsmith JR. "Epidemiologic evidence relevant to radar (microwave) effects."

Environmental Health Perspectives, 1997, 105 (supplement 6): 1579–1587.
53. Wartenberg D. "Residential magnetic fields and childhood leukemia: a meta-analysis." *American Journal of Public Health*, 1998; 88 (12): 1787–1794.
54. Henshaw DL, and Reiter RJ. "Do magnetic fields cause increased risk of childhood leukemia via melatonin disruption?" *Bioelectromagnetics*, 2005 (supplement 7): 86–97.
55. Stevens RG. "Electric power use and breast cancer: a hypothesis." *American Journal of Epidemiology*, 1987; 125 (4): 556–561.
56. Stevens RG, Davis S, Thomas DB, Anderson LE, and Wilson BW. "Electric power, pineal function and the risk of breast cancer." *The FASEB* (Federation of American Societies for Experimental Biology) *Journal*, 1992; 6 (3): 853–860.
57. Stevens RG, and Davis S. "The melatonin hypothesis: electric power and breast cancer." *Environmental Health Perspectives*, 1996; 104 (supplement 1): 135–140.
58. Caplan LS, Schoenfeld ER, O'Leary ES, and Leske MC. "Breast cancer and electromagnetic fields: a review." *Annals of Epidemiology*, 2000; 10 (1): 31–44.
59. Liburdy RP, Sloma TR, Sokolic R, and Yaswen P. "ELF magnetic fields, breast cancer, and melatonin: 60 Hz fields block melatonin's oncostatic action on ER+ breast cancer cell proliferation." *Journal of Pineal Research*, 1993; 14 (2): 89–97.
60. Osmundsen JA. "Radio waves found to affect cell behavior." *New York Times*, March 30, 1959, p. 1.
61. Teixeira-Pinto AA, Nejelski LL Jr, Cutler JL, and Heller JH. "The behavior of unicellular organisms in an electromagnetic field." *Experimental Cell Research*, 1960, 20: 548–564.
62. Heller JH, and Teixeira-Pinto AA. "A new physical method of creating chromosomal aberrations." *Nature*, 1959; 183 (4665): 905–906.
63. Nordenson I, Mild KH, Nordstrom S, Sweins S, and Birke E. "Clastogenic effects in human lymphocytes of power frequency electric fields: in vivo and in vitro studies." *Radiation and Environmental Biophysics*, 1984; 23 (3): 191–201.
64. Nordstrom S, Birke E, and Gustavsson L. "Reproductive hazards among workers at high voltage substations." *Bioelectromagnetics*, 1983; 4 (1): 91–101.
65. Theriault G, Goldberg M, Miller AB, Armstrong B, Guenel P, Deadman J, Imbernon E, To T, Chevalier A, Cyr D, and Wall C. "Cancer risks associated with occupational exposure to magnetic fields among electric utility workers in Ontario and Quebec, Canada, and France: 1970–1989." *American Journal of Epidemiology*, 1994, 139 (6): 550–572.
66. Preston-Martin S, Lewis S, Winkelmann R, Borman B, Auld J, and Pearce N. "Descriptive epidemiology of primary cancer of the brain, cranial nerves, and cranial meninges in New Zealand, 1948–88." *Cancer Causes and Control*, 1993; 4 (6): 529–538.
67. Speers MA, Dobbins JG, and Mills VS. "Occupational exposures and brain cancer mortality: a preliminary study of east Texas residents." *American Journal of Industrial Medicine*, 1988; 13 (6): 629–638.
68. Spitz MR, and Johnson CC. "Neuroblastoma and paternal occupation. A case-control analysis." *American Journal of Epidemiology*, 1985; 121 (6): 924–929.
69. Lin RS, Dischinger PC, Conde J, and Farrell KP. "Occupational exposure to electromagnetic fields and the occurrence of brain tumors. An analysis of possible associations." *Journal of Occupational Medicine*, 1985; 27 (6): 413–419.
70. Brown HD, and Chattopadhyay SK. "Electromagnetic-field exposure and cancer." *Cancer Biochemistry Biophysics*, 1988; 9 (4): 295–342.
71. Tornqvist S, Knave B, Ahlbom A, and Persson T. "Incidence of leukaemia and brain tumours in some 'electrical occupations'." *British Journal of Industrial Medicine*, 1991; 48 (9): 597–603.

72. Beall C, Delzell E, Cole P, and Brill I. "Brain tumors among electronics industry workers." *Epidemiology*, 1996; 7 (2): 125–130.
73. Villeneuve PJ, Agnew DA, Johnson KC, Mao Y; Canadian Cancer Registries Epidemiology Research Group. "Brain cancer and occupational exposure to magnetic fields among men: results from a Canadian population-based case-control study." *International Journal of Epidemiology*, 2002; 31 (1): 210–217.
74. Milham S Jr. "Mortality in workers exposed to electromagnetic fields." *Environmental Health Perspectives*, 1985; 62: 297–300.
75. Savitz DA, and Calle EE. "Leukemia and occupational exposure to electromagnetic fields: review of epidemiologic surveys." Journal of Occupational Medicine, 1987; 29 (1): 47–51.
76. Schroeder JC, and Savitz DA. "Lymphoma and multiple myeloma mortality in relation to magnetic field exposure among electric utility workers." *American Journal of Industrial Medicine*, 1997; 32 (4): 392–402.
77. Villeneuve PJ, Agnew DA, Miller AB, and Corey PN. "Non-Hodgkin's lymphoma among electric utility workers in Ontario: the evaluation of alternate indices of exposure to 60 Hz electric and magnetic fields." *Occupational and Environmental Medicine*, 2000: 57 (4): 249–257.
78. Deapen DM, and Henderson BE. "A case-control study of amyotrophic lateral sclerosis." *American Journal of Epidemiology*, 1986; 123 (5):790–799.
79. Davanipour Z, Sobel E, Bowman JD, Qian Z, and Will AD. "Amyotrophic lateral sclerosis and occupational exposure to electromagnetic fields." *Bioelectromagnetics*, 1997; 18 (1): 28–35.
80. Savitz DA, Checkoway H, and Loomis DP. "Magnetic field exposure and neurodegenerative disease mortality among electric utility workers." *Epidemiology*, 1998; 9 (4):398–404.
81. Savitz DA, Loomis DP, and Tse C-K. "Electrical occupations and neurodegenerative disease: analysis of US mortality data." *Archives of Environmental Health*, 1998; 53 (1): 71–74.
82. Johansen C, and Olsen JH. "Mortality from amyotrophic lateral sclerosis, other chronic disorders, and electric shocks among utility workers." *American Journal of Epidemiology*, 1998; 148 (4): 362–368.
83. Hakansson N, Gustavsson P, Johansen C, and Floderus B. "Neurodegenerative diseases in welders and other workers exposed to high levels of magnetic fields." *Epidemiology*, 2003; 14 (4): 420–426; discussion 427–428.
84. Sobel E, Davanipour Z, Sulkava R, Erkinjuntti T, Wikstrom J, Henderson VW, Buckwalter G, Bowman JD, and Lee PJ. "Occupations with exposure to electromagnetic fields: a possible risk factor for Alzheimer's disease." *American Journal of Epidemiology*, 1995; 142 (5): 515–524.
85. Sobel E, Dunn M, Davanipour Z, Qian Z, and Chui HC. "Elevated risk of Alzheimer's disease among workers with likely electromagnetic field exposure." *Neurology*, 1996; 47 (6): 1477–1481.
86. Noonan CW, Reif JS, Yost M, and Touchstone J. "Occupational exposure to magnetic fields in case-referent studies of neurodegenerative diseases." *Scandinavian Journal of Work, Environment and Health*, 2002; 28 (1): 42–48.
87. Baris D, Armstrong BG, Deadman J, and Theriault G. "A mortality study of electrical utility workers in Quebec." *Occupational and Environmental Medicine*, 1996; 53 (1): 25–31.
88. Baris D, Armstrong B G, Deadman J, and Theriault G. "A case cohort study of suicide in relation to exposure to electric and magnetic fields among electrical utility workers."

Occupational and Environmental Medicine, 1996; 53 (1): 17–24.

89. Loomis DP, Savitz DA, and Ananth CV. "Breast cancer mortality among female electrical workers in the United States." *Journal of the National Cancer Institute*, 1994; 86 (12): 921–925.
90. Cantor KP, Stewart PA, Brinton LA, and Dosemeci M. "Occupational exposures and female breast cancer mortality in the United States." *Journal of Occupational and Environmental Medicine*, 1995; 37 (3): 336–348.
91. Coogan PF, Clapp RW, Newcomb PA, Wenzl TB, Bogdan G, Mittendorf R, Baron JA, and Longnecker MP. "Occupational exposure to 60-hertz magnetic fields and risk of breast cancer in women." *Epidemiology*, 1996; 7 (5): 459–464.
92. Pollen M, and Gustavsson P. "High-risk occupations for breast cancer in the Swedish female working population." *American Journal of Public Health*, 1999; 89 (6); 875–881.
93. Caplan LS, Schoenfeld ER, O'Leary ES, and Leske MC. "Breast cancer and electromagnetic fields: a review." *Annals of Epidemiology*, 2000; 10 (1): 31–44.
94. Forssen UM, Feychting M, Rutqvist LE. Floderus B, and Ahlbom H. "Occupational and residential magnetic field exposure and breast cancer in females." *Epidemiology*, 2000; 1 (1): 24–29.
95. Gardner KM, Ou Shu X, Jin F, Dai Q, Ruan Z, Thompson SJ, Hussey JR, Gao YT, and Zheng W. "Occupations and breast cancer risk among Chinese women in urban Shanghai." *American Journal of Industrial Medicine*, 2002; 42 (4): 296–308.
96. Kliukiene J, Tynes T, and Andersen A. "Follow-up of radio and telegraph operators with exposure to electromagnetic fields and risk of breast cancer." *European Journal of Cancer Prevention*, 2003; 12 (4): 301–307.
97. Kliukiene, J., Tynes, T., and Andersen, A. "Residential and occupational exposures to 50-Hz magnetic fields and breast cancer in women: a population-based study." *American Journal of Epidemiology*, 2004; 159 (9): 852–861.
98. Demers PA, Thomas DB, Rosenblatt KA, Jimenez LM, McTiernan A, Stalsberg H, Stemhagen A, Thompson WD, Curnen MG, Satariano W, Austin DF, Isacson P, Greenberg RS, Key C, Kolonel LN, and West DW. "Occupational exposure to electromagnetic fields and breast cancer in men." *American Journal of Epidemiology*, 1991; 134 (4): 340–347.
99. Goldsmith JR. "Epidemiologic evidence of radiofrequency radiation (microwave) effects in health in military, broadcasting and occupational studies." *International Journal of Occupational and Environmental Health*, 1995; 1 (1): 47–57.
100. Lin RS, Dischinger PC, Conde J, and Farrell KP. "Occupational exposure to electromagnetic fields and the occurrence of brain tumors: an analysis of possible associations." *Journal of Occupational Medicine*, 1985; 27 (6): 413–419.
101. Grayson JK. "Radiation exposure, socioeconomic status, and brain tumor risk in the US Air Force: a nested case-control study." *American Journal of Epidemiology*, 1996; 143 (5): 480–486.
102. Szmigielski S. "Cancer mortality in subjects occupationally exposed to high frequency (radiofrequency and microwave) electromagnetic radiation." *Science of the Total Environment*, 1996; 180: 9–17.
103. Sigler AT, Lilienfeld AM, Cohen BH, and Westlake JE. "Radiation exposure in parents of children with mongolism (Down's Syndrome)." *Bulletin of John Hopkins Hospital*, 1965; 117: 374–399.
104. Ouellet-Hellstrom R, and Stewart WF. "Miscarriages among female physical therapists who report using radio- and microwave-frequency electromagnetic radiation." *American Journal of Epidemiology*, 1993; 138 (10): 775–786.

105. Kallen B, Malmquist G, and Moritz U. "Delivery outcome among physiotherapists in Sweden: is non-ionizing radiation a fetal hazard?" *Archives of Environmental Health*, 1982; 37 (2): 81–85.
106. Larsen AI, Olsen JH, and Svane O. "Gender-specific reproductive outcome and exposure to high-frequency electromagnetic radiation among physiotherapists." *Scandinavian Journal of Work, Environment and Health*, 1991; 17 (5): 324–329.
107. Wertheimer N, and Leeper E. "Electrical wiring configuration and childhood cancer." *American Journal of Epidemiology*, 1979; 109 (3): 273–284.
108. Wertheimer N, and Leeper E. "Adult cancer related to electrical wires near the home." *International Journal of Epidemiology*, 1982; 11 (4): 345–355.
109. Savitz DA, Wachtel H, Barnes FA, John EM, and Tvrdik JG. "Case-control study of childhood cancer and exposure to 60-Hz magnetic fields." *American Journal of Epidemiology*, 1988; 128 (1): 21–38.
110. Li C-Y, Lee W-C, and Lin RS. "Risk of leukemia in children living near high-voltage transmission lines." *Journal of Occupational and Environmental Medicine*, 1998; 40 (2): 144–147.
111. Feychting M, and Ahlbom A. "Magnetic fields and cancer in children residing near Swedish high-voltage power lines." *American Journal of Epidemiology*, 1993; 138 (7): 467–481.
112. Draper G, Vincent T, Kroll ME, and Swanson J. "Childhood cancer in relation to distance from high voltage power lines in England and Wales: a case-control study." *British Medical Journal* (Clinical Research Edition), 2005; 330 (7503): 1290.
113. Washburn EP, Orza MJ, Berlin, JA, Nicholson WJ, Todd AC, Frumkin H, and Chalmers TC. "Residential proximity to electricity transmission and distribution equipment and risk of childhood leukemia, childhood lymphoma, and childhood nervous system tumors: systematic review, evaluation, and meta-analysis," *Cancer Causes and Control*, 1994; 5 (4): 299–309.
114. Linet MS, Hatch EE, Kleinerman RA, Robison LL, Kaune WT, Friedman DR, Severson RK, Haines CM, Hartsock CT, Niwa S, Wacholder S, and Tarone RE. "Residential exposure to magnetic fields and acute lymphoblastic leukemia in children." *The New England Journal of Medicine*, 1997; 337 (1): 1–7.
115. Ahlbom A, Albert EN, Fraser-Smith AC, Grodzinsky AJ, Marron MT, Martin AO, Persinger MA, Shelanski ML, and Wopow ER. *Biological Effects of Power Line Fields*, New York State Power Lines Project, Scientific Advisory Panel Final Report, New York, NY, USA, July 1, 1987.
116. Lowenthal RM, Tuck DM, and Bray IC. "Residential exposure to electric power transmission lines and risk of lymphproliferative and myeloproliferative disorders: a case-control study." *Internal Medicine Journal*, 2007, 37 (9): 614–619.
117. Feychting M, Forssen U, Rutqvist LE, and Ahlbom A. "Magnetic fields and breast cancer in Swedish adults residing near high-voltage power lines." *Epidemiology*, 1998; 9 (4): 392–397.
118. Tynes T, Klaeboe L, and Haldorsen T. "Residential and occupational exposure to 50 Hz magnetic fields and malignant melanoma: a population based study." *Occupational and Environmental Medicine*, 2003; 60 (5): 343–347.
119. Zyss T. "Epidemiological studies on neurotic disturbances, anxiety and depressive disorders in a population living near an overhead high voltage transmission line (400 kV)." [In Polish]. *Psychiatria Polska* (Poland), 1999; 33 (4): 535–551.
120. Poole C, Kavet R, Funch DP, Donelan K, Charry JM, and Dreyer NA. "Depressive

symptoms and headaches in relation to proximity of residence to alternating-current transmission line right-of-way." *American Journal of Epidemiology*, 1993; 137 (3): 318–330.

121. Cherry N. *ICNIRP Critique 2000: Criticism of the Health Assessment in the ICNIRP Guidelines for Radiofrequency and Microwave Radiation (100kHz–300 GHz)*, 31 January, 2000. [Online, accessed 2nd August, 2009]. URL:http://www.neilcherry.com/cart/cart/?mode=show_category&catid=1&page=1

122. Zhu K, Hunter S, Payne-Wilks K, Roland CL, and Forbes DS. "Use of electric bedding devices and risk of breast cancer in African-American women." *American Journal of Epidemiology*, 2003; 158 (8): 798–806.

123. Dockerty JD, Elwood JM, Skegg DC, and Herbison GP. "Electromagnetic field exposures and childhood cancers in New Zealand." *Cancer Causes and Control*, 1998; 9 (3): 299–309.

124. Hocking B, Gordon IR, Grain HL, and Hatfield GE. "Cancer incidence and mortality and proximity to TV towers." *Medical Journal of Australia*, 1996; 165 (11–12): 601–605.

125. Hocking B, and Gordon I. "Decreased survival for childhood leukemia in proximity to TV towers." *Archives of Environmental Health*, 2003; 58 (90): 560–564.

126. Anderson BS, and Henderson AK. *Cancer Incidence in Census Tracts with Broadcasting Towers in Honolulu, Hawaii*, Report submitted to the Environmental and Epidemiology Program, Honolulu City Council, Honolulu, Hawaii, October 27, 1986. Cited in: JR Goldsmith, (editor), "Epidemiological status of radio-frequency radiation: current status and areas of concern." *The Science of the Total Environment*, 1996; 180 (1): 3–8.

127. Michelozzi P, Capon A, Kirchmayer U, Forastiere F, Biggeri A, Barca A, and Perucci CA. "Adult and childhood leukemia near a high-power radio station in Rome, Italy." *American Journal of Epidemiology*, 2002; 155 (12): 1096–1103.

128. Neutra RR, DelPizzo V, and Lee GM. *An Evaluation of the Possible Risks from Electric and Magnetic Fields (EMFs) from Power Lines, Internal Wiring, Electrical Occupations and Appliances*, California EMF Risk Program, California Department of Health and Human Services, Oakland, California, USA, Final Report, June 2002.

129. Morton W, and Phillips D. "Cancer promotion by radiowave emissions." [2000 Annual Conference of the ISEE]. *Epidemiology*, 2000; 11 (4): 57.

130. Dolk H, Shaddick G, Walls P, Grundy C, Thakrar B, Kleinschmidt I, and Elliott P. "Cancer incidence near radio and television transmitters in Great Britain, 1. Sutton Coldfield transmitter." *American Journal of Epidemiology*, 1997; 145 (1): 1–9.

131. Park SK, Ha M, Im HJ. "Ecological study on residences in the vicinity of AM radio broadcasting towers and cancer death: preliminary observations in Korea." *International Archives of Occupational and Environmental Health*, 2004; 77 (6): 387–394.

132. Selvin S, Schulman J, and Merrill DW. "Distance and risk measures for the analysis of spatial data: a study of childhood cancers." *Social Science and Medicine*, 1992; 34 (7): 769–777.

133. Dolk H, Elliott P, Shaddick G, Walls P, and Thakrar B. "Cancer incidence near radio and television transmitters in Great Britain, II. All high power transmitters." *American Journal of Epidemiology*, 1997; 145 (1): 10–17.

134. Cherry N. *Childhood Cancer in the Vicinity of the Sutro Tower, San Francisco*, 10 October, 2002.
[Online, accessed 2nd August, 2009]. URL:http://www.neil.cherry.com

135. Cherry N. Re: "Cancer incidence near radio and television transmitters in Great Britain, 1–Sutton Coldfield transmitter; II–All high power transmitters." Letter, *American Journal of Epidemiology*, 2001; 153 (2): 204–205.

136. Hallberg O, and Johansson O. "Melanoma incidence and frequency modulation (FM)

broadcasting." *Archives of Environmental Health*, 2002; 57 (1): 32–40.
137. Hallberg O, and Johansson O. "Malignant melanoma of the skin–not a sunshine story!" *Medical Science Monitor*, 2004; 10 (7): CR336–340.
138. Hallberg O. "A theory and model to explain the skin melanoma epidemic." *Melanoma Research*, 2006; 16 (2): 115–118.
139. Kolodynski AA, and Kolodynska VV. "Motor and psychological functions of school children living in an area of the Skrunda Radio Location Station in Latvia." *The Science of the Total Environment*, 1996; 180 (1): 87–93.
140. Altpeter ES, Roosli M, Battaglia M, Pfluger D, Minder CE, and Abelin T. "Effects of short-wave (6–22 MHz) magnetic fields on sleep quality and melatonin cycle in humans: the Schwarzenburg shut-down study." *Bioelectromagnetics*, 2006; 27 (2): 142–150.
141. Bawin SM, Kaczmarek LK, and Adey WR. "Effects of modulated VHF fields on the central nervous system." *Annals of the New York Academy of Sciences*, 1975; 247: 74–81.
142. Bawin SM, and Adey WR. "Sensitivity of calcium binding in cerebral tissue to weak environmental electric fields oscillating at low frequency." *Proceedings of National Academy of Sciences of the United States of America*, 1976; 73 (6): 1999–2003.
143. Adey WR, Bawin SM, and Lawrence AF. "Effects of weak amplitude-modulated microwave fields on calcium efflux from awake cat cerebral cortex." *Bioelectromagnetics*, 1982; 3 (3): 295–307.
144. Blackman CF, Benane SG, Elliot DJ, House DE, and Pollack MM. "Influence of electromagnetic fields on the efflux of calcium ions from brain tissue in vitro: a three-model analysis consistent with the frequency response up to 510 Hz". *Bioelectromagnetics*, 1988; 9 (3): 215–227.
145. Blackman CF. "ELF effects on calcium homeostasis." In: *Extremely Low Frequency Electromagnetic Fields: The Question of Cancer*. BW Wilson, RG Stevens, and LE Anderson (editors). Battelle Press, Columbus, Ohio, USA, 1990: pp. 187–208.
146. Schwartz JL, House DE, and Mealing GA. "Exposure of frog hearts to CW or amplitude-modulated VHF fields: selective efflux of calcium ions at 16 Hz." *Bioelectromagnetics*, 1990; 11 (4): 349–358.
147. Becker RO, and Selden G, ibid reference 2, 296 ff.
148. Wilson BW, Anderson LE, Hilton DI, and Phillips RD. "Chronic exposure to 60-Hz electric fields: effects on pineal function in the rat." *Bioelectromagnetics*, 1981; 2 (4): 371–380.
149. Reiter RJ, Anderson LE, Buschbom RL, and Wilson BW. "Reduction of the nocturnal rise in pineal melatonin levels in rats exposed to 60-Hz electric fields in utero and for 23 days after birth." *Life Sciences*, 1988; 42 (22): 2203–2206.
150. Vasquez BJ, Anderson LE, Lowery CI, and Adey WR. "Diurnal patterns in brain biogenic amines of rats exposed to 60-Hz electric fields." *Bioelectromagnetics*, 1988; 9 (3): 229–236.
151. Free MJ, Kaune WT, Phillips RD, and Cheng HC. "Endocrinological effects of strong 60-Hz electric fields on rats." *Bioelectromagnetics*, 1981; 2 (2): 105–121.
152. Al-Akhras M-A, Darmani H, and Elbetieha A. "Influence of 50 Hz magnetic field on sex hormones and other fertility parameters of adult male rats." *Bioelectromagnetics*, 2006; 27 (2): 127–131.
153. Editorial: "Serotonin, suicidal behaviour, and impulsivity." *The Lancet*, 1987; 330 (8565): 949–950.
154. Seegal RF, Wolpaw JR, and Dowman R. "Chronic exposure of primates to 60-Hz electric and magnetic fields: II. Neurochemical effects." *Bioelectromagnetics*, 1989; 10 (3): 289–301.
155. Delgado JM, Leal J, Monteagudo JL, and Gracia MG. "Embryological changes induced by

weak, extremely low frequency electromagnetic fields." *Journal of Anatomy*, 1982; 134 (3): 533–551.

156. Phillips RD, Anderson LB, and Kaune WT. *Biological Effects of High-strength Electric Fields on Small Laboratory Animals*, Pacific Northwest Laboratories, Richland, Washington, USA, DOE/TIC-10084, DOE Contract No: E4-76-C-06-1830, December 1, 1979.

157. Lai H, and Singh NP. "Acute exposure to a 60 Hz magnetic field increases DNA strand breaks in rat brain cells." *Bioelectromagnetics*, 1997; 18 (2): 156–165.

158. Lai H, and Singh NP. "Magnetic-field-induced DNA strand breaks in brain cells of the rat." *Environmental Health Perspectives*, 2004; 112 (6): 687–694.

159. Salford LG, Brun A, Sturesson K, Eberhardt JL, and Persson BR. "Permeability of the blood-brain barrier induced by 915 MHz electromagnetic radiation, continuous wave and modulated at 8, 16, 50, and 200 Hz." *Microscopy Research and Technique*, 1994; 27 (6): 535–542.

160. Salford LG, Brun AE, Eberhardt JL, Malmgren L, and Persson BR. "Nerve cell damage in mammalian brain after exposure to microwaves from GSM mobile phones." *Environmental Health Perspectives*, 2003; 111 (7): 881–883.

161. Aitken RJ, Bennetts LE, Sawyer D, Wiklendt AM, and King BV. "Impact of radio frequency electromagnetic radiation on DNA integrity in the male germline." *International Journal of Andrology*; 2005; 28 (3): 171–9.

162. Diem D, Schwarz C, Adlkofer F, Jahn O, and Rudiger H. "Non-thermal DNA breakage by mobile-phone radiation (1800 MHz) in human fibroblasts and in transformed GFSH-R17 rat granulosa cells in vitro", *Mutation Research*, 2005; 583 (2): 178–183.

163. Verschaeve L, Slaets D, Van Gorp U, Maes A, and Vanderkom J. "In vitro and in vivo genetic effects of microwaves from mobile phone frequencies in human and rat peripheral blood lymphocytes." *Proceedings of Cost 244 Meetings on Mobile Communication and Extremely Low Frequency Field: Instrumentation and Measurements in Bioelectromagnetics Research*, D Simunic (editor), Information Ventures Inc, Plzen, Czech Republic, 1994, pp. 74–83.

164. Tice RR, Hook GG, Donner M, McRee DI, and Guy AW. "Genotoxicity of radiofrequency signals. 1. Investigation of DNA damage and micronuclei induction in cultured human blood cells." *Bioelectromagnetics*, 2002; 23 (2): 113–126.

165. Lai H, and Singh NP. "Acute low-intensity microwave exposure increases DNA single-strand breaks in rat brain cells." *Bioelectromagnetics*, 1995; 16 (3): 207–210.

166. Lai H, and Singh NP. "Single- and double-strand DNA breaks in rat brain cells after acute exposure to radiofrequency electromagnetic radiation." *International Journal of Radiation Biology*, 1996; 69 (4): 513–521.

167. Sarkar S, Ali S, and Behari J. "Effect of low power microwave on the mouse genome: a direct DNA analysis." *Mutation Research*, 1994; 320 (1–2): 141–147.

168. Lee S, Johnson D, Dunbar K, Dong H, Ge X, Kim YC, Wing C, Jayathilaka N, Emmanuel N, Zhou CQ, Gerber HL, Tseng CC, and Wang SM. "2.45 GHz radiofrequency fields alter gene expression in cultured human cells." *FEBS* (Federation of European Biochemical Societies) *Letters*, 2005; 579 (21): 4829–4836.

169. Phillips JL, Ivaschuk O, Ishida-Jones T, Jones RA, Campbell-Beachler M, and Haggren W. "DNA damage in Molt-4 T-lymphoblastoid cells exposed to cellular telephone radiofrequency fields in vitro."
Bioelectrochemistry and Bioenergetics, 1998; 45 (1): 103–110.

170. Repacholi MH, Basten A, Gebski V, Noonan D, Finnie J, and Harris AW. "Lymphomas in E mu-Pim1 transgenic mice exposed to pulsed 900 MHz electromagnetic fields." *Radiation

Research, 1997; 147 (5): 631–640.
171. Chou C-K, Guy AW, Kunz LL, Johnson RB, Crowley JJ, and Krupp JH. "Long-term, low-level microwave irradiation of rats." *Bioelectromagnetics*, 1992; 13 (6): 469–496.
172. Frey AH. "Effects of microwaves and radar frequency energy on the central nervous system." In: *Biological Effects and Health Implications of Microwave Radiation*, S Cleary (editor), PB193898, Food and Drug Administration, Washington, D.C., USA, 1969: 134–139
173. Silverman C. "Nervous and behavioral effects of microwave radiation in humans." *American Journal of Epidemiology*, 1973; 97 (4): 219–224.
174. Djordjevic Z, Kolak A, and Stojkovic M, Rankovic N, and Ristic P. "A study of the health status of radar workers." *Aviation, Space and Environmental Medicine*, 1979; 50 (4): 396–398.
175. Forman SA, Holmes CK, McManamon TV, and Wedding WR. "Psychological symptoms and intermittent hypertension following acute microwave exposure." *Journal of Occupational Medicine*, 1982; 24 (11): 932–934.
176. Johnson Liakouris AG. "Radiofrequency (RF) sickness in the Lilienfeld Study: an effect of modulated microwaves?" *Archives of Environmental Health*, 1998; 53 (3): 236–238.
177. Independent Expert Group on Mobile Phones, Sir William Stewart Chairman. *The Stewart Report: Mobile Phones and Health*, National Radiological Protection Board, Oxford, UK, 28 April, 2000: pp. 35–36.
[Online, accessed 2nd August, 2009]. URL:http://www.iegmp.drg.uk/report/index.htm
178. Frey AH. "Headaches from cellular telephones: are they real and what are the implications?" *Environmental Health Perspectives*, 1998; 106 (3): 101–103.
179. Braune S, Wrocklage C, Raczek J. Gailus T, and Lucking CH. "Resting blood pressure increase during exposure to a radio-frequency electromagnetic field." *The Lancet*, 1998; 351 (9119): 1857–1858.
180. Mann K, and Roschke J. "Effects of pulsed high-frequency electromagnetic fields on human sleep." *Neuropsychobiology*, 1996; 33 (1): 41–47.
181. Borbely AA, Huber R, Graf T, Fuchs B, Gallmann E, and Achermann P. "Pulsed high-frequency electromagnetic field affects human sleep and sleep electroencephalogram." *Neuroscience Letters*, 1999; 275 (3): 207–210.
182. Von Klitzing L. "Low frequency pulsed electromagnetic fields influence EEG of man." *Physica Medica*, 1995; 11 (2): 77–80.
183. Reiser H, Dimpfel W, and Schober F. "The influence of electromagnetic fields on human brain activity." *European Journal of Medical Research*, 1995; 1 (1): 27–32.
184. Freude G, Ullsperger P, Eggert S, and Ruppe I. "Microwaves emitted by cellular telephones affect human slow brain potentials." *European Journal of Applied Physiology*, 2000; 81 (1–2): 18–27.
185. Huber R, Treyer V, Schuderer J, Berthold T, Buck A, Kuster N, Landolt HP, and Achermann P. "Exposure to pulse-modulated radio frequency electromagnetic fields affects regional cerebral blood flow." *European Journal of Neuroscience*, 2005; 21 (4): 1000–1006.
186. Curcio G, Ferrara M, Moroni F, D'Inzeo G, Bertini M, and De Gennaro L. "Is the brain influenced by a phone call? An EEG study of resting wakefulness." *Neuroscience Research*, 2005; 53 (3): 265–270.
187. Hardell L, Mild KH, and Carlberg M. "Case-control study on the use of cellular and cordless phones and the risk for malignant brain tumours." *International Journal of Radiation Biology*, 2002; 78 (10: 931–936.
188. Hardell L, Mild KH, and Carlberg M. "Further aspects on cellular and cordless telephones

and brain tumours." *International Journal of Oncology*, 2003; 22 (2): 399–407.

189. Hardell L, Mild KH, Carlberg M, and Hallquist A. "Cellular and cordless telephone use and the association with brain tumours in different age groups." *Archives of Environmental Health*, 2004; 59 (3): 132–137.

190. Hardell L, Carlberg M, and Mild KH. "Case-control study of cellular and cordless telephones and the risk for acoustic neuroma or meningioma in patients diagnosed in 2000–2003." *Neuroepidemiology*, 2005; 25 (3): 120–128.

191. Hardell L, Carlberg M, and Mild KH, "Case-control study of the association between the use of cellular and cordless telephones and malignant brain tumours diagnosed during 2000–2003." *Environmental Research*, 2006; 100 (2): 232–241.

192. Hardell L, Mild KH, Carlberg M, and Soderqvist F. "Tumour risk associated with use of cellular or cordless desktop telephones." *World Journal of Surgical Oncology*, 2006; 4: 74.

193. Hardell L, Carlberg M, and Mild KH. "Pooled analysis of two case-control studies on the use of cellular and cordless telephones and the risk of benign brain tumours diagnosed during 1997–2003." *International Journal of Oncology*, 2006; 28 (2): 509–518.

194. Hardell L, Carlberg M., and Mild KH. "Pooled analysis of two case-control studies on use of cellular and cordless telephones and the risk for malignant brain tumours diagnosed in 1997–2003." *International Archives of Occupational and Environmental Health*, 2006; 79 (8): 630–639.

195. Hardell LO, Carlberg M, Soderqvist F, Mild KH, and Morgan LL. "Long-term use of cellular phones and brain tumours: increased risk associated with use for 10 or more years." *Occupational and Environmental Medicine*, 2007, 64 (9): 626–632.

196. Barnes DE, and Bero LA. "Industry-funded research and conflict of interest: an analysis of research sponsored by the tobacco industry through the Centre for Indoor Air Research." *Journal of Health Politics, Policy and Law*, 1996; 21 (3): 515–542.

197. Barnes DE, and Bero LA. "Why review articles on the health effects of passive smoking reach different conclusions." *Journal of the American Medical Association*, 1998; 279 (19): 1566–1570.

198. Bero LA. "Tobacco industry manipulation of research." *Public Health Reports*, 2005; 120 (2): 200–208.

199. Stelfox HT, Chua G, O'Rourke K, and Detsky AS. "Conflict of interest in the debate over calcium-channel antagonists." *The New England Journal of Medicine*, 1998; 338 (2): 101–106.

200. Yaphe J, Edman R, Knishkowy B, and Hermand J. "The association between funding by commercial interests and study outcome in randomized controlled drug trials." *Family Practice*, 2001; 18 (6): 565–568.

201. Bekelman JE, Li Y, and Gross CP. "Scope and impact of financial conflicts of interest in biomedical research: a systematic review." *Journal of the American Medical Association*, 2003; 289 (4): 454–465.

202. Lexchin J, Bero LA, Djulbegovic B, and Clark O. "Pharmaceutical industry sponsorship and research outcome and quality: systematic review." *British Medical Journal*, 2003; 326 (7400): 1167–1170.

203. Huss A, Egger M, Hug K, Huwiler-Muntener K, and Roosli M. "Source of funding and results of studies of health effects of mobile phone use: systematic review of experimental studies." *Environmental Health Perspectives*, 2007; 115 (1): 1–4.

204. Schoemaker MJ, Swerdlow AJ, Ahlbom A, Auvinen A, Blaasaas KG, Cardis E, Christensen HC, Feychting M, Hepworth SJ, Johansen C, Klaeboe L, Lonn S, McKinney PA, Muir K, Raitanen J, Salminen T, Thomsen J, and Tynes T. "Mobile phone use and risk of acoustic neuroma: results of the Interphone case-control study in five North European

countries." *British Journal of Cancer*, 2005; 93 (7): 842–848.
205. Lonn S, Ahlbom A, Hall P, and Feychting M. "Mobile phone use and the risk of acoustic neuroma." *Epidemiology*, 2004; 15 (6): 653–659.
206. Schuz J, Bohler, E., Berg, G., Schlehofer, B., Hettinger, I., Schlaefer, K., Wahrendorf, J., Kunna-Grass K, and Blettner M. "Cellular phones, cordless phones, and the risks of glioma and meningioma (Interphone Study Group, Germany). *American Journal of Epidemiology*, 2006; 163 (6): 512–520.
207. Fejes I, Zavaczki Z, Szollosi J, Koloszar S, Daru J, Kovacs L, and Pal A. "Is there a relationship between cell phone use and semen quality?" *Archives of Andrology*, 2005; 51 (5): 385–393.
208. Agarwal A, Deepinder F, Sharma RK, Ranga G, and Li J. "Effect of cell phone usage on semen analysis in men attending infertility clinic: an observational study." *Fertiliy and Sterility*, 2008, 89 (1): 124–128.
209. Desoil M, Gillis P, Gossuin Y, Pankhurst QA, and Hautot D. "Definitive identification of magnetite nanoparticles in the abdomen of the honey bee *Apis mellifera*." *Journal of Physics: Conference Series*, 2005; 17 (1): 45–49.
210. Kuhn J, and Stever H. "Effects of high frequency electromagnetic fields on bee populations." [In German]. *Deutsches Bienen Journal* (German Bee Journal), 2002; 10 (4): 9–14.
211. Kirschvink J, Padmanabha S, Boyce C, and Oglesby J. "Measurement of the threshold sensitivity of honeybees to weak, extremely low-frequency magnetic fields." *Journal of Experimental Biology*, 1997; 200 (9): 1363–1368.
212. Warnke U. Bees, *Birds and Mankind. Destroying Nature by Electrosmog: Effects of Wireless Communication Technologies*. M von Luttichau (translator), a brochure series by the Competence Initiative for the Protection of Humanity, Environment and Democracy, Brochure 1. Stuttgart, Germany, March 2009.
[Online, accessed 2nd August, 2009].
URL:http://www.broshcuerenreihe.de/international/bees-birds-and-mankind/index.html
213. Warnke U. "Effects of electric charges on honeybees." *Bienenwelt* (Bee World), 1976; 57 (2): 50–56.
214. Altmann G, and Warnke U. "The metabolism of bees (*Apis mellifera* L) in 50 cycles per second high-voltage area." [In German]. *Zeitschrift fuer angewandte Entomologie* (Magazine for Applied Entomology: Germany), 1976; 80 (3): 267–271.
215. Korall H, Leucht T, and Martin H. "Bursts of magnetic fields induce jumps of misdirection in bees by a mechanism of magnetic resonance." *Journal of Comparative Physiology A: Neuroethology, Sensory, Neural and Behavioral Physiology*, 1988; 162 (3): 279–284.
216. Harst W, Kuhn J, and Stever H. "Can electromagnetic exposure cause a change in behaviour? Studying possible non-thermal influences on honey bees: an approach within the framework of educational informatics." *Acta Systemica*, 2006; 6 (1): 1–6.
217. Kimmel S, Kuhn J, Harst W, and Stever H. *Electromagnetic Radiation: Influences on Honeybees (Apis mellifera)*, Institute for Environmental Sciences, University of Koblenz, Landau Campus, Landau in der Pfalz, Germany, 2007.
[Online, accessed 2nd August 2009].
URL:http://agbi.uni-landau.de/material_download/preprint_IAAS_2007_pdf
218. Biesmeijer J, Roberts SPM, Reemer M, Ohlemueller R, Edwards M, Peeters T, Schaffers AP, Potts SG, Kleukers R, Thomas CD, Settele J, and Kunin WE. "Parallel declines in

pollinators and insect-pollinated plants in Britain and the Netherlands." *Science*, 2006; 313 (5785): 351–354.

219. Everaert J, and Bauwens D. "A possible effect of electromagnetic radiation from mobile phone base stations on the number of breeding house sparrows (*Passer domesticus*)." *Electromagnetic Biology and Medicine*, 2007; 26 (1): 63–72.

220. Balmori A. *The Effects of Microwave Radiation on the Wildlife: Preliminary Results*, Feb, 2003. [Online, accessed 2nd August, 2009]. URL:http//:www.buergerwelle.de/pdf/micro_waves_effects_on_wildlife _animals.pdf

221. Balmori A. "Possible effects of electromagnetic fields from phone masts on a population of white stork (Ciconia ciconia)." *Electromagnetic Biology and Medicine*, 2005; 24 (2): 109–119.

222. British Trust for Ornithology. *Missing! Ten Million House Sparrows*, Thetford, Norfolk, UK, 2003/2004, updated July, 2009.
[Online, accessed 2nd August, 2009].
URL: http://www.bto.org/appeals/house_sparrows.htm

223. Kelbie P. "Fall in sparrow numbers is reversed in Scotland." *The Independent*, UK, November 10, 2001.

224. Tanner JA. "Effect of microwave radiation on birds." *Nature*, 1966; 210 (5036): 636.

225. Tanner JA, Romero-Sierra C, and Davie SJ. "Non-thermal effects of microwave radiation on birds." *Nature*, Letters, 1967; 216 (5120): 1139.

226. Oberfeld G, Schimke H, and Bernatzky G. "Radiation from mobile phone base stations influences brain waves." [In German]. *Salzburger Landeskorrespondenz*, Salzburg District Government, Department of Environmental Medicine, Salzburg, Austria, 27 April, 2005.

227. Wolf R. and Wolf D. "Increased incidence of cancer near a cellphone transmitter station." *International Journal of Cancer Prevention*, 2004; 1 (2): 123–128.

228. Eber H, Hagen KU, Lucas B, Vogel P, and Voit H. "Influence of proximity to mobile telephony on the incidence of cancer." [In German].*Umwelt-Medizin-Gesellshaft* (Environmental Medicine Society, Germany) 2004; 17 (4): 326–332.

229. United States Environment Protection Agency. *An Evaluation of the Potential Carcinogenicity of Electromagnetic Fields (EMFs)*, June, 1990. Summary and conclusions of the draft report re-published by *Microwave News*, May/June 1990.
[Online, accessed 2nd August, 2009]. URL:http://www.microwavenews.com/epa.html

230. Portier CJ, and Wolfe MS (editors). *Assessment of Health Effects from Exposure to Power-line Frequency Electric and Magnetic Fields: Working Group Report*, National Institute for Environmental Health Science, Research Triangle Park, North Carolina, USA. National Institutes of Health, publication no. 98-3981, 16-24 June, 1998.
[Online, accessed 2nd August, 2009].
URL:http://www.niehs.nih.gov/health/topics/agents/emf/

231. World Health Organization, International Agency for Research on Cancer, *Non-ionizing Radiation, Part 1: Static and Extremely Low-Frequency (ELF) Electric and Magnetic Fields*, IARC Monographs on the Evaluation of Carcinogenic Risks to Humans, IARC Press, Lyon, France, 2002; volume 80, p. 338.

232. Elmer-Dewitt P. "Technology: hidden hazards of the airwaves." *Time* Magazine, 1990; 136 (5): 53.

233. Adey R, Linda L, Anderson L, Blackman C, Carpenter D, Feero W, Frazier M, Lovely R, Luben R, Misakien M, O'Connor ME, and Stevens R, (members of the NRCP Scientific Committee 89-3),*Extremely Low Frequency Electric and Magnetic Fields (Draft Report)*, 13 June, 1995. Summary and conclusions re-published in *Microwave News*, "Draft NCRP

report seeks strong action to curb EMFs: committee cites 2mG limit as goal." And, "Special report: NCRP draft recommendations on EMF exposure guidelines." July/August, 1995; 15 (4): 1, 11–15.
[Online, accessed 2nd August, 2009]. URL:http://www.microwavenews.com/ncrp1.html
234. Edwards R. "Leak links power lines to cancer." *New Scientist*, 7 October, 1995; p. 4.

CHAPTER 15—The Rape of Life

Quote of Abraham Lincoln: made in 1858, attributed to Abraham Lincoln by Fred Wheeler, cited in the *New York Times*, 26 August, 1887.

1. Food and Agriculture Organization (FAO) of the United Nations (UN). *The State of the World's Plant Genetic Resources for Food and Agriculture, Rome*, Italy, 1997, p. 14.
2. Penso G. *Inventory of Medicinal Plants and Compilation of a List of the Most Widely Used Plants*, World Health Organization document DPM/WP/78.2., Geneva, Switzerland, 1978.
3. FAO, ibid reference 1, p. 35.
4. Mooney P. "The massacre of Apple Lincoln." *New Internationalist*, October, 1990, issue 212.
5. Center for Biodiversity and Conservation, American Museum of Natural History, *Living with Biodiversity: Biodiversity and Your Food, A Guide for Green Consumers*, "Did you known that:", 1998.
[Online, accessed 8th August, 2009].
URL:http://cbc.amnh.org/center.pubs/pdfs/LivingWithBiodiversity-1998.pdf
6. FAO, ibid reference 1, p. 34.
7. Wilson EO. *The Diversity of Life*, Harvard University Press, Cambridge, Massachusetts, USA, 1992.
8. Cervigni R. *Biodiversity in the Balance: Land Use, National Development and Global Welfare*, Edgar Elgar Publishing Ltd, Cheltenham, Gloucestershire, UK, 2001.
9. Gaud WS. *The Green Revolution: Accomplishments and Apprehensions*, Address by the Honorable William S Gaud, Administrator, Agency for International Development, US Department of State, before the Society for International Development, Shorehan Hotel, Washington, DC, USA, on March 8, 1968, AgBioWorld, 2005.
[Online, accessed 8th August, 2009].
URL:http://www.agbioworld.org/biotech-info/topics/borlaug/borlaug-green.html
10. Dowie M. *American Foundations: An Investigative History*, The MIT Press, Cambridge, Massachusetts, USA, 2001: pp. 109–114.
11. Shand H. *Human Nature: Agricultural Biodiversity and Farm-Based Food Security*, an independent study prepared by Rural Advancement Foundation International (RAFI)—today, the Action Group on Erosion, Technology and Concentration (ETC Group)—for the Food and Agriculture Organization of the United Nations; Ottawa, Canada, December, 1997.
12. Food and Agriculture Organization (FAO) of the United Nations (UN). *Biological Diversity in Food and Agriculture: Domestic Animal Genetic Diversity*, D Pilling and B Rischkowsky (editors), Rome, Italy, 2007.
13. Seymour J. "Hungry for a new revolution," *New Scientist*, 1996; 149: 32–37.
14. Welch RM, Combs GF Jr, Duxbury JM. "Toward a 'Greener' Revolution." *Issues in Science and Technology*, 1997; 14 (1): 50–58.
15. Schroder B, Marks N. "The retailer-driven UK food industry: structure, performance and

implications for Australia" *Australasian Agribusiness Review*: vol 4, no. 2, 1996.
[Online, accessed 8th August, 2009].
URL:http://www.agrifood.info/review/1996/Shroder.html

16. ETC Group (Action Group on Erosion, Technology and Concentration [formerly, Rural Advancement Foundation International [RAFI]). "Global seed concentration." *ETC Group Communique,* Ottawa, Canada, September/October 2005; Issue 90.
[Online, accessed 8th August, 2009].
URL:http://www.etcgroup.org/documents/Comm90GlobalSeed.pdf

17. Cañada E. "Food sovereignty: the people's alternative." *Progressio*, Catholic Institute for International Relations, London, UK, October, 2006.
[Online, accessed 8th August, 2009].
URL:http://ciin.org/progressio/s/basket/93391/food_sovereignty/

18. Delforce R, Dickson A, and Hogan J. "Australia's food industry: recent changes and challenges." *Australian Commodities*, 2005; 12 (2): 379–390.

19. National Association of Retail Grocers of Australia (NARGA). Editorial: *Who determines grocery market shares?* 5 August, 2005.
[Online, accessed 8th August, 2009]. URL:http://www.narga.net.au/index.php?paged=2

20. Halweil B. "Home-grown: the case for local food in a global market." *Worldwatch Paper*, no. 163, Worldwatch Institute, Washington, DC, USA, November, 2002.

21. Hawtin GC. "Maintaining a diversity of crops and varieties is a key to survival for millions of farmers living on impoverished land." *UNESCO Courier*, 1 May, 2000.

22. Siddle HV, Kreiss A, Eldridge MD, Noonan E, Clarke CJ, Pyecroft S, Woods GM, and Belov K. "Transmission of a fatal clonal tumour by biting occurs due to depleted MHC diversity in a threatened carnivorous marsupial." *Proceedings of the National Academy of Sciences of the United States of America*, 2007; 104 (41): 16221–6.

23. Nettle D, and Romaine S. *Vanishing Voices: The Extinction of the World's Languages*, Oxford University Press, New York, NY, USA, 2000.

24. M Walsh and C Yallop (editors). *Language and Culture in Aboriginal Australia*, Aboriginal Studies Press, Canberra, ACT, Australia, 1993.

25. US Supreme Court. *Diamond v. Chakrabarty: Diamond, Commissioner of Patents and Trademarks v. Chakrabarty, Certiorari to the United States Court of Customs and Patent Appeals. 447 United States Reports*, 1980; 303, no. 79-136. Argued March 17, 1980; decided June 16, 1980.
[Online, accessed 8th August, 2009].
URL:http://caselaw.lp.findlaw.com/scripts/getcase.pl?court=us&vol=447&invol=303

26. United Kingdom Parliament, House of Commons Select Committee on Environmental Audit, Appendix to the Minutes of Evidence (Appendix 7), *Trade Related Intellectual Property Rights (TRIPS) and Farmers' Rights, Session 1998-99*.
[Online, accessed 8th August, 2009].
URL:http://www.publications.parliament.uk.pa.cm199900/cmselect/cmenaud/45/45ap08.htm

27. United Nations Development Programme, Global Policy Forum, Human Development Report: *Reducing the Gap between the Knows and the Know-Nots*, New York, NY, USA, July 12, 1999.

28. Watkins K, and Fowler P. *Rigged Rules and Double Standards: Trade, Globalisation and the Fight Against Poverty*, Oxfam Publishing, Oxfam International, Oxford, UK; Chapter 8: "International rules as an obstacle to development", 2002, pp. 222–231.

29. Meek J. "The race to buy life." *The Guardian* (UK), 15 November, 2000. Cited in: *The Ethics*

of Patenting DNA: A Discussion Paper, Nuffield Council on Bioethics, London, UK, July, 2002, p. 5.

30. Torrance AW. "After the Gene Rush." *Bio-IT World*, Cambridge Healthtech Institute, Cambridge, Massachusetts, USA; November 12, 2002.
[Online, accessed 8th August, 2009].
URL:http://www.bio-itworld.com/archive/111202/insights_rush.html

31. Jensen K, and Murray F. "Intellectual property landscape of the human genome." *Science*, 2005; 310 (5746): 239–240.

32. "Patents on life: the facts." *New Internationalist*. September 2002; issue 349.

33. Martin-Rendon E, and Blake DJ. "Patenting human genes and stem cells." *Recent Patents on DNA and Gene Sequences*, 2007; 1 (1): 25–34.

34. Yanez RJ, and Porter ACG. "A chromosomal position effect on gene targeting in human cells." *Nucleic Acid Research*, 2002; 30 (22): 4892–4901.

35. Ho M-W, Ryan A, and Cummins J. "Cauliflower mosaic viral promoter: a recipe for disaster?" *Microbial Ecology in Health and Disease*, 1999; 11 (4): 194–197.

36. Alliance for Bio-Integrity. *Key FDA Documents Revealing: (1) Hazards of Genetically Engineered Foods, and (2) Flaws With How the Agency Made Its Policy*, Fairfield, Iowa, USA, 2000.
[Online, accessed 8th August, 2009]. URL:http://www.biointegrity.org/list.htm

37. Druker SM. Executive Summary: *How the US Food and Drug Administration Approved Genetically Engineered Foods Despite the Deaths One Had Caused and the Warnings of Its Own Scientists About Their Unique Risks*, Alliance for Bio-Integrity, Fairfield, Iowa, USA, 2000.
[Online, accessed 8th August, 2009].,URL:
http://www.biointegrity.org/execsummaryoecd.html

38. Maryanski J. "Genetically engineered foods: fears and facts." *FDA Consumer*, January-February, 1993, p.14.

39. MacKay AW (Judge). *Monsanto Canada Inc. and Monsanto Company, and, Percy Schmeiser and Schmeiser Enterprises Ltd*, "Reasons for Judgment", Federal Court of Canada, Ottawa, Ontario, Canada. Neutral citation: 2001FCT256; March 29, 2001.
[Online, accessed 8th August, 2009].
URL: http://www.percyschmeiser.com/T1593-98-%20 Decision.pdf

40. Phillips PWB, and Corkindale D. "Marketing GM foods: the way forward." *AgBioForum*, 2003; 5 (3): 113–121.

41. Greenpeace Canada. *Life is not a commodity: plants, animals, humans and genes should not be patented*, Toronto, Ontario, Canada, 2006.
[Online, accessed 3rd March, 2010].
URL: http://www.greenpeace.org/canada/en/campaigns/ge

42. Southwood R, Epstein MA, Martin WB, and Walton J. *Report of the Working Party on Bovine Spongiform Encephalopathy (the 'Southwood Report')*." UK Department of Health, and the Ministry of Agriculture, Fisheries and Food, published by HMSO, London, UK, 1989.

43. Arpad Pusztai's homepage, 2000. *Correspondence with the Royal Society*.
[Online, accessed 8th August, 2009].
URL:http://www.freenetpages.co.uk/hp/A.Pusztai/index.htm

44. Editorial, *The Lancet*, 29 May, 1999; 353 (9167): 1811.

45. British Medical Association, Board of Education and Science. *Impact of Genetic Modfication on Agriculture, Food and Health: An Interim Statement*. 18 May, 1999.
[Online, accessed 8th August, 2009].
URL:http://www.globalreality.com/biotech/articles/othernews012.htm

46. *Open Letter from World Scientists to All Governments Concerning Genetically Modified Organisms (GMOs)*. Institute of Science in Society, London, UK, 2000.
    [Online, accessed 8th August, 2009].
    URL:http://www.i-sis.org.uk/list.php
47. Barnett A. "GM genes 'jump species barrier' ". *The Observer* (UK), May 28, 2000.
48. Reiche R, Horn U, Wolfl S, Dorn W, Kaatz HH. "The bee as a vector of gene transfer from transgenic plants into the environment." [In French], *Apidologie* (France), 1998; 29 (5): 401–403.
49. Gebhard F, and Smalla K. "Monitoring field releases of genetically modified sugar beets for persistence of transgenic plant DNA and horizontal gene transfer." *FEMS Microbiology Ecology*, 1999; 28 (3): 261–272.
50. Fulponi L. "Ethics and economics of labelling: the case of genetically engineered foods." Directorate for Food, Agriculture and Fisheries, Organisation for Economic Co-operation and Development, Paris, France. In: *Eursafe 2001: Food Safety, Food Quality, and Food Ethics*, The Third Congress of the European Society for Agricultural and Food Ethics, 3–5 October, 2001, Florence, Italy, pp. 234–237.
51. Food Standards Australia New Zealand (FZANZ). *Australia New Zealand Food Standards Code*, "Standard 1.5.2., Food Produced Using Gene Technology", issue 103, and issue 114, Commonwealth of Australia, and Anstat Pty Ltd, South Melbourne, Victoria, Australia, 2010.
52. Australia and New Zealand Food Authority. ANZFA Occasional Papers, Series No. 1; *GM Foods and the Consumer*, ANZFA, Canberra, ACT, Australia, June 2000.
53. Gene-Ethics Network Northern Rivers, *Australian GE Food Guide*, February 2000.
    [Online, accessed 1st May, 2001].
    URL:http://www.nor.com.au/environment/genethic/foodguide.html
54. Ho M-W. *GM Soya Fed Rats: Stunted, Dead, or Sterile*. Institute of Science in Society (ISIS), London, UK. ISIS press release, 28 November, 2006.
    [Online, accessed 8th August, 2009].
    URL:http//:www.i-sis.org.uk/GM_Soya_Fed_Rats.php
55. Fagan JB. *Tryptophan Summary*, Website of Physicians and Scientists for Responsible Application of Science and Technology (PSRAST), 1997.
    [Online, accessed 8th August, 2009]. URL:http://www.psrast.org/jftrypt.htm
56. Physicians and Scientists for Responsible Application of Science and Technology (PSRAST). *The Showa Denko Tryptophan Disaster: New Evidence Indicates That Genetic Engineering Was The Most Probable Cause*, 2007.
    [Online, accessed 8th August, 2009]. URL:http://www.psrast.org/demsd.htm
57. Raphals P. "Does medical mystery threaten biotech?" *Science*, 1990; 250 (4981): 619.
58. Crist WE. *Deadly Toxic L-Tryptophan: Shedding Light on a Mysterious Epidemic*, 2005. On website of: Institute for Responsible Technology, Fairfield, Iowa, USA.
    [Online, accessed 8th August, 2009].
    URL:http://www.seedsofdeception.com/Public/Ltryptophan/1Introduction/index.cfm
59. Nowak R. "Killer virus: an engineered mouse virus leaves us one step away from the ultimate bioweapon." *New Scientist*, 2001; January 13: 4–5.
60. Ho M-W, Cummins J, and Bartlett J. *The Killing Fields: Terminator Crops At Large*, Institute of Science in Society, London, UK, 1999.
    [Online, accessed 8th August, 2009].
    URL:http://www.i-sis.org.uk/terminatorstory-pr.php?printing=yes
61. Wald G. "The case against genetic engineering." In: DA Jackson and SP Stitch (editors),

The Recombinant DNA Debate, Prentice Hall, Englewood Cliffs, New Jersey, USA, 1979, pp. 127–128. (Reprinted from *Sciences*, 1976; 16: 6–11).

62. Jha A (presenter), Duckworth A (producer). Podcast, "Science Weekly: The world's first artificial life form." *The Guardian* (UK), Friday 21 May, 2010.
    [Online, accessed 23rd May, 2010].
    URL:http://www.guardian.co.uk/science/blog/audio/2010/may/21/science-weekly-podcast-artificial-life-form

63. Food and Agriculture Organization of the United Nations (FAO). *World Agriculture: Towards 2015/30,* Interim Report, Prospects for Food, Nutrition, Agriculture and Major Commodity Groups, Global Perspectives Studies Unit, FAO, Rome, Italy, 2006, pp. 1–15.

64. Food and Water Watch. *Status of food irradiation around the world.* November 2006.
    [Online, accessed 8th August, 2009].
    URL:http://documents.foodandwaterwatch.org/World%20Irradiation%20Report.pdf

65. European Union. "List of Member States' authorisations of food and food ingredients which may be treated with ionising radiation." *Official Journal of the European Union*, 24 November, 2009, C283/5.
    [Online, accessed 8th August, 2009].
    URL:http://eur-lex.europa.eu/LexUriServ/LexUriServ.do?uri=OJ:C:2009:283:0005:0005:EN:PDF

66. Carslaw N. "Shops breaking irradiation food laws." *BBC News*, 23 March, 2001.
    [Online, accessed 8th August, 2009].
    URL:http://news.bbc.co.uk/2/hi/uk_news/1236485.stm

67. UK Food Standards Agency. *Irradiated food supplements: enforcement exercise.* Wednesday 1 February, 2006. [Online, accessed 9th August, 2009].
    URL:http://www.food.gov.uk/multimedia/pdfs/ifsenforcementexercise.pdf

68. Food Safety Authority of Ireland. Survey of Noodle Products for Evidence of Irradiation 2005, March 2006.
    [Online, accessed 9th August, 2009].
    URL:http://www.fsai.ie/uploadedFiles/Irradiation_Noodle_2005.PDF

69. US Food and Drug Administration. *Foods Permitted to be Irradiated under FDA Regulations (21 CFR 179.26).* September 2008.
    [Online, accessed 9th August, 2009].
    URL:http://www.fda.gov/Food/FoodIngredientsPackaging/IrradiatedFoodPackaging/ucm074734.htm

70. Commonwealth of Australia, Food Standards Australia New Zealand (FSANZ). *Australia New Zealand Food Standards Code*, Chapter 1, Part 1.5, Standard 1.5.3. "Irradiation of Food", FSANZ, Barton, Canberra, ACT, Australia. Published by Anstat Pty Ltd, South Melbourne, Victoria, Australia, 2010.

71. Worth M, and Jenkins P. *Hidden Harm: How the FDA is Ignoring the Potential Dangers of Unique Chemicals in Irradiated Food*, A special report by Public Citizen and the Center for Food Safety, Washington, D.C. USA, December, 2001.
    [Online, accessed 8th August, 2009].
    URL:http://www.citizen.org/cmep/foodsafety/foodirrad/index.cfm?=18catID=1148secID=1269

72. LeTellier PR, and Nawar WW. "2-alkylcyclobutanones from the radiolysis of triglycerides." *Lipids*, 1972; 7: 75–76. Cited in Worth M, and Jenkins P, ibid reference 70.

73. Stevenson MH, Crone AVJ, and Hamilton JTG. "Irradiation detection." *Nature*, March 15, 1990; 344 (6263) : 202–203. Cited in Worth M, and Jenkins P, ibid reference 70.

74. Victoria A, Crone AVJ, Hamilton JTG, and Stevenson MH. "Detection of 2-

dodecylcyclobutanone in radiation-sterilized chicken meat stored for several years." *International Journal of Food Science and Technology*, December 17, 1992; 27 (6): 691–696. Cited in Worth M, and Jenkins P, ibid reference 70.

75. Stevenson MH. "Progress in the identification of irradiated foods." *Trends in Food Science and Technology*, 1992; 3: 257–262. Cited in Worth M, and Jenkins P, ibid reference 70.
76. Crone AVJ, Hand MV, Hamilton JTG, Sharma ND, Boyd DR, and Stevenson MH. "Synthesis, characterization and use of 2-tetradecylcyclobutanone together with other cyclobutanones as markers for irradiated liquid whole egg." *Journal of the Science of Food and Agriculture*, 1993; 62 (4): 361–367. Cited in Worth M, and Jenkins P, ibid reference 70.
77. Stevenson MH, Crone AVJ, Hamilton JTG, and McMurray CH. "The use of 2-dodecylcylobutanone for the identification of irradiated chicken meat and eggs." *Radiation Physics and Chemistry*, 1993; 42 (1–3): 363–366.
78. Stevenson MH. "Identification of irradiated foods." *Food Technology*, 1994; 48 (5): 141–144, 1993.
79. Stewart EM, Moore S, Graham WD, McRoberts WC, and Hamilton JTG. "2-alkylcylobutanonees as markers for the detection of irradiated   mango, papaya, Camembert cheese and salmon meat." *Journal of the Science of Food and Agriculture*, 80 (1): 121–130, 2000.
80. Lembke P, Boernert J, and Engelhardt H. "Characterization of irradiated food by SFE and GC-MSD." *Journal of Agricultural and Food Chemistry*, 43 (1): 38–45, 1995.
81. Delincee H, and Pool-Zobel B-L. "Genotoxic properties of 2-dodecylcyclobutanone, a compound formed on irradiation of food containing fat." *Radiation Physics and Chemistry*, 52 (1–6): 39–42, 1998.
82. Delincee H, Pool-Zobel BL, and Rechkemmer G. "Genotoxicity of 2-dodecylcyclobutanone." *Food Irradiation: Fifth German Conference*, Report EFE-R-99-01, Federal Nutrition Research Institute, Karlsruhe, Germany, November 11–13, 1998.
83. Delincee H, Soika C, Horvatovich P, Rechkemmer G, and Marchioni E. "Genotoxicity of 2-alkylcyclobutanones, markers for an irradiation   treatment in fat-containing food. Part 1: Cyto-and genotoxic potential of 2-tetradecylcyclobutanone." *Radiation Physics and Chemistry*, 2002; 63 (3–6): 431–435.
84. Public Citizen, and the Global Resource Action Center for the Environment (GRACE). *Bad Taste: The Disturbing Truth About the World Health Organization's Endorsement of Food Irradiation*, A special report by Public Citizen (Washington, DC) and GRACE (New York, NY, USA)), prepared by M Worth, October 2002.
[Online, accessed 8th August, 2009].
URL:http://www.citizen.org/documents/BadTaste.pdf
85. Poling CE, Warner WD, Humburg FR, Reber EF, Urbain WM, and Rice EE. "Growth, reproduction, survival and histopathology of rats fed beef irradiated with electrons." *Food Research*, 1955; 20 (3): 193–214.
86. Metta VC, Marmeesh MS, and Johnson BC. "Vitamin K deficiency in rats induced by feeding of irradiated beef." *Journal of Nutrition*, 1959; 69: 18–21.
87. Mellette SJ, and Leone LA. "Influence of age, sex, strain of rat and fat soluble vitamins on hemorrhagic syndromes in rats fed irradiated beef." *Federation Proceedings* [Federation of American Societies for Experimental Biology], 1960; 19 (4): 1045–1049.
88. Swaminathan MS, Nirula S, Natarajan AT, and Sharma RP. "Mutations: Incidence in *Drosophila melanogaster* reared on irradiated medium." *Science*, 1963; 141 (3581): 637–638.
89. Rinehart RR, and Ratty FJ. "Mutation in *Drosophila melanogaster* cultured on irradiated food." *Genetics*, 1965; 52 (6): 1119–1126.

90. Lofroth G, Hanngren K, Ehrenberg L, and Ehrenberg A. "Biological effects of irradiated food. II: Chemical and biological studies of compounds distilled from irradiated food." [In German]. *Arkiv Zoologie* (Germany), 1966; 18: 529–547.
91. Rinehart RR, and Ratty FJ. "Mutation in *Drosophila melanogaster* cultured on irradiated whole food or food components." *International Journal of Radiation Biology*, 1967; 12 (4): 347–354.
92. Spiher AT. "Food irradiation: An FDA report." *FDA Papers*, October, 1968.
93. Schubert J. "Mutagenicity and cytotoxicity of irradiated foods and food components." *Bulletin of the World Health Organization*, 1969; 41: 873–904.
94. Moutschen-Dahmen M, Moutschen J, and Ehrenberg L. "Pre-implantation death of mouse eggs caused by irradiated food." *International Journal of Radiation Biology*, 1970; 18 (3): 201–216.
95. Tinsley IJ, Bone FJ, and Bubl EC. "The growth , reproduction, longevity, and histopathology of rats fed gamma-irradiated carrots." *Toxicology and Applied Pharmacology*, 1970; 16 (7): 306–317.
96. Kesavan PC, and Swaminathan MS. "Cytotoxic and mutagenic effects of irradiated substrates and food material." *Radiation Biology* (India), 1971; 11 (4): 253–281.
97. Reichelt D, Renner HW, and Diehl JF. *Long-term Animal Feeding Study for Testing the Wholesomeness of an Irradiated Diet With a High Content of Free Radicals*, [In German]. Federal Research Institute for Food Preservation, Technical Report No. BFL-3/1972, Institute for Radiation Technology, Karlsruhe, Gemany, 1 January, 1972.
98. Bhaskaran C, and Sadasivan G. "Effects of irradiated wheat to malnourished children." *American Journal of Clinical Nutrition*, 1975; 28: 130–135.
99. Vijayalaxmi, and Sadasivan G. "Chromosomal aberrations in rats fed irradiated wheat." *International Journal of Radiation Biology*, 1975; 27 (2): 135–142.
100. Johnson-Arthur T, Brena-Valle M, Turanitz K, Hruby R, and Stehlik G. "Mutagenicity of irradiated food in the host mediated assay system." [In German]. *Studia Biophyica* (Germany), 1975; 50: 137–141.
101. Vijayalaxmi. "Genetic effects of feeding irradiated wheat to mice." *Canadian Journal of Genetics and Cytology*, 1976; 18 (2): 231–238.
102. Vijayalaxmi, and Rao KV. "Dominant lethal mutations in rats fed on irradiated wheat." *International Journal of Radiation Biology*, 1976; 29 (1): 93–98.
103. Renner HW. "Chromosome studies on bone marrow cells of Chinese hamsters fed a radiosterilized diet." *Toxicology*, 1977; 8 (2): 213–222.
104. Vijayalaxmi,. Cytogenic studies in monkeys fed irradiated wheat." *Toxicology*, 1978; 9: 181–184.
105. Vijayalaxmi. "Immune response in rats given irradiated wheat." *British Journal of Nutrition*, 1978; 40: 535–541.
106. Lusskin RM. *Evaluation of the Mutagenicity of Irradiated Sterilized Chicken by the Sex-linked Recessive Lethal Test in Drosophila melanogaster*, Raltech Scientific Services Inc, Madison, Wisconsin, USA, Final report submitted to the US Army Medical Research and Development Command, Fort Detrick, Maryland, USA, 15 June, 1979.
107. Anderson D, Clapp MJ, Hodge MC, and Weight TM. "Irradiated laboratory animal diets: Dominant lethal studies in the mouse." *Mutation Research*, 1981; 80 (2): 333–345.
108. Renner HW, Graf U, Wurgler FE, Altmann H, Asquith JC, and Elias PS. "An investigation of the genetic toxicology of irradiated foodstuffs using short-term test systems. III: In vivo tests in small rodents and in *Drosophila melanogaster*." *Food Chemistry and Toxicology*, 1982; 20 (6): 867–878.

109. Raul F, Gosse F, Delincee H, Hartwig A, Marchioni E, Mische H, and Werner D. "Food-borne radiolytic compounds (2-alkylcyclobutanones) may promote experimental colon carcinogenesis." *Nutrition and Cancer*, 2002; 44 (2): 198–191.
110. FAO/WHO/Codex Alimentarius Commission. *Report of the 33rd Session of the Codex Committee on Food Additives and Contaminants*, Joint report of the FAO/WHO Food Standards Programme, Rome, Italy, and the Codex Alimentarius Commission, Rome, Italy, Report No. FAO-ESN-ALINORM 01/12A, The Hague, The Netherlands, March 12–16, 2001, p. 11.
111. FAO/IAEA/WHO. *Wholesomeness of Irradiated Food. Report of a Joint FAO/IAEA/WHO Expert Committee*, World Health Organization Technical Report No. 659. Geneva, Switzerland, 1981.
112. FAO/IAEA/WHO. *High-dose Irradiation: Wholesomeness of Food Irradiated With Doses Above 10 kGy. Report of a Joint FAO/IAEA/WHO Study Group*, World Health Organization Technical Report Series No. 890, Geneva, Switzerland, 1999, p. 48.
113. Food Irradiation Watch. "Irradiation of cat food banned: call for total ban on food irradiation." Food Irradiation Watch, (affiliated with Friends of the Earth Australia), West End, Brisbane, Queensland, Australia, 2008.
    [Online, accessed March 15th, 2010].
    URL:http://www.foodirradiationinfo.org/index.html
114. Burke K. "Cat deaths linked to pet food." *Sydney Morning Herald*, November 24, 2008.
115. Burke K. "Cat-food irradiation banned as pet theory proved." *Sydney Morning Herald*, May 30, 2009.
116. Feynman RP. "There's plenty of room at the bottom." Talk presented to the American Physical Society at the California Institute of Technology (Caltech) on 29 December, 1959. First published in Caltech's *Engineering and Science*, 1960; 23 (5): 22–36.
117. Woodrow Wilson International Center for Scholars, and the Pew Charitable Trusts. *An Inventory of Nanotechnology-Based Consumer Products Currently on the Market*, The Project on Emerging Nanotechnologies, Washington, DC, USA, October, 2007.
    [Online, accessed 8th August, 2009].
    URL:http://www.nanotechnproject.org/inventories/consumer
118. Borm PJ, Robbins D, Haubold S, Kuhlbusch T, Fissan H, Donaldson K, Schins R, Stone V, Kreyling W, Lademann J, Krutmann J, Warheit D, and Oberdorster E. "The potential risks of nanomaterials: a review carried out for ECETOC [European Centre for Ecotoxicology and Toxicology of Chemicals, Brussels, Belgium]." *Particle and Fibre Toxicology*, 2006; 3: 11.
119. Hardman R. "A toxicologic review of quantum dots: toxicity depends on physicochemical and environmental factors." *Environmental Health Perspectives*, 2006; 114 (2): 165–172.
120. Oberdorster G, Sharp Z, Atudorei V, Elder A, Gelein R, Kreyling W, and Cox C. "Translocation of inhaled ultrafine particles to the brain." *Inhalation Toxicology*, 2004; 16 (6–7): 437–445.
121. Elder A, Gelein R, Silva V, Feikert T, Opanashuk L, Carter J, Potter R, Maynard A, Ito Y, Finkelstein J, and Oberdorster G. "Translocation of inhaled ultrafine manganese oxide particles to the central nervous system." *Environmental Health Perspectives*, 2006; 114 (8): 1172–1178.
122. Sample I. "Research on tiny particles could damage brain, scientists warn." *The Guardian* (UK), 9 January, 2004.
123. ETC Group. *Down on the Farm: The Impact of Nano-Scale Technologies on Food and Agriculture*, Action Group on Erosion, Technology and Concentration (ETC Group), Ottawa, Ontario, Canada; November 2004: p. 63.

[Online, accessed 8th August, 2009].
URL:http://www.etcgroup.org/en/materials/publications.html?.pub_id=80
124. Rinehart RR, and Ratty FJ, ibid reference 90, pp. 11–13.

Index

Aboriginal people, 20, 43, 100, 101, 177, 178, 240
  before European invasion, 177, 178
  diseases of, 43, 100, 101, 177, 178
  health of, 100, 101
  languages of, 177, 178
  psychosocial health of, 178
abortions, therapeutic, 71, 72
acausal connections, 77, 104, 129–139
Access Economics, 18
acid/alkaline balance, 166
acute illnesses, 35, 102, 147, 148, 151
adaptation, human
  to foods, 185
  to micro-organisms, 185, 186
  to milk, 185
  to sunlight, 185
Addison's disease, 187
adrenal exhaustion, 207
Aeschylus, 115
Africa, 20, 59, 61, 63, 68, 79, 85–87, 95, 104, 105, 124, 181, 182, 185, 186, 238
aging of the population, 167,
Agrarian Revolution, 177,
  benefits of, 181, 182
  costs of, 182–185
  diseases of, 177, 185, 186
  human roles in, 182,
  staple foods of, 182
agro-chemical industry, 188, 244,
Ahold, 227,
AIDS (*see also* HIV), 103–107
air, 21, 60, 77, 115, 128, 131, 132, 143, 147, 151, 155, 157, 159, 165, 170, 176, 180, 188, 189, 191, 195, 197, 199, 200, 218, 219, 243
Alaska Department of Health and Social Services, 67
Albertsons, 227
Algorithms, 161
Allan, Dr Beverley, 71
allergies (*see also* anaphylaxis), 18, 97, 102, 103
  statistics on, 18
Alliance for Bio-Integrity, 232
Altman, Dr, 76
aluminium, 197
  aluminium sulphate (alum), 78
Alzheimer's disease, 61, 188, 209
American Academy of Pediatrics, 79, 99

American Medical Association, 26, 86, 99
American Public Health Association, 84
Amish, 40, 73
amyotrophic lateral sclerosis (Lou Gerig's disease), 97, 108, 109, 188, 209, 221
anabolic/catabolic processes, 165, 166
anaemia, 177, 186, 226
  iron-deficiency, 177
  sickle-cell, 186
anaphylaxis, statistics on, 18, 97
ancient civilisations and communities, 125
  Akkadia, 183
  Assyria, 183
  Babylonia, 183
  Crete, 183
  Egypt, 28, 44
  Greece, 114, 115, 118, 132, 151, 219, 221
  Indus Valley, 183
  Mediaeval Europe, 122, 184
  Norte Chico (Peru), 183
  Rome, 44, 183, 212
  Skara Brae (Orkney), 183
  Sumer, 132, 183
Andersen, Hans Christian, 221
Angell, Professor Marcia, 38
antibiotics (*see* drugs, antibiotics)
Anticancer Research, 94
antimony, 29
anxiety (*see* mental health, anxiety)
appendicitis, 20
apples, 128, 190, 223–225, 239
Archer Daniels Midland, 227
Argentina, 73
Aristotle, 112–116, 125, 137, 161, 172
arsenic (*see also* drugs, arsenic), 27, 29, 37, 76, 80
arthritis, 18, 34, 39, 103, 108, 149, 177, 186, 187
  in hunters and gatherers, 177, 186
  osteoarthritis, 177, 186
  rheumatoid arthritis, 187
  statistics on, 18
Arysta LifeScience Corp, 227
ascorbic acid (*see* vitamins, vitamin C)
Asia, 61, 69, 79, 95, 181, 182, 185, 224
aspartame, 96
Asperger's syndrome, 18, 98
aspirin (*see* drugs, aspirin)

asthenic (*see* sthenic/asthenic responses)
asthma, 18, 20, 29, 35, 39, 40, 76, 97, 99, 102, 103
   statistics on, 18
astrology, 129, 132, 136
attention deficit/ hyperactivity disorder (ADHD), 39, 40, 41
aubergine (*see* egg plants)
Australia, 17–26, 30, 31, 47, 52, 63, 64, 69, 71, 73, 76, 78, 84, 87–92, 94, 100
AusDiab study, 17,
Australasian Society of Clinical Immunology, 18
Australian Bureau of Statistics, 19,
Australian High Court Ruling: Rogers v. Whitaker, 47
Austria, 220, 221
autism, 18, 39 –41, 47, 61, 72, 90, 97–99, 188, 198
   statistics on, 18
autoimmune disease (*see also* arthritis–rheumatoid, type I diabetes, multiple sclerosis, systemic lupus erythematosus), 18, 97, 102, 103, 108, 198
   statistics on, 18
Avicenna (Ibn Sina), 172
Ayurveda (*see* medical systems)
babies, 34, 44, 64, 69–73, 100, 103, 172, 176, 179, 180, 185, 194, 195, 210
   as a reference point for health, 176,
   instincts of, 171–173, 176
Backster, Dr Cleve, 154
Bacon, Francis, 118, 172
Baker, Professor Robin, 157
balance problems, 101, 144, 146
Balmori, Dr Alfonso, 219
Bantu, 20
BASF, 244
Bateson, Professor Gregory, 127, 160
Bayer, 227
Bayer CropScience, 227, 224
Becker, Professor Robert, 203, 204, 208
beef, 189, 234, 239, 240
bees, 189, 218, 219, 235
   population decline of, 218,
beets, 224
Behaviourism, 171
Belgium, 55, 219, 221, 224, 238
Bellis, Professor Mark, 157
benzethonium chloride, 96
Berkeley, Bishop George, 172
beta-propiolactone, 96
Big Bang, 121, 141, 159, 160
bio-monitoring studies, 190, 193–195

biopiracy, 235
birds, 153, 154, 169, 204, 218
   population decline of, 219
birth defects (*see* foetal abnormalities)
birthweight, low, 210
Biskind, Dr Morton, 77
bladder, 123, 133, 157, 166
Blair, Prime Minister Tony, 49
blood-brain barrier, 207, 214, 215
blood cell disturbances, 186, 207, 208, 241
blood sugar disturbances (*see also* diabetes), 207
Bohm, Professor David, 160
Boerhaave, Dr Herman, 76
Bohr, Professor Niels, 20
Bolivians, 20
Boltzmann, Professor Ludwig, 160
Bonaparte, Napoleon, 74, 76
Bonine, Professor John, 196
borax, 96
boron, 226
bovine spongiform encephalopathy (BSE), 234
bowels (*see* gastro-intestinal tract), 74
brain damage, 190, 242
brain waves (*see* electromagnetism, effect on brain waves), 220, 216
Brazil, 20, 73, 104, 238
Bright's disease, 137
British Association for the Advancement of Science, 45
British Medical Association, 234
British Medical Journal, The, 24, 78, 246
British Minstry of Defence, 108
British Ministry of Health, 78
Brodie, Dr Maurice, 80
brominated flame retardants, 180, 194
Brunet, Dr Laura, 102
Bruno, Dr Richard, 89, 90
Buddhism, 113
   Buddha nature, 162
bubonic plague, 44, 184
Bulletin of the American Association of Public Health Physicians, 85
Bunge, 227
Burnet, Dr Frank Macfarlane, 107
Bush, President George Herbert Walker, 222, 232
Byron, Lord George Gordon, 128
cabbages, 223
cadmium, 193
Calgene,233
California Department of Health Services, 221

camelpox, 52
Cameroon, 52
Campbell, Professor Joseph, 115
Campbell Soup, 244
Canada, 17, 20, 26, 49, 53, 69, 70, 72, 82, 83, 86, 106, 108, 233, 234
cancer
   acoustic neuroma, 216, 217
   bowel cancer, 17, 19–21, 241
   brain cancer, 17, 85, 91–93, 97, 98, 189, 209, 210, 212, 216, 217, 221
      astrocytoma, 92, 98
      glioblastoma, 92, 93, 209, 216, 217
      ependymoma, 91
      medulloblastoma, 91–93
   breast cancer
      in women, 17, 21, 103, 191, 207, 209, 211
      in men, 209, 210
   childhood cancer, 17, 98, 210, 211, 212, 221
   Kaposi's sarcoma, 105
   leukaemia, 97, 98, 189, 207, 209–212, 221
   lung cancer, 17, 92, 217
   melanoma, 17, 103, 211, 212
   mesothelioma, 92, 217
   myeloma, 17, 103
   neuroblastoma, 98
   non-Hodgkin's lymphoma, 17, 92, 93, 95, 97, 209, 210, 212, 214, 215
   osteosarcoma, 92, 98
   ovarian cancer, 102, 103
   prostate cancer, 17, 103
   retinoblastoma, 98
   rhabdomyosarcoma, 98
   sarcoma, 210, 215
   squamous cell carcinoma, 215
   statistics on various cancers, 17
Cancer Council of South Australia, 17
canola 233 - 235
Cantwell, Dr Alan, 107
Carbone, Professor Michele, 92, 95
carbon monoxide, 76
carbon tetrachloride, 77
cardiovascular disease/ disturbances, 17, 19, 21, 22, 36, 96, 220
Cargill, 227, 244
Carrefour, 227
Carson, Dr Rachel, 189
CAS (Chemical Abstracts Service) Registry, 192
catabolic processes (*see* anabolic/catabolic processes), 165, 166
cataracts, 69, 72, 208

cauliflower mosaic virus, (CaMV 35S) 230, 231
Caverly, Dr Charles, 74, 75
cereals (*see also* maize, millet, oats, rice, sorghum, wheat), 225, 227, 228, 238
cerebral palsy, 97
Chakravarty, Professor Ananda, 229
chance, blind, 130
   in evolution of life, 158–160
   in formation of insulin, 159
   in formation of proteins, 159
   in formation of DNA, 159
   in universe evolving, 160, 161
chaos theory, 121, 125, 140
cheese (*see* dairy products), 192, 240
chemical- and drug-resistant micro-organisms, 107, 129, 165, 166, 183, 236
chemicals
   carcinogenic, 54, 86, 96, 190, 196
   mutagenic, 39, 96
   neurotoxic, 96, 184
chemicals, synthetic/ man-made, 192, 197
   children's vulnerability to, 36, 194, 195, 197, 198
   in food, 21, 165, 180, 188–197, 231, 239–242, 244
   in water, 180, 187, 195–197
   number of, 20, 192, 193, 197
   safety of, 193–198
   synergy of, 96, 196
   tests on, 193–197
chemical weapons, 108, 190
Cherry, Professor Niel, 211, 212, 222
chickenpox, 48, 69, 185
Chile, 73
chimpanzees, 28, 104, 182
China, 19, 28, 33, 56, 60, 68, 92, 132, 182, 221, 224, 238
chloral benzene, 77
chlorinated compounds, 188
cholera, 44, 45, 80, 184
Chomsky, Professor Noam, 173
Chopra, Dr Deepak, 128,
Christian Church, 106, 115, 116, 122, 124, 130, 183, 184
chromosomal abnormalities, 190, 208
chronic diseases, 147, 177
chronic fatigue syndrome (*see* myalgic encephalomyelitis: ME)
circadian rhythms, 204
Classen, Dr J Barthelow, 99
clinical trials, 29, 30, 36, 38, 40
Clinton, President William Jefferson, (Bill), 222,

closed systems, 121
Coalition for Informed Choice, (NY), 89
Coca-Cola, 227
Cochrane Collaboration, 39, 73
Codex Alimentarius, 240
coincidence (*see* acausal connections)
Coles, 227
collagen vascular disease (*see also* polyarteritis nodosa, rheumatoid arthritis, systemic lupus erythematosus), 108
collective unconscious, 173
commerce, 120, 195
communication, 153–156, 158, 200, 218
   between animals, birds and insects, 153
   between humans, 153, 154
   between organs, cells and DNA, 154, 155
   between plants, 154
Conagra Foods, 244
concentration problems, 219
Confucius, 44
congenital rubella syndrome, 69, 71–73
Cooke, Dr John, 73
Copernicus, 116, 122
Coppedge, Dr James, 159
copper, 225, 226
correspondences, 155
Costco, 227
cot death (*see* sudden infant death syndrome)
cotton seed, 235
Coxsackie virus, 81, 84, 89, 103
Creighton, Dr Charles, 51,
Crick, Professor Francis, 229
crisis, 19, 151, 164, 167
Crohn's disease, 34, 97, 103, 188
Crookshank, Professor Edward M, 51
Crowley, Dr T, 54
Cutter incident, the, 82, 83
cuttlefish, 171
cyanide, 76
cytomegalovirus, 69, 81, 87, 90
Czech Republic, 69, 238
dairy products, 77, 234
Darwin, Charles, 50, 158, 159, 171
Das Deutsch Center Clinic for Special Needs Children, Ohio, 40
Davies, Professor Paul, 121, 125, 159–162
Davis, Ann-Warren, 175,
Da Vinci, Leonardo, 116
deductive reasoning (*see also* inductive reasoning), 113, 117
deep vein thromboses, 20
degenerative diseases, 35, 103, 106, 145, 167, 209
Denmark, 55, 70, 83

dental caries, 20
Department of Health and Social Security (DHSS) UK, 67, 72
depression (*see* mental health, depression)
Descartes, René, 116–120, 124, 172
Dettman, Dr Glen, 101
developmental problems, 97, 99, 172, 193, 198, 213
dextrin, 235
diabetes, 17–19, 34, 100, 177, 178, 226
   type I, 18, 72, 97, 100
   type II, 20, 21
Diabetes UK, 18
Diamond, Professor Jared, 176,
diet, 20, 33, 34, 36, 45, 70, 79, 101, 144, 146–148, 182, 184, 185, 197, 223, 226, 234, 235, 238, 239
   according to seasons, 182, 184
Dingle, Professor Peter, 197
dioxins, 194, 221
diphtheria, 44, 45, 47–49, 53–59, 61, 64, 67, 78, 80
disease
   catabolic processes in, 166
   classifications of, 164
   meaning of, 164, 165
   negative processes of, 167
   positive processes of, 166, 167
   the two phases of, 165, 166
   tolerant processes of, 167
Ditchburn, Dr Robert, 62
diverticular disease, 20
divinity, 114, 125, 128, 151, 161
dizziness, 108, 148, 215
DLF-Trifolium, 227
DNA, 75, 90, 92, 96, 154, 155, 159, 170, 191, 213, 214, 229–231, 233, 236, 237
Doctrine of Signatures, 176
Doll, Regius Professor Sir Richard, 197
Dow Chemical Company, 227
Down's syndrome, 210
Dowsett, Dr Betty, 89
Drefus, 227
drugs
   antibiotics, 35, 36, 43, 45, 60, 102, 146, 159, 191, 230
   anticoagulants, 37
   arsenic, 27, 29, 76
   aspirin, 36, 38, 64, 146, 187
   cardiovascular drugs, 36
   chemotherapy, 36, 93, 166
   mutagens, 39, 96
   parcetamol, 64, 146
   penicillin, 37, 38, 191, 208

sulphonamides, 60
teratogens, 37, 38
thalidomide, 37
vaccines (see vaccines)
drug interactions, 37
drug reactions, 25, 36
dualism, 114, 119
Dupont, 227
ear, 35, 166, 215–217
ECHO virus, 84, 89, 103
Ecologist, 75, 174
Eddington, Professor Arthur, 141
Eddy, Dr Bernice, 81–83, 85–87
Edeka Zentrale AG & Co, 227
Edison, Thomas, 199, 203
eggplants, 224
eggs, 96, 239, 240
Egypt, 28, 44, 73, 128, 175, 183, 220
Egyptian medicine (see medical systems, Egyptian)
Ehrlich, Professor Paul, 27
Eisenstein, Dr Mayer, 40
Einstein, Professor Albert, 130, 132, 014, 140, 147, 152
elders, 43, 194
electromagnetic radiation, 21, 177, 199–222, 244
  at home, 202, 205, 210, 211,
  at work, 202, 209, 210
  difference between AC and DC currents, 199, 200
  effect on bacteria, 204, 208
  effect on brain-waves, 209, 216, 220
  effect on cows, 205, 212, 213
  effect on garlic, 208
  effect on physiology, 205, 206, 213–215
  effect on sleep, 203, 205, 213, 216, 220
  effect on wildlife, 205, 206, 218, 219
  extra-low frequencies (ELFs), 200, 203, 204, 207–209, 211, 213, 214, 218, 221, 222
  from mobile phones, 201, 202, 205, 215–218
  from mobile phone towers, 201, 205, 219–221
  from power lines, 202, 206, 210, 211
  from radar, 200, 201
  from radiostation masts, 201, 212
  from television masts, 201, 205, 211, 212
  harm from, 203–222
  Interphone International Study, 217
  levels today, 203
  microwaves, 200, 201, 204, 205, 208, 210, 214–216, 218–221
  microwave sickness, 207, 215
  natural, 199, 201, 202, 205
  radiofrequency (RF), 201, 205, 221
  radiofrequency syndrome, 207, 215
  standards for, 221, 222
  Stewart Report: Mobile Phones and Health, 215
  synergistic effects of, 204
Eli Lilly, 82
empiricism (see observation and experience/experiment)
emotions (see also communication, emotions), 131, 132, 154, 156
encephalitis, 39
Encyclopaedia Britannica, 159, 242
Enders, Dr John, 81
endocarditis, 108
endurance problems, 212
energy, 125, 132, 133, 140, 141, 143, 145–147, 149, 151, 152, 156, 157, 161, 165, 192, 199, 200, 203, 219, 239, 241, 244
entropy, 121, 162
Environmental Defense Fund (US), 195
Environment Protection and Heritage Council (Australia), 194
Environmental Working Group (EWG, US), 194
enzymes, 154, 158
eosinophilia myalgia, 236
epidemics, 17, 19, 24, 44, 45, 51–54, 56, 57, 59, 62–64, 66, 68, 69, 71, 77–80, 83, 89, 169, 183, 184, 187, 237
  American Civil War, 59, 82
  Boer War, 59
  Crimean War, 59
  during peacetime, 59
  Franco-Prussian War, 59
  Napoleonic Wars, 53
  Peninsula War, 59
  World War I, 58–60, 78, 79, 98
  World War II, 58, 60, 78, 79, 98
epilepsy, 97, 103
Ecuador, 20
ergot poisoning, 184
Ermakova, Dr Irina, 235
Estonia, 86
exercise, 21, 29, 33, 34, 38, 144, 160
Euripides, 115
European Union (EU), 238
evolution, 50, 74, 130, 158–160, 171–173, 177, 182
  micro-evolution, 159
  the chances of, 158–160
exanthema subitum (roseola rash), 103

eyes, 64, 133, 143, 152, 162, 166, 170, 176, 200, 215, 223
Fantz, Dr Robert, 172
farming, 102, 181, 192, 226, 228
   crop and animal diversity in 19th century, 181
   crop and animal diversity today, 218, 223, 224, 227, 228
   crop losses in, 224, 228, 229
   crop rotation in, 44, 45, 226
   energy expenditure in, 192
   impact of transnational corporations on, 227, 230
   monoculture in, 226, 229
   plant breeding in, 224, 228, 236
Farr, Dr William, 51
fatigue, 84, 89, 108, 147, 207, 213, 215, 216, 220
Federal Research Centre for Nutrition and Food (Germany), 241
fertilisers, chemical, 188, 226, 244,
fertility (*see* infertility)
fever, 29, 44, 54, 56, 64, 69, 74, 76, 99, 102, 146, 148, 149, 151, 165, 166, 186
   metabolic rate in, 165
Feynman, Professor Richard, 242, 243
fibre, dietary, 226
fibromyalgia, 90, 108
Finland, 18, 70, 81, 92, 211
fish, 43, 159, 171, 191, 238, 239, 242
Flexner, Dr Simon, 75
fluorides, 21, 149, 197
foetal abnormalities, 19, 37, 38, 109, 190, 194, 196, 197, 208–210, 213, 239, 241
folate, 225
food intolerance, 188
Food Standards Australia New Zealand (FSANZ), 239
food miles, 223, 228
foods (specifics)
   additives in, 21, 37, 76, 193–197
   impact of transnational corporations on, 224–227, 232, 244
   labelling of (*see* government standards, for food labelling)
   number of foods in bonobo chimpanzee diet, 182
   number of foods in hunter/gatherer diet, 182, 225
   number of foods in modern diet, 182, 228
   nutritient deficiencies in, 76, 238, 241
   the influence of colours on selection of, 131, 175, 176
   the influence of smells on selection of, 131, 175, 176
   the influence of tastes on selection of, 131, 175, 176
Ford Foundation, 225
formaldehyde, 54, 58, 78, 81, 83, 85, 221
Foucault's pendulum, 129, 130, 132, 143, 152
France, 55, 68, 74, 92, 184, 209, 238
Francis, Dr Thomas Jr., 81–83
Frey, Professor Allan, 216
flight or fright responses, 207
fruit, 52, 146, 190, 225, 238, 239
fruit fly, 155
fungal infections, 36
fungicides (*see* pesticides)
Gallilei, Galileo, 116
gallstones, 20
Gambia, 63, 68
Gard, Professor Sven, 81, 83
Gardner, Professor Howard, 172
garlic (*see also* herbal medicines, garlic), 37, 208, 238, 239
gas gangrene, 59, 60
gastro-intestinal tract, 28, 35, 44, 96, 166
Geffen, Dr Dennis, 78
General Mills, 244
genes, 16, 39, 90, 117, 124, 155, 158–160, 169, 186, 191, 210, 214, 223, 229–231, 235–237, 241
genetic engineering (GE)
   dangers of, 235, 236, 241
   deaths from, 235, 236
   labelling laws for, 231, 234, 235, 236
   of foods, 223, 227, 229, 231–238
   procedure of, 230, 232, 233
Georgia, 57, 65, 71, 95, 99
German measles (*see* rubella)
Germany, 51, 54–56, 184, 189, 219, 235, 240
germs, 16, 57, 59, 74, 75, 77, 96, 102, 103, 124, 169, 170, 176, 178, 179, 183, 185, 188, 191
gestalt, 118, 160
gingivitis, 108
Giorbran, Gevin, 141
giraffes, 154
glucose, 17, 20, 235
glucose metabolism, impaired, 17
glutaraldehyde, 96
GM (*see* genetic engineering)
God, 107, 114, 116, 117, 119, 123, 124, 128, 141, 160, 161, 176, 183, 229, 236–238
Gold, Dr Julian, 25
Goldman, Dr Gary, 97
Goldsmith, Dr Edward, 174

Goodall, Professor Jane, 182
Goodman Fielder, 244
government standards
   for chemicals, 195–198
   for electromagnetism, 208
   for food labelling, 234, 238, 239, 242
Graham, Dr David, 26
gravity, 130, 150, 161, 173
Gray, Dr Harold Farnsworth, 183
Greece, 44, 114, 115, 118, 132, 151, 219, 221
Greek civilisation, 28, 114, 115
Greek medicine (see medical systems, Greek)
Green Revolution, 189, 223, 225, 238, 242
Greenberg, Dr Bernard, 84, 85
Greene, Professor Brian, 161
Greenpeace, 190
Gregg, Dr Norman, 69
Grote, Dr J, 107
Groupe Danone, 227
Groupe Limagrain, 227
Guillain Barré syndrome, 39
Gulf War syndrome, 103, 108, 109
Hadwen, Dr Walter R, 50, 54, 62, 102
haemorrhoids, 20
hair loss, 108
Haiti, 104, 105
Hardell, Professor Lennart, 216
Harris, Robert, 106
Hawaii State Department of Health, 212
hayfever, 102, 103, 187
headaches, 76, 108, 119, 207, 215, 216, 220
health
   origins of word, 125, 163
   meaning of, 125, 163–165
heart disease, 19, 21, 178, 226
heart rate, 207, 215
Hedrich, Dr Arthur, 57
Heisenberg, Professor Werner, 120, 140, 141
Heller, Dr John, 208
hepatitis A, 103
hepatitis B, 49, 96, 100, 105–107
Heraclitus, 113
herbal lore/medicine, 28, 176
herbal medicines
   alfalfa, 239
   aloe vera, 239
   bitter leaf, 28
   brazzein berries, 230
   cascara, 37
   dong quai, 37
   garlic, 37, 203, 238, 239
   ginkgo, 37
   guarana, 239
   honey, 60, 175, 218, 219
   Korean ginseng, 239
   Neanderthal use of, 28, 177
   neem, 230
   psyllium seeds, 37
   saw palmetto, 239
   senna, 37
   Siberian ginseng, 239
   turmeric, 230, 239
herbal poisons, 175
herbicides, 180, 190–192, 195, 226, 233, 244
   Agent Orange, 190
   atachlor, 191
   atrazine, 191
   carbon tetrachloride, 77
   crop losses from resistance to, 192
   effect on human health, 190, 191
   glyphosate, 191
   resistance to, 191
   2,4-D, 190
   2,4,5-T, 190
herd protection, 57, 58, 63, 67
Hermeticism, 128
high blood pressure, 19, 21, 31, 35, 38, 226
high cholesterol levels, 19, 21, 31
High-Frequency Active Auroral Research
   Project (HAARP), 219
Hilleman, Dr Maurice, 85
Hinduism, 23, 113, 114
Hippocrates, 115, 129
Hippocratic Oath, 23
HIV (see also AIDS), 69, 1041–08
H.J. Heinz, 244
Ho, Professor Mae-Wan, 155
Hobby, Oveta Culp, US Secretary of the
   Department of Health, Education and
   Welfare, 82
Hocking, Dr Bruce, 211
holism, 124, 125
homoeostasis, 156–158
   of atmospheric oxygen, 129, 155, 157
   of the environment, 118, 121, 125, 153,
      155–158, 160–165, 170, 171, 244
Homo erectus, 27, 170, 173
Homo habilis, 27, 170, 173
Homo Neanderthalis, 173
Homo sapiens, 170, 173
homoeopathy, 34, 48
Horowitz, Dr Leonard G, 107
hormones, 154, 158, 190, 193, 194, 197, 210,
   240
Horwin, Alexander, Michael and Raphaele,
   93, 94
Hoyle, Professor Fred, 153, 160
Huffman, Professor Mike, 28, 177

human continuum, 162, 169, 170, 176–181, 186, 223, 229, 244
  meaning of, 162, 169
  time spent in, 169, 199, 222
Human Genome Project, 16,
human papilloma virus, 70
Hume, David, 172
humoral medicine, 131, 132
hundredth monkey phenomenon, 130, 160, 181,
hunters and gatherers
  as a reference point for health, 170
  diseases of, 20
  health of, 21, 43, 177–179
  in comparison with modern lifestyles, 28, 44, 182
  longevity of, 43, 44
  modern day, 20
Hunzakuts, 20
Hussein, Saddam, 108
hygiene, 16, 45, 54, 57, 102, 169, 183
hygiene hypothesis of atopy, 102
iatrogenic disease, 23–25, 35
Ibn Sina (*see* Avicenna)
Ibn Tufayl, 172
Illich, Professor Ivan, 24
illness, 15, 16, 33–35, 43, 48, 62, 67, 78, 100, 102, 123, 124, 129, 144, 147–149, 151, 161, 162, 164, 165, 167, 169, 185
immunity, 53, 56, 57, 58, 61, 63, 64, 68–71, 73, 79, 86, 108, 185
Immunology Today, 102
India, 20, 65, 123, 132, 151, 182, 183, 185, 224, 230, 234, 238, 241
indigenous peoples, 20, 30, 43, 112–114, 177, 178, 185, 186
  Pima Indians, 20
inductive reasoning (*see also* deductive reasoning), 118
Industrial Revolution, 74, 182, 186, 243,
inertia, 129, 130, 173
infant mortality, 17, 45, 100, 101
infertility, 18, 39, 96, 192, 198
  statistics on, 18, 19
inflammation, 35, 64, 84, 148, 151, 165–167
influenza, 35, 44, 48, 49, 69, 96, 100, 109
insecticides (*see* pesticides)
instincts, 112, 113, 127, 156, 157, 172–176,
  of babies, 176
  of wild animals, 131, 171, 173, 175, 177
intelligence, 125, 153, 156, 157, 159, 161, 162, 172–174, 185
  cognitive (intellect), 174, 175, 180
  general purpose intelligence (*see* trial and error)
  human, 153, 174, 175
  innate (*see* instincts)
  in the universe, 121, 122, 125, 127
  language, 115, 120, 131, 153, 173
  of animals, 28, 122, 153, 171, 173
  of Homo habilis and Homo erectus, 27, 173
  of life, 157, 161
  of natural history, 173
  of physics, 140, 147, 152, 173
  social, 128, 173
  technical, 173
International Agency for Research on Cancer (IARC), 92, 222
International Atomic Energy Agency (IAEA), 241
International Committee on Non-ionizing Radiation Protection (ICNIRP), 210
Interphone International Study, 217
intuition (*see* instincts)
Inuit, 20
iodine, 225
Iran, 238
Iraq, 108, 109, 132, 177
iron, 73, 128, 177, 218, 225, 226
irradiation of foods, 237, 239, 241
  harm from eating irradiated foods, 242
  labelling laws for, 237
  novel chemicals from irradiation, 240
irritability, 148, 207, 215, 216
Islam, 114, 160, 161, 172
Israel, 24, 64, 72, 221
Italy, 51, 68, 92, 115, 116, 184, 219, 221, 238
ITM Enterprises, 227,
Ivory Coast (Côte d'Ivoire), 52
Jackson, Peter, 200
Japan, 23, 28, 52, 67, 72, 103, 130, 234, 236
Jeans, Professor James, 141
Jenner, Dr Edward, 49, 52, 102
jing, 162
Journal of the American Medical Association, 26, 86
Journal of the Royal Society of Medicine, 107
Judaism, 114, 160, 161
Jung, Professor Carl, 130, 151, 173
Kalokerinos, Dr Archie, 100, 101
Kaatz, Professor Heinrich, 235
Kazakhstan, 57, 86
Keats, John, 128
Kennedy, President John Fitzgerald (JFK), 122
Kent, Dr Christopher, 88

kidney disease, 20
kidneys, 37, 81, 87, 94, 96, 133, 166, 189
King Charles II, 23
King, Dr Paul, 97
King, Dr Truby, 45
Klenner, Dr Frederick, 79
knowledge, 24, 28, 29, 43, 56, 66, 72, 97, 106, 107, 112–122, 127, 129, 169, 171–173, 175, 232
Koestler, Arthur, 130, 158
Kolmer, Dr John, 80
Koor Trade International, 227
Kops, Stanley, 93, 94
Kosovo, 237
Kraft Foods Inc, 227, 244
Krasner, Gary, 39
Kroger, 227
Kuwait, 108
KWS AG, 227
lactose intolerance, 185
Lai, Professor Henry, 213
lamb, 239, 240
Lancet, The, 50, 234
Land O'Lakes, 227
Landsteiner, Dr Karl, 75
Landré-Beauvais, Professor Augustin Jacob, 187
Landrigan, Professor Philip, 195
languages
   Aboriginal, 177, 178
   world, 115, 119, 151, 154, 163, 177, 178, 229
Latvia, 57, 86, 212
lead, 76, 77, 80, 186, 193
Leape, Professor Lucian, 24, 25
learning (*see* trial and error)
lecithin, 235
Lederle, 87, 88, 93–95
Leeper, Dr Edward, 210
Leibniz, Dr Gottfried Wilhelm, 172
Lewis, Dr Paul, 75
Liberia, 52
libido, 157, 162, 220
   decrease in, 207, 215
lie detectors, 154
Liedloff, Jean, 178
life expectancy, 17, 44, 45
life force (*see* vital force)
life span (*see* longevity)
light, 18, 20, 105, 143, 145, 151, 152, 170
lightning strikes, 61, 158
livestock breeds, 225
liver, 34, 36, 96, 133, 154, 166, 189
Loat, Lily, 54, 79

Locke, Dr John, 172
locomotor ataxia, 187
longevity, 45, 177
   in hunters and gatherers, 177
   in modern times, 45
Los Angeles County–University of Southern California Medical Center, 49
Lou Gerig's disease (*see* amyotrophic lateral sclerosis)
lungs, 64, 73, 129, 131, 133, 143, 166, 191,
lymphocyte abnormalities, 209, 241
MacArthur, Dr Donald, 107
McCain Foods, 244
McCloskey, Dr Bertram, 78
mad cow disease (*see* bovine spongiform encephalopathy)
maize, 182, 223–225, 228, 229
malaria, 44, 76, 103, 186
malformed babies (*see* foetal abnormalities)
maltodextrin, 235
manganese, 186, 234
mangoes, 239, 240
Maoris, 20
Marconi, Guglielmo, 200
Mars Inc, 227
Martin, Harry V, 107
Martin, Professor John, 87, 90, 91
Martin, JK, 78
mass extinction, 170
Matrix, The, 112
Matsumoto, Gary, 108
measles, 44, 45, 47–49, 54, 56, 57, 61, 62, 64–70, 102, 103, 164, 185
meat (*see also* beef, lamb, pork, poultry), 146, 191, 234, 239
Medawar, Professor Sir Peter, 160
medical science, 16, 22, 29, 30, 34–36, 97, 111, 119, 120, 127, 140, 161, 169
medical systems,
   Ayurveda, 132, 135, 139, 151
   Egyptian, 175
   Greek, 134, 138, 151
   Traditional Chinese (TCM), 120, 131, 133, 138, 146, 152
medical treatment, 17, 24, 43, 73
   contraries, 35, 36
   of anxiety, 148, 211
   of deficient conditions, 147–149, 167, 226
   of fevers, 29, 146, 166
   of measles, 57
   of polio, 45, 47, 49, 56, 73–95, 104
   of rubella, 48, 49, 61, 64, 69, 70–73
   of wounds, 59, 60, 180, 228
   root treatment, 111, 120

stem treatment, 35, 120
Medical Veritas, 97
Medin, Dr Oskar, 74, 75
melatonin, 207, 213–216
memory problems, 108, 207, 212, 215, 216, 230
meningitis, 35, 39, 56, 64, 84, 88, 89
mental health
  anxiety, 133, 148, 211
  depression, 21, 35, 54, 149, 207, 211, 213, 220
  mental retardation, 97
  social violence, 97
  suicide, 19, 129, 236
  temporary psychosis, 216
mercury, 29, 58, 61, 76, 78, 80, 96, 133, 186, 193
Metro AG, 227
Mexico, 224, 238
micoplasmas, 75, 96
micro-organisms, 107, 129, 165, 166, 183, 236
  antibiotic resistance in, 35,36, 159, 191,192, 230
Microwave News, 221, 222
milk (*see* dairy products)
Miller, Professor Stanley, 158, 159
millet, 182, 228
mind/body split, 113, 114, 117, 119
miscarriage, 19, 207, 210, 221
Mithen, Professor Steven, 172–174
Mitzer, Dr Albert, 81, 83
mobile phones (*see* electromagnetism, from mobile phones)
mobile phone towers (*see* electromagnetism, from mobile phone towers)
Moldova, 69
monkeypox, 52
monosodium glutamate (MSG), 96
Monsanto, 227, 232–234, 244
morphogenetic fields, 160
Moser, Lt Col Robert H, 23, 25
Mother Goddess, 183
Mount Sinai School of Medicine, 193, 195
mousepox virus, 236
mucous membranes, 166
multiple sclerosis, 18, 20, 39, 97, 108, 186
mumps, 48, 49, 56, 61, 64, 68–70, 102, 103, 185
Murray Darling River, 195
mylagic encephalomyelitis (ME), 84, 89, 108, 213, 215
mystics, 113, 120, 121, 128, 141, 161
nanotechnology, 242, 243

National Anti-Vaccination League of Great Britain, 54, 79
National Cervical Screening Program (Australia), 17
National Council on Radiation Protection and Measurements (NCRP, US), 222
National Foundation for Infantile Paralysis (US), 80, 82, 85
National Heart Foundation of Australia, 17
National Institute of Medical Herbalists (NIMH, UK), 175
National Toxics Network (Australia), 194
nature/nurture debate, 171
nasal passages, 166
Nestlé, 227, 244
Netherlands, The, 55, 63, 70, 218, 238
New England Journal of Medicine, The, 38, 99
Newport Daily News, The, 109
New Scientist, 236
Newton, Isaac, 119, 129, 130
New York Power Lines Project, 210
New York Times, 83, 86, 99, 106, 109
New Zealand, 17, 18, 20, 26, 45, 67, 68, 78, 90, 100, 190, 209, 211, 222, 235, 239
Nigeria, 52
nitrates, 226
Nixon, President Richard Milhous, 122
Noon, Dr Geoffrey, 60
Norway, 18, 55, 68, 74, 76, 189
Nufarm, 227
nutrition, 21, 44, 45, 52–54, 59, 168, 197, 225, 228, 234, 238, 241
nutritional deficiencies, 76, 226, 228, 241
  beriberi, 76
  pellagra, 76
  scurvy, 76, 101
oats, 182, 228
obesity (*see also* over-weight), 19, 31, 38, 226
Obi-Wan Kenobi, 150
observation and experience/experiment, 29, 118, 125, 127, 171, 172, 176
octopuses, 171
O'Dea, Professor Kerin, 20, 178
Organisation for Economic Co-operation and Development (OECD), 196, 235
Offit, Dr Paul A, 83, 99
Olmstead, Dan, 40
Oman, 88
onions, 238
Oppenheimer, Professor Julius Robert, 120
order (*see* homoeostasis)
Orwell, George, 183, 197, 199
osteomalacia, 185
osteoporosis, 18

over-weight (*see also* obesity), 20, 21
Oxford English Dictionary, 125, 152
pagans, 161
Papua New Guinean highlanders, 19, 20
pain, 18, 19, 33, 36, 84, 123, 148, 161, 165, 167
  importance of, 123, 165
  statistics on, 19
Pakistan, 132, 238
palaeopathology, 177
papaya, 239, 240
Paracelsus, 29
parasitic worms, 103
Parke-Davis & Co, 82, 86, 87
Parkinson's disease, 103, 187, 209
Parr, Thomas, 44
Parsifal, 163
Pasteur, Professor Louis, 16, 30, 75, 102
Pasteur Institute, 54
patents, 30
  on foods, 230, 236
  on genes, 229, 230
  on life, 230
Paxman, Jeremy, 106
peanuts, 240
peas, 223
pears, 223
Penrose, Professor Roger, 160
PepsiCo, 227, 244
perfluorinated compounds (PFCs), 194
Peru, 182, 183
pesticides, 76, 77, 92, 109, 180, 188–196, 220, 233, 234, 244
  aldrin, 189
  carbon tetrachloride, 77
  chloral benzene, 77
  chlordane, 189, 193
  chlorpyrifos, 189, 193
  DDT, 189, 193
  diazinon, 189
  dichlorvos, 189
  dieldrin, 189
  fenitrothion, 189
  heptachlor, 189
  hexachlorobenzene (HCB), 189
  malathion, 189
  maldison, 189
  parathion, 189, 190, 193
  Paris Green, 76
  Permethrin193
  poisoning from, 76, 77, 186, 190
  synthetic pyrethroids, 190, 193
Pesticide Action Network North America (PANNA), 190, 193

pet food irradiation, 239, 242
Pfizer, 31, 87
Pharmaceutical Benefits Scheme (PBS) (Australia), 21
pharmaceutical industry, 31, 188, 217
  drug trials (*see also* clinical trials), 217
  marketing, 31, 36
  profits, 30, 196
phenol, 96
2-phenoxyethanol, 96
Pheidias, 115
Philippines, The, 44, 51, 78, 238
Phipps, James, 52
phosphate compounds, 96
phthalates, 193, 194
Physicians' Desk Reference, The
phytoplankton, 155
pigeons, 171
Pimentel, Professor David, 192
pineal gland, 204, 207
Pioneer Hi-bred International (*see* Dupont)
pistachio nuts, 240
Pitcairn, John, 52
Plato, 44, 112–116, 172
pneuma, 151
Pneumocystis carinii pneumonia, 35, 105
poisonous plants, 173, 175
Poland, 69, 211, 238
Poling, Dr John, Terry and Hannah, 98, 99
polio, 45, 47, 49, 56, 73–95, 98, 104
polyarteritis nodosa, 108
polychlorinated biphenyls (PCBs), 193, 194, 221
polyethylene 9–10 nonyl phenol, 96
polysorbate 20/80, 86
Popow, Professor, 76
Popper, Dr Erwin, 75
pork, 96, 191, 239, 240
Portugal, 56, 59, 69
Post-Polio Institute (NJ, USA), 89
potassium, 226
potatoes, 228, 229, 234, 235, 238
Poulos, Professor Alfred, 195, 196
poultry, 191, 238
poverty, 31, 45, 54, 111, 129, 183, 226, 238
prana, 151
prions, 75, 96, 234
provocation polio, 78, 88
psoriasis, 103
psychology, 112, 118, 171
Public Citizen (US), 241
public sanitation, 45, 50, 57, 184
  sewage disposal, 45, 183
  water (*see* water)

pulses (see also peas), 225, 238
Pusztai, Professor Arpad, 234
Pygmies, 104
Pythagorus, 115, 129
quantum physics, 114, 119–121, 125, 127, 140, 141, 155
Queen Elizabeth I, 44
qi, 145, 147, 151
quinoa, 182, 230
Quit Campaign (the National Tobacco Campaign–Australia), 17
Rath, Dr Matthias, 25, 26
Ratner, Dr Herbert, 80, 85, 95
rats, 30, 37, 171, 173, 184, 213–215, 233–235
reaction times, 207, 212
Reagan, President Ronald Wilson, 232
Red Cross, 194
reductionism, 117, 122
religion, 114, 115, 118, 123, 160, 161, 163, 244
Renaissance, 115, 116, 129
Repacholi, Professor Michael, 214
Rescue Generation, 40
Reye's syndrome, 36
rice, 182, 190, 224, 225, 228, 230, 235
Richter, Professor Carl, 174
rickets, 185
Roberts, Janine, 75, 81
Robbins, Dr Frederick, 81
Rockefeller Foundation, 225
Rockefeller Institute for Medical Research, 75
Roman civilization, 28, 115, 183, 184
Romania, 88
Rook, Professor Graham, 102
Roosevelt, President Franklin Delano, 80, 84
root vegetables, 45, 146, 148, 182
Rosen, Professor Robert, 121, 127, 162, 187
roseola rash (see exanthema subitum)
rotavirus colitis, 103
Rowett Institute of Nutrition and Health, 234
Royal Commission on Vaccinations, 1889 – 1896, 50
Royal Society (UK), The, 234
Ruata, Professor Carlos, 51
rubella (German measles), 48, 49, 61, 64, 69–73
Rudolf Steiner schools, 102, 220
Rumsfeld, Secretary of Defense Donald, 47, 100
Russia, 57, 58, 60, 221, 261
Russian Academy of Sciences, 235
Sabin, Dr Albert, 81
safety guidelines (see government standards)
Sagan, Professor Carl, 170

St Anthony's fire, 184
St Helena, 74
St Louis Post-Dispatch, 197
Sakata, 227
Salk, Dr Jonas, 81–88, 93, 105
Samoa, 76
Sandler, Dr Benjamin, 79
Sara Lee, 244
Savitz, Professor David, 210
scarlet fever , 44, 54, 56
Schmeiser, Percy, 233
Scobey, Dr Ralph, 76, 77
Scott, Professor Donald W, and William, 106
Scheibner, Dr Viera, 84, 89
Schrödinger, Professor Erwin, 158
Schumann resonances, 199, 203, 204
seasons, 115, 131, 180
selenium, 225
Seminis (see Monsanto)
sexual behavior, 104, 105, 154, 157
sewage (see public sanitation)
Shakespeare, William, 44, 89, 113, 116, 127
Sheldrake, Professor Rupert, 127, 160
Shelley, Percy Bysshe, 128
shen, 152
Showa Denko KK, 236
Schrödinger, Professor Erwin, 158
shellfish, 238, 239
Sierra Leone, 52
signs from the universe (see acausal connections)
simian cytomegalovirus (SCMV), 81, 87, 90
simian immunodeficiency virus (SIV), 81, 104
simian virus 40 (SV40), 81, 87, 93–95
Singh, Professor Narendra, 213, 214
skin, 37, 64, 96, 128, 131, 133, 146, 147, 152, 165, 166, 170, 185
  complaints, 29, 76, 103
Skinner, Professor Burrhus Frederic, 171
Skywalker, Luke, 156
sleep, 113, 123, 143, 180, 207, 213, 216, 220
  animals' posture in, 176
  human posture in, 176, 180
Slesin, Dr Louis, 221
smallpox, 43, 47, 49–54, 62, 80, 102–104, 106, 108, 184, 236
Smithells, Professor Dick, 38
Smuts, Jan Christian, 124
Socrates, 172
sodium, 197, 226
sorbitol, 96
sorghum, 182, 228
Sorokin, Professor Pitirim, 115
South Africa, 20, 63, 68, 124, 238

soy, 228, 234, 325, 237
Spain, 59, 69, 184, 219
sperm abnormalities, 18, 19, 191, 207, 217, 218
sperm wars, 157
spina bifida, 38
Spinoza, Baruch de, 172
sugar cane/sugar beet, 79, 86, 207, 228, 235
Szmuness, Professor Wolf, 105
stability (*see* homoeostasis)
standardization, 39, 228
Star Wars, 156
stealth viruses, 90, 91
Stewart, Emeritus Professor Gordon, 62
Stewart, Dr Sarah, 85
Stewart, Professor Sir William, 215
sthenic/asthenic responses, 151, 166, 167
stillbirths (*see also* miscarriage), 207
Still's disease, 103, 187
stomach, 28, 133, 166, 233
Stone Age (*see* hunters and gatherers)
Strecker, Dr Robert, 107, 108
stress, 22, 57, 67, 109, 154, 164, 167, 175, 183, 207
strokes, 226
subacute illnesses, 167
sudden infant death syndrome (SIDS), 97, 100, 176, 207
suicide genes, 236
sulphate compounds, 78, 96
Sumitomo, 227
supermarkets, 228, 234
superstring theory, 161
suppression of disease, 106, 167
Suzuki, Professor David, 117, 189
Swan, Dr Norman, 6, 24
Sweden, 18, 51, 55, 56, 74, 209, 211
Sweet, Dr Ben, 85
sweet potatoes, 130, 228
Switzerland, 55, 69–71, 213, 215, 221
Sydenham, Dr Thomas, 50
synchronicity (*see* acausal connections)
Syngenta, 227, 244
syphilis, 27, 106, 184
systemic lupus erythematosus, 97, 108, 187
tabula rasa, 172
Takii & Co Ltd, 227
talking trees, 154
Taoism, 113
Tasmanian devil, 228
Taylor, Professor Michael R, 232
Tempest, The, 113
Tesco, 227

Tesla, Nikola, 199, 200, 210, 211, 213, 214, 222
tetanus, 48, 49, 59, 60, 61
Thailand, 56, 238
thiomersal (in vaccines), 61, 78, 96
Third World, 38, 45, 225, 226
thirst, 146, 148, 157, 174
Thorndike, Professor Edward Lee, 171
thyroid gland, 207
thyroiditis, 108
Times, The (London), 104
tobacco industry, 217
tobacco smoking, 21
Tognon, Professor Mauro, 92
Tolkien, Professor John Ronald Reuel, 141, 260
Tolman, Professor Edward, 173
tomatoes, 223, 233
Tongwe people of west Tanzania, 28, 177
Tonkin, Professor Andrew, 17
Toomey, Dr John, 79
toxoplasmosis, 69
Trade Related Aspects of Intellectual Property Rights (TRIPS), 230
Traditional Chinese Medicine (*see* medical systems, Traditional Chinese), 131, 133–135
trial and error, 27, 64, 160, 171–174, 176, 207, 216
triorthocresyl phosphate, 76
tryptophan, 236
Trobriand Islanders, 19
tuberculosis, 31, 43–45, 49, 52, 103
Turkey, 80, 92
Tuskagee experiment, 106
typhoid, 44, 56, 134
typhus, 44
Tyson Foods, 227
Ukraine, 57, 239
Unani Medicine (*see* medical systems, Greek)
Underwood, Dr Michael, 74
Unilever, 244
UK Committee on the Safety of Medicines, 38
United Kingdom, 18, 26, 62, 98, 238
United Nations, 55, 108, 104, 108, 241, 238
 Children's Fund (UNICEF), 19, 101
 Food and Agriculture Organisation (FAO), 240, 241
 World Food Programme (WFP), 238
 World Health Organisation (WHO), 28, 45, 56, 57, 61, 68, 69, 75, 84, 101, 107, 186, 190, 240
  Traditional Medicine Programme, 28

United States, 17, 26, 31, 53, 63, 65–68, 70–74, 77, 78, 82, 83, 88, 93, 98, 100, 105, 106, 108, 172, 218, 234, 236
unity, 2, 113, 125, 128, 140, 161
universe, 111, 115, 116, 121, 122, 125, 127, 130, 132, 140, 141, 143, 152, 158, 160, 161
   fundamental constants of, 161
   theories about
Urey, Professor Harold, 158, 159
urinary tract, 191
USSR, 55, 95
US Agency for International Development (USAID), 225
US Centers for Disease Control and Prevention (CDC), 39, 40, 56, 57, 63, 65–67, 71, 88, 89, 91, 93, 94, 97, 99, 105
US Department of Health and Human Services (DHHS), 94, 99
US Department of Defense (USDoD), 108, 109
US Environmental Protection Agency (EPA), 193, 197, 221
US Food and Drug Administration (FDA), 94, 97–99, 231–236, 239
US House of Representatives, 76, 77, 94
US Institute of Medicine (IOM), 24, 94, 95
US National Academy of Sciences (NAS), 195
US National Cancer Institute (NCI), 85, 86, 95, 107
US National Institutes of Health (NIH), 81, 85–87, 99, 100, 105
   Division of Biologics Standards, 87
US National Institute of Environmental Health Sciences (NIEH), 221
US National Institutes of Science (NIS), 18
US National Research Council (NRC), 196
US Patent and Trademark Office (USPTO), 230
US Public Health Service (PHS), 86, 106
US Vaccine Adverse Events Reporting System (VAERS), 96
uterus, 166
vaccines, 21, 39–41, 47–109, 169, 180, 188, 217
   association with autism, 39–41
   constituents of, 96
   for diphtheria, 53–58
   for haemophilus influenza type B, 48, 96–100, 109
   for hepatitis B, 49
   for human papilloma virus, 70
   for measles, 64–68
   for mumps, 68, 69
   for polio, 73–95
   for rubella, 69–73
   for smallpox, 49–52
   for tetanus, 59–61
   for whooping cough, 61–64
   non-compliance of doctors on, 48, 49
   squalene in, 108, 109
   testing of, 39
vaccination programmes, 18, 33, 40, 41, 43, 45, 47–109
vaccinia virus, 104
vagina, 157, 166
Vankin, Jonathon, 107
varicose veins, 20
vis medicatrix naturae, 125
vital force, 46, 111, 113, 124, 125, 127–141, 143–162, 164–167, 169
vitamins
   vitamin A, 54, 70, 225, 226
   vitamin B1, 76
   vitamin B3, 76
   vitamin C, 54, 76, 79, 100, 101
   vitamin D, 185
   vitamin E, 235
Von Heine, Dr Jakob, 74
Von Saal, Professor Frederick, 197
Vulpian, Dr Alfred, 76
Wade, Dr Nicholas, 109
Waddington, Professor Conrad Hal, 158, 160
Wald, Professor George, 236
Wallace, Professor Alfred Russel, 50, 51
Wal-Mart, 227
Wang, Dr Heng, 40
war
   American Civil War, 59, 82
   Boer War, 59
   Crimean War, 59
   First Gulf War (Iraq), 108, 109
   Franco-Prussian War, 59
   Napoleonic Wars, 53
   Peninsula War, 59
   Vietnam, 190
   World War I, 54, 59, 190
   World War II, 58, 60, 78, 79, 98, 188
Warren-Davis, Ann, 175
Washington, President George, 23
water, 2, 21, 45, 64, 75, 102, 128, 129, 131–133, 145, 149, 157, 158, 165, 170, 174, 180, 181, 183, 185, 186, 194, 197, 243
Watson, Professor James Dewey, 229
Watson, Professor John Broadus, 171
weakness, 84, 148, 207–215
wellbeing, 115, 156, 163, 166, 174, 176, 220
Weller, Dr Thomas, 81

Wertheimer, Dr Nancy, 210
West, Jim, 77, 80
wheat, 45, 182, 190, 224, 225, 228, 229, 239, 241
white pox, 52
whistle-blowers, 86, 97–102
whooping cough, 44, 45, 47–49, 54, 56, 61–64, 78
Wickman, Dr Ivar, 75
Wildebeest, 154
witches, 123
Wittgenstein, Professor Ludwig, 122
Woodrow Wilson International Center for Scholars, 243
Woolworths, 227
Wordsworth, William, 128
Workman, Dr William, 82
World Trade Organisation (WTO), 229
World Watch Institute (WWI), 192
World Wildlife Fund (WWF), 194
worm (helminth) infection (*see* parasitic worms)
Wyeth, 82, 87
xanthum gum, 235
xenoestrogens, 21, 180
yaws, 76
Yellowlees, Dr Henry, 72
Yekuana, psychosocial health of, 175–179, 143–149
yin/yang, 113, 121, 122, 143–149, 151, 164–167
Youngner, Dr Julius, 81
Zaire, 52
zeitgeist, 124
Zimbabwe, 237
zinc, 225, 226

www.ingramcontent.com/pod-product-compliance
Ingram Content Group UK Ltd.
Pitfield, Milton Keynes, MK11 3LW, UK
UKHW051257180426
11947UKWH00020B/1751